Medicare

Medicare

Preparing for the
Challenges of the
21st Century

Robert D. Reischauer
Stuart Butler
Judith Lave
Editors

NATIONAL ACADEMY OF SOCIAL INSURANCE
Washington, D.C.

Medicare: Preparing for the Challenges of the 21st Century
may be ordered from:

BROOKINGS INSTITUTION PRESS
1775 Massachusetts Avenue N.W.
Washington, D.C. 20036
Tel: 1-800-275-1447
     (202)-797-6258
Fax: (202) 797-6004

Library of Congress Cataloging-in-Publication Data

Medicare : preparing for the challenges of the 21st century / Robert D. Reischauer . . .
  [et al.], editors.
    p. cm.
  Includes bibliographical references and index.
  ISBN 0-8157-7399-4 (alk. paper)
  1. Medicare—Congresses.   2. Medicare—Forecasting—Congresses.
I. Reischauer, Robert D. (Robert Danton), 1941– .
RA412.3.M43   1997   97-33931
368.4′26′00973—dc21   CIP

9 8 7 6 5 4 3 2 1

Typeset in Palatino

Composition by AlphaWebTech
  Mechanicsville, Maryland

Printed by Kirby Lithographic Co.
  Arlington, Virginia

Preface

THE PRIMARY PURPOSE of the ninth annual conference of the National Academy of Social Insurance, which was held in Washington, D.C., on January 23–24, 1997, was to provide a forum at which the major issues that confront Medicare over the long run could be addressed in a dispassionate and informed manner. Those who spoke and presented papers identified a wide range of options that Congress and the president could consider as they debated ways to strengthen the program. They also offered a number of principles that could be used to guide the restructuring effort.

Many of these issues and options were debated when Congress and the president devised the Medicare titles of the Balanced Budget Act of 1997. That act, which together with the Taxpayer Relief Act of 1997 promises to balance the budget by 2002, will reduce the growth of Medicare spending by between $112 billion (Congressional Budget Office estimate) and nearly $150 billion (Office of Management and Budget estimate) by fiscal year 2002 and change the structure of the program in many significant ways. Nevertheless, more fundamental changes will be required if Medicare is to cope successfully with the retirement of the baby boom generation and the continued escalation of health care costs.

These changes will be the focus of the seventeen-member National Commission on the Future of Medicare that was established by the Balanced Budget Act. This volume and the other reports of the Academy's Restructuring Medicare for the Long Term project are intended to provide useful information for the commission and policymakers as they consider how best to restructure and strengthen Medicare for the long term.

Those who presented papers and spoke at the conference were chosen for their expertise and with eye to providing different disciplinary and ideological perspectives on the problems. Given time constraints and other commitments, not all were able to transform their remarks into a form suitable for publication. Those that are contained in this volume reflect the views of the authors and do not necessarily reflect those of the officers, board, staff, or members of the Academy nor its funders. The Academy does, however, assume responsibility for ensuring the independence of this volume.

The Robert Wood Johnson Foundation, the Henry J. Kaiser Family Foundation, The Pew Charitable Trusts, and the Kaiser Permanente Foundation provided generous support for the conference.

The editors thank the conference participants for lively discussion and debate. We also gratefully acknowledge Pamela J. Larson, Terry T. Nixon and the Academy staff for their smooth and skillful management of the conference. In addition to their work on the conference, Michael E. Gluck and Dwayne L. Smith are thanked for the significant contribution they have made to help transform the conference proceedings into this volume.

We appreciate the efforts of Jim Schneider, who edited the manuscript, and the rest of the staff of the Brookings Institution Press. The book was proofread by Ellen Garshick and indexed by Mary Mortenson.

ROBERT D. REISCHAUER
STUART BUTLER
JUDITH R. LAVE

Contents

1

Introduction

Karen Matherlee

THE NINTH ANNUAL conference of the National Academy of Social Insurance focused on the challenge of sustaining and strengthening the Medicare program over the long term in the face of the severe fiscal and demographic pressures the program will face in the twenty-first century. The conference, which opened on January 23, 1997, was convened at a time when Medicare reform was a major policy issue. Different visions of the program's future had been a major focus of disagreement during the budget battles of 1995 and 1996. The presidential and congressional elections of 1996 were significantly shaped by competing claims and charges about what each party might do to Medicare. Heightening the sense of urgency was the official actuaries' prediction that the Hospital Insurance (HI) Trust Fund would become insolvent as early as 2001.

The conference, Medicare: Preparing for the Challenges of the 21st Century, drew some 350 participants. For two days, experts drawn from the ranks of academics, policymakers, health practitioners, and affected interests examined the social contract that underlies Medicare, probed the program's financial viability, analyzed the political forces that support and constrain it, and investigated the various forces that influence efforts to bring about change.

The conference was an integral part of the academy's project, Restructuring Medicare for the Long Term. In late 1995 the project's steering committee and three study panels began to consider the problems likely to face Medicare in the first half of the next century. The conference's cochairs—Stuart Butler, vice president and director of domestic and economic policy studies at the Heritage Foundation; Judith R. Lave, professor of health economics at the University of Pittsburgh's School of Public Health; and Robert D. Reischauer, senior fellow in economics at the Brookings Institution—serve on the project's steering committee and study panels. The structure of the conference followed that of the project, which has one study panel examining Medicare's larger social role, another looking into issues of capitation and choice, and a third exploring how fee-for-service Medicare might be strengthened and modernized for the next century. A fourth study panel, scheduled to begin work in late 1997, will examine options for financing Medicare over the long term.

Medicare's Social Contract

A significant concern at the conference was the nature of the commitment between the Medicare program and those whom the program was designed to serve. Looking back over Medicare's thirty-plus years, observers had different perspectives on the nature of its social contract. Leading off, Stuart Butler said that the social contract is the same now as it was when the program was created. It assures elderly and disabled recipients that they have modern health care benefits comparable to those available to the rest of the insured population at a reasonable cost to them and to society. But, he said, the structure set up to carry out that contract is inherently flawed. He described the system's creation as a 1960s-style compromise consisting, on the one hand, of mandatory part A hospital and home health care funded by a payroll tax (a social insurance model) and, on the other hand, voluntary part B physician and other nonhospital services funded by beneficiary premiums subsidized by government (a subsidized model).

Butler contended that it would be difficult to use administered pricing and organizational changes to correct the program's financial problems and such benefit shortfalls as lack of catastrophic coverage and out-of-hospital pharmaceutical coverage. To make the program more equitable between rich and poor, he suggested imposing income-related changes in part A deductibles and copayments and means-testing beneficiaries' part B premiums. He also put forth the idea of beneficiaries' using vouchers based on the financial value of their Medicare benefits to obtain health coverage from a wide range of plans in the private sector—in other words, a change to a "defined contribution" plan.

Butler's suggestions drew sharp opposition from Theda Skocpol, professor of government and sociology at Harvard University. Referring to the Medicare social contract as a "national commitment to fund a consistent set of health services with maximum choice of providers," she criticized "elites" for attempting to erode the contract by shifting it from a defined benefit to a defined contribution. She contended instead that most Americans favor modest structural reforms, such as making cuts or reducing the rates of increase in payments to hospitals and physicians and raising taxes and premiums on richer beneficiaries. "My message is: look before you leap," she warned. "Trained (in most cases) as economists, health care experts are accustomed to arguing in terms of static technical design and rational claims about cost efficiency. But histori-cally grounded moral understandings are much more important for regular citizens."

Former Social Security Commissioner Robert M. Ball, now a consultant on Social Security, health, and welfare matters, drew on his personal experience to explore the history and original goals of the Medicare program. He explained that the social contract targeted the elderly, the most costly group to serve, because they were ill suited to obtain voluntary private insurance and offered the best political opportunity for enacting the initial piece in what some hoped would be universal coverage. Basing part A on the Blue Cross system available to the privately insured and part B on an Aetna policy offered to federal workers under the Federal Employees Health Benefits Program (FEHBP), the Johnson administration and Congress put in place the compromise system that endures today. Following a pragmatic political approach, the program's fram-ers intended "to put Medicare patients in an equal position with those already covered under private insurance or those who could pay their own way." In Ball's view, the program currently falls short of such goals, both in its benefit package and in its failure to adopt the cost-containment techniques used by private health plans.

Syndicated columnist E. J. Dionne looked back to the turn of the century, when social insurance was a vision, and to the late 1930s, when it first became a reality in the form of both Social Security retirement benefits. He expressed concern that social insurance, in terms of both Social Security retirement and Medicare benefits, is under pressure. He identified some of the major forces threatening social insurance: efforts to trim benefits in the global economy, a declining proportion of unionized workers, a growing population of elderly, and widening economic inequalities in a technology-driven environment that highly prizes skills and education. He remained optimistic, however, that social insurance would be preserved because of the support of the American people for the retirement and health programs, which he indicated are the underpin-nings of social stability and justice.

Financing Medicare

Of the threat to the original Medicare social contract that is posed by the size of the baby boom, Joseph R. Antos, assistant director for health and human resources at the Congressional Budget Office, said that now is the calm before the storm. Commenting on the projected depletion of the Hospital Insurance Trust Fund early in the next century, he said that the greatest stress on the program would occur from 2010 through 2030 as increasing numbers of baby boomers enter the Medicare program. Key sources of Medicare spending growth, he said, would be fee-for-service payment methods and unrestrained expenditures for home health and skilled nursing facility care. As the volume and intensity of services continue to increase, Medicare's cost per beneficiary will continue to spiral upward, placing an enormous burden on the federal budget and the economy. He reviewed some options that could be implemented over the long term: moving from a defined benefit to a defined contribution, reducing payments to providers, increasing beneficiary cost sharing, and raising the payroll tax or premiums or both.

David B. Kendall, senior analyst for health policy for the Progressive Policy Institute, generally agreed with Antos on the need for financing reforms to make the program sustainable. He said that the options Antos mentioned are consistent with Medicare's social contract: having a geographically uniform set of benefits, operating a program that is consistent with the private marketplace, and ensuring equal access for rich and poor. He recommended modernizing the program by tying the Medicare subsidy to a package of uniform benefits that are competitively priced, by setting performance measures, by updating and indexing the benefits to inflation and increases in lifespan, and by reducing subsidization of the well-off.

Charles N. (Chip) Kahn III, staff director of the Health Subcommittee of the House Ways and Means Committee and a member of the Academy's Medicare project steering committee, noted that for political reasons the current Congress could only make short-term fixes. He argued that it would have to consider long-term options to sustain the Medicare program for the baby boom generation. Restructuring and capitation proposals may be on the table (if the goals are to preserve the basic benefit structure and quality of services), but he warned that new taxes to solve the funding problem would meet considerable opposition. He stressed that the earlier long-term options are addressed, the better it would be for beneficiaries.

Judith Feder, professor of public policy at Georgetown University's Institute for Health Care Policy and Research, contended that there are two major risks to be avoided in the consideration of Medicare reform options. One is to look at Medicare financing solely as a budgetary problem. The other is to take a social engineering, rather than an incremental, approach. Opposed to capping Medicare and turning it from a defined benefit entitlement to a defined contribution program, Feder argued for making its operation more efficient. In line with some earlier recommendations, she supported slowing growth of payments to hospitals and physicians and addressing problems in home health and skilled nursing facility expenditures. Although she was against opening the program to adverse risk selection and other problems of an unbridled marketplace, she advocated broadening the range of choices and informing consumers about them.

Building a Sound Infrastructure for Choice

If beneficiaries have the option to choose among health plans, they need to develop new attitudes and gain new skills, according to Stanley B. Jones, director of the Health Insurance Reform Project at George Washington University. Pointing out that 80,000 beneficiaries a month left traditional Medicare for risk-bearing health plans in 1996, he contrasted the old with the new realities of the emerging Medicare program. For example, the program is moving from standard to varying premiums and benefits, from free to limited choice of provider, and from being politically motivated to being market driven. Beneficiaries are moving from coordinating their own care to having primary care doctors do it and from choosing a physician to selecting a health plan. Government is changing from paying for health services to offering health plans and from giving a good deal to certifying a good plan.

Expressing special concern for those with chronic illness and disability, he warned that they may discover physicians and plans do not want to serve them and they may find it harder to predict what kinds of services they would receive after they had chosen a health plan. Jones suggested four ways in which such beneficiaries might be helped: through fair premiums for their coverage, assistance from purchasing agents, education, and retention of traditional Medicare as an option.

After Jones discussed choice from a Medicare consumer's perspective, Roger D. Feldman and Bryan Dowd outlined various ways of structuring choice under the Medicare program. Feldman is Blue Cross professor of health insurance and professor of economics at the University of Minnesota, where Dowd is a professor in the Division of Health Services Research and Policy in the School of Public Health. Contending that Medicare is unfair in its subsidies and inefficient in the prices it pays for benefits, they focused on health maintenance organizations in the Medicare market. They described competitive pricing proposals in which Medicare would specify a basic benefit package, put it out for bid, and set the program's contribution equal to the price of the cheapest qualified plan in the market area. They discussed various types of problems that might arise and ways of dealing with them. They also provided some models drawn from the state of Minnesota's Buyers' Health Care Action Group (BHCAG) and from the FEHBP for limiting the number of plans made available, looking at open enrollment and lock-in issues, and addressing administrative concerns.

James C. Robinson, professor of health economics at the School of Public Health, University of California at Berkeley, and Patricia E. Powers, executive director of the Pacific Business Group on Health (PBGH), discussed the role public and private purchasing alliances might have in restructuring Medicare. Drawing on PBGH's experiences with HMOs in California as well as lessons from state and federal models, they explored the pros and cons of using purchasing alliances to act as sponsors for Medicare beneficiaries, particularly those who are under alliance sponsorship when they move from the work force to coverage under Medicare.

First, Robinson and Powers considered the Department of Health and Human Services' Health Care Financing Administration (HCFA) as a sole sponsor. Next, they examined multiple sponsors (both large firms with retiree programs and a wide range of organizations, including, in addition to employers, associations and labor unions). They went on to describe examples of sponsoring organizations: the California Public Employees Retirement System (CalPERS), the Health Insurance Plan of California, BHCAG in Minnesota, and FEHBP. They also looked at criteria for multiple sponsors, for employers as well as competing public agencies, business groups, industry or union purchasing pools, senior citizen or consumer organizations, and private brokerages. Moreover, they explored other relevant sponsorship issues: for-profit and not-for-profit status, geographic scope, administrative fees, and selection and management of health plans. Finally, they reviewed some ground rules for competition, such as criteria for participation, premium negotiation and enrollment procedures, risk-measurement and risk-adjustment concerns, and customer service and quality standards.

In addressing choice, Melinda Beeukes Buntin, a graduate student in the Department of Health Care Policy, Harvard University, and David Blumenthal, chief of the Health Policy Research and Development Unit at the Medical Practices Evaluation Center of Massachusetts General Hospital and member of the Academy project's steering committee, examined carve-outs, which pay for specific types of care under arrangements that are separate from other services a patient receives. They described different types of carve-outs, assessed their advantages and disadvantages, and provided an initial evaluation of their effectiveness. They found that carve-outs vary a great deal but those that work best show some resemblances. They focused on a condition that tends to be relatively high cost and common, is best cared for in a specialized setting, is not associated with interacting comorbid conditions, is best treated by a provider who experiences a high volume of patients with the condition, and develops gradually and is not hard to pinpoint.

Buntin and Blumenthal argued that carve-outs' major strengths and weaknesses relate to the same variables: quality of care and cost containment, with problems arising also from maintaining confidentiality and the segregation of vulnerable populations. They identified pharmaceutical services, dental and vision care, behavioral health services, and management of diseases such as diabetes and end-stage renal disease (ESRD) as appropriate for carve-outs. They also discussed some specifics of the HCFA's ESRD managed care demonstration under which four health plans have risk contracts for ESRD patients: SalickNet, a capitated contract with Physician Corporation of America for provision of cancer care; Community Medical Alliance, a capitated agreement with the Massachusetts Medicaid program for care of severely disabled and end-stage AIDS patients; and Control Diabetes, provision of disease management services to persons with diabetes. They concluded that specialty and population carve-outs seem suited to Medicare beneficiaries.

Fee-for-Service Medicare in a Managed Care World

While others focused on putting providers at risk for providing services to Medicare beneficiaries, Peter D. Fox examined the Medicare fee-for-service system. Fox, president of the consulting firm PDF, Inc., examined opportunities for applying managed-care techniques to the traditional system to address concerns about utilization and quality. He commented that a broad definition of managed care might be any measure by a health plan or purchaser that affects the cost, use, or quality of health services. He excluded from its purview measures relying on price per unit of service or use of a voucher (or defined contribution).

Contending that the bulk of Medicare beneficiaries will remain in the fee-for-service system (despite increases in enrollees in HMOs under risk contracts), Fox examined techniques used by HMOs, preferred provider organizations (PPOs), and point-of-service (POS) plans (which combine HMO and indemnity insurance options) that might apply to the traditional system. Data- and claims-analysis techniques might include using performance data to compare quality among providers; examining use-claims data to identify underservice; using improved provider—especially physician—profiling; conducting studies of areawide variations in use; and developing PPO arrangements based on practice profiles. He also suggested using administrative techniques, such as employing prior authorization and concurrent review, and encouraging beneficiaries to elect primary care gatekeepers. He added that bundling or packaging services (such as facility and physician payments), including skilled nursing facility services in payments to hospital diagnosis-related-groups, and paying for home health services on a per-episode basis would also save money. Prevention and case management techniques involving self-care at home, efforts by community agencies, and primary care in nursing homes may be other options.

Although he agreed that Medicare needs to adopt some of the practices of the private sector, David G. Smith, professor emeritus of political science at Swarthmore College, focused on different organizational models for restructuring fee-for-service Medicare. Saying that there needs to be "a period of sustained development," he examined four models. The first, *incrementalism,* would build on the current powers of the Department of Health and Human Services—in detecting fraud and abuse, improving purchasing procedures, and reforming home health and skilled nursing facility services—to improve the program and add new authority to enable the HCFA to make it more competitive. The second model, *consumer choice,* would entail adapting FEHBP to the Medicare population. The third, *prudent purchasing,* would reinvent HCFA to give it authority to develop both fee-for-service Medicare and procompetition managed care options. The fourth, *independent agency,* would spin the HCFA off from DHHS so that it would be free to contract for and purchase services for beneficiaries. Different models are suggested for the new HCFA: the independent agency, such as the Social Security Administration; the quasi-public U.S. Postal Service model; and the partial privatization approach of the Institute of Medicine.

In response to Fox and Smith, Alan R. Nelson, chief executive officer of the American Society of Internal Medicine and a member of the Study Panel on Fee-for-Service Medicare, stressed that fee-for-service medicine and managed care are not mutually exclusive. He pointed out that a capitation payment may be distributed on a fee-for-service basis within a medical group. Looking at the techniques and structures offered by other observers, he rejected a bureaucratic approach to controlling use and costs and chose instead to restrain them through the group at the local level. He also underscored the need for choice in beneficiaries' relationships with physicians and in their access to approved drugs and devices. Moreover, he supported the use of a risk-adjusted voucher, with beneficiaries able to purchase a POS rider.

Also addressing the question of whether fee-for-service Medicare can survive in a managed care world, Kathleen Ann Buto, the HCFA's associate administrator for policy, emphatically answered yes. In responding, she reflected on the nature of Medicare managed care, which she called "an administered-price capitation program set with a very detailed formula in statute." She also expressed faith in fee-for-service Medicare's changing and evolving to become more cost effective and in its providing for larger and larger shares of beneficiaries who are older than age 85 and are disabled. Commenting on the growth of Medicare managed care, she said that participating health plans are leading the HCFA's efforts to examine quality measurement and health outcomes; she noted that they are using their savings to offer extra benefits. Distinguishing between cost savings and restructuring, she indicated that savings for fee-for-service Medicare might come from adopting prospective payment for home health and skilled nursing facility care, competitive purchasing of durable medical equipment and laboratory services, and bundling of postacute services. Restructuring is being demonstrated by the Medicare Choices program, with experimentation of risk sharing, total risk, and capped fee-for-service. At the same time, she underscored the importance of consumer information to the success of both the fee-for-service and Medicare Choices programs.

President and chief executive officer of the Federation of American Health Systems and member of the Study Panel on Fee-for-Service Medicare, Thomas A. Scully had his own definition of managed care: "the ability to not pay every provider the same amount." Contending that the flaw of the fee-for-service system is that every provider has to be paid the same amount in each community, he emphasized that the HCFA will survive, regardless of the policy direction that Medicare takes. He endorsed reshaping the agency, however, along the lines of the U.S. Postal Service, Fannie Mae, or FEHBP. But the bottom line for him was budget legislation. He praised the reform package that passed in 1995, although he objected to the extent of its budget cuts. He expressed faith that the president and Congress would "agree on the numbers" in reconciling the budget this year: "Let us take $100 billion [in Medicare savings] and reform the system."

Leadership and Politics

Anthony C. Beilenson, who was a member of Congress representing California's Twenty-Fourth District from 1977 to 1996, set the tone for a discussion of political factors that influence efforts to change Medicare by asking: "Is there some way we can fix this problem, either wholly or in part, without hurting ourselves politically in the process?" Citing the costs of political campaigns, he stressed that congressional fund-raising from political action committees, special-interest groups, and single-issue advocates was a barrier to change because supporting reform might affect contributions. The number of politically active organizations has increased tremendously over the past few decades; their ability to use technology and generate grassroots support for their positions reflects their power. Beilenson also noted that negative campaigning contributes to members' reluctance to support reforms because their votes are used as weapons against them. Few people back home, perhaps 10 to 15 percent, really know the issues. He said that leadership is important and pointed to the bipartisan leadership that seemed to be developing in the current Congress for some politically palatable budgetary reforms.

Sheila Burke, executive dean of the Kennedy School of Government at Harvard University and chief of staff to former Senate Majority Leader Robert Dole, looked at some legislative successes of the past to illustrate the factors needed to bring about change. Public support, bipartisan commitment, risk taking, honesty in dealing, early establishment of trust, a common language, and common goals all contributed to the passage of the Tax Equity and Fiscal Responsibility Act of 1982, the Kassebaum-Kennedy health insurance portability bill, and other successful measures. They were missing in the case of Medicare catastrophic insurance and other failures. She counseled that, if Medicare reforms are to come about, the press and the American Association of Retired Persons (AARP) need to agree on a common language and a common goal to save the program. All parties need to start with what they can agree on, devote time to building trust, engage in a bipartisan effort, educate the public to gain support, and confront any failure to deal honestly.

Washington Post reporter Haynes Johnson, who coauthored *The System* with David Broder, reflected on the health system reform initiative that was the topic of their book. Saying that acceptance of the Clinton health reform plan was a political, not a policy, question, he said that it reached perfection in its failure. It was not bipartisan, it tried to do too much too fast, and it did not have public support. Agreeing with Burke about bipartisanship, incremental change, and pace, he cited the Marshall Plan and the space program as initiatives that succeeded with public consensus. Pointing to division and discord in the country, he said a new governing party might emerge that would form around fiscal discipline and generational equity and tackle not only the question of entitlement but also fiscal responsibility and money in politics.

John C. Rother, director of legislation and public policy at the AARP and member of the Study Panel on Capitation and Choice, underlined Burke's point about the need for public education on Medicare, Medicaid, and their interactions with income support and maintenance programs. He also said that any reform effort must be gradual. Referring to concerns about fraud and abuse in the Medicare program mentioned by previous commentators, he applauded Operation Restore Trust, the antifraud, antiabuse initiative that had received a funding boost from the previous Congress. He also advocated making clear the difference between a program cut and a saving, agreeing to common language, seeking bipartisanship, and perhaps separating reform legislation from the budget process. For him, language was a vital part of leadership in the politics of Medicare reform.

Public Opinion and Medicare Restructuring

The need for public support of Medicare restructuring was stressed again and again, as were the importance of gauging public opinion and bringing the public along in any effort to reform the program. Karlyn H. Bowman, a resident fellow at the American Enterprise Institute, discussed survey data compiled by the Roper Center of the University of Connecticut during the last three months of 1996 and found sixty-nine questions on Medicare. Respondents were overwhelmingly positive about the program: 72 percent viewed it favorably in a survey done by Public Opinion Strategies. But when questions were posed about the political tug-of-war over the program, the public was skeptical about whether there really is a crisis. People did recognize that the program has problems and, according to an NBC News/*Wall Street Journal* poll, tended to support some means-testing of higher-income beneficiaries but resisted raising the eligibility age and increasing the payroll tax. Only 30 percent of those polled were in favor of a voucher system, but respondents were evenly divided on providing incentives to participate in HMOs.

For Robert J. Blendon, professor and chairman of the Department of Health Policy and Management in the School of Public Health at Harvard University, "Medicare is both a public opinion issue and a voting issue." Pointing out that there are significant differences in voting behavior relative to Medicare between those over the age of 60 and those under the age of 30, he noted that people in the older group gave high priority to Medicare and Social Security and those in the younger group "chose not to concern themselves with this set of problems." He also said that many people do not see Medicare and Social Security as part of the consolidated federal budget and oppose balancing the budget with benefit reductions. He noted that public misconceptions over Medicare's share of the budget (that it is smaller than it really is) and the number of elderly in poverty (that it is larger than it really is) are barriers to making budget or benefit changes. Blendon's advice to politicians was to focus on the short term: to pay providers less, means-test benefits for upper-income people, and make some administrative changes. In the long term, they should consider managed care. He insisted, however, that public education be part of the process for political legitimacy.

William McInturff, a partner and cofounder of Public Opinion Strategies, reflected on the dangers of taking on Medicare reform in the face of public resistance. Because the public resisted cutting the program to balance the budget and because the elderly wanted more Medicare benefits and were suspicious of Republican efforts to lead reform, he advocated that Republicans take a "preserve, protect, and strengthen" approach. But off-the-cuff comments from Republican leaders and television ads undermined that strategy. In the future, McInturff said that the president should take the lead in recommending restructuring changes. Although he doubted that the president would follow that course, he observed that, for both political parties, dealing with reform before the 2000 election would be most prudent.

Celinda Lake, president of Lake Research, looked at polls taken in 1995 and in 1996 and agreed with McInturff that policy people need to separate the senior vote from the nonsenior vote. She contended that senior voters showed volatility in the extent to which they supported the president and uncertainty in their congressional voting intentions. They also tended to be suspicious of talk about Medicare changes, although all age groups opposed cuts in the program. However, only 23 percent of persons 18 to 35, 20 percent of those 36 to 50, and 35 percent of those 51 to 64 thought that Medicare would have funding available to provide benefits for them in their retirement (as opposed to 54 percent of those 65 and older). Reductions in the program gained support only if they were intended to protect it. Lake thought that Republican campaign strategy had been successful in raising interest in matters affecting health care and retirement before the election; however, around the time of the election, that interest had declined, resulting in a Democratic president and Republican Congress.

Lake also noted that health care, Medicare, and Social Security issues tended to move in tandem. In addition, she commented on gender differences, that women tend to be more concerned about health care and Social Security while men are more focused on the deficit, taxes, and campaign reform. These differences were reflected in women's tilt toward the president on Election Day. She believed that Medicare reform remained the Democrats' "most powerful issue." Moreover, she was convinced that "it will be hard to create the political will for the kinds of changes we need in Medicare."

The conference concluded in agreement that restructuring Medicare will be one of the most difficult tasks facing the nation because of the nature of the original contract; the mixed payroll tax, premium, and general revenue financing, as well as cost-containment concerns; the challenge of aligning Medicare with a reconfiguring health marketplace; the program's fee-for-service tradition; the difficulty of gaining political leadership; and the complexities of getting public support. The conference brought together veterans and new thinkers to consider options to contribute to the deliberations of the National Academy of Social Insurance's Medicare Steering Committee and in part to encourage attendees and those who read this volume to think about the shape the program should take in the twenty-first century.

2

Medicare's Social Contract

S EVERAL AUTHORS in this chapter address the Medicare
social contract created between the federal government
and the program beneficiaries more than thirty years ago. Although the authors
agree on the significance of the contract to discussions of Medicare reform,
they disagree on whether specific changes would preserve or destroy the
program.

The Contract and Medicare Reform
Stuart Butler

WHEN THE MEDICARE SYSTEM was created in the mid-
1960s, the social contract generally promised to provide the elderly with
medical services that were similar to those enjoyed by the typical worker and
to do so at reasonable cost to the elderly and to society. What the United States
achieved in trying to fulfill the contract was, unfortunately, badly flawed.
Medicare was a compromise that reflected the politics of the Vietnam War and
Johnson administration years. Now the system is frozen in time according to
the politics of thirty years ago.

Medicare has a mandatory social insurance component, principally to pay
for hospital care (and other institutional care and home health care), that is
funded by a payroll system. In addition, it has a heavily subsidized system of
voluntary insurance run by the government. This covers and subsidizes
physicians' and other nonhospital services without regard to the income of the
people receiving the services. So, the arrangement in place is a hybrid and not
one a policymaker would initially think of to carry out the contract.

First, the system promised specific benefits irrespective of cost. The cost
was going to be paid mostly by society. Unlike Social Security, which prom-

ised specific levels of income, Medicare promised specific benefits. Second, Medicare used central planning to deliver services at a cost affordable to patients and society. This meant using administered prices, regulation, and centralization to try to bring about the contract itself at reasonable cost. Third, the system was not means tested, although a person's payroll taxes were linked to his income. The subsidy for the delivery of hospital services and the voluntary physician payments were and remain not linked to income. Fourth, no limit was placed on the total financial exposure of the patients, the elderly themselves.

The problems that have arisen as a result of the way Medicare was designed are now demanding to be addressed. The one that attracts the most attention in Washington during the budget cycle is that the program has chronic financial problems that are related both to the public's perception of it and to the means established to discharge the social contract.

Most people have the notion that Medicare is a true social insurance program, that whether one is rich or poor, one has paid for the benefits. Therefore, any attempt to adjust premium costs, such as raising those paid by the very affluent, leads to righteous indignation among people who feel that they are merely getting back what they paid. Anybody who knows anything about the finances of the program knows, of course, that it is not true social insurance, but a large segment of the population that is not poor resists changing it.

But government, with the means currently used to fulfill the social contract, is failing to deliver. The quality and quantity of benefits are more similar to those of private plans in the 1960s than those of the 1990s. Medicare does not cover people for the cost of pharmaceuticals out of hospital. Surgery is covered, but drugs used during recovery at home are not. A surgical patient has to buy medigap coverage or pay for the necessary drugs himself. Finally, there is no true catastrophic coverage.

Moreover, Medicare no longer effectively protects society from high costs. Not only is there no effective means of making sure that costs to the elderly are reasonable, but the funding of part B has also given unlimited exposure to the ordinary taxpayer in order to provide heavy subsidies to people who, in many cases, do not need it.

If one looks fairly at the problems, it is not unreasonable to say, "Maybe we should start reevaluating the system." Are there better ways to achieve the contract and provide a better program for the elderly? This does not mean destroying the system and the social contract itself. This means improving Medicare.

One of the basic flaws is centralization. Central planning and its price controls and regulations did not work in Soviet agriculture, and they do not work in Medicare. The program has used price controls, or administered pricing, since its inception in an attempt to keep costs down. Policymakers had hoped this would not lead to distortions and inefficiency, but that is exactly what has happened. So more and more controls have been added, which means more and more intrusion and more and more cheating by care providers. The providers always have better computers and experts to figure out ways of using the system than the Health Care and Finance Administration has computers and experts to stop them. There is a continuous cat-and-mouse game in which the providers always seem to win and the taxpayers always seem to lose.

Another feature of this highly centralized administered agreement is the barriers encountered in trying to make any fundamental changes in the price structure. Those who would change the program must mount an enormous campaign over many years and obtain statutes in Congress by taking on all the lobbyists to effect a change that a corporation and its union can agree on in one Friday afternoon meeting. That is the result of a system that is centralized, one that the Congress of the United States is essentially designing every detail of and running. It necessarily follows that it is extremely difficult to make any reasonable adjustment of the system.

The system of benefits is inefficient for the same reason. Every change is resisted by those who believe they would lose something. So it is extremely difficult to make even the most subtle and reasonable change to allow Medicare to catch up with the private sector. And that is why, when people go into Medicare, in many ways they feel they are entering a time warp and why it is so difficult to introduce reasonable changes to improve the program.

In considering all this, it becomes clear that America needs a public debate to figure out ways, first of all, to reaffirm the original social contract itself, but then to look at more effective ways of fulfilling it.

I believe the social contract today should assure the elderly and the disabled that they will have a modern health care system, including modern benefits, comparable to that available to the rest of the population. We should deliver health care at an affordable cost to all the elderly, rich or poor, and at a reasonable cost to society. That should be our contract.

Two broad steps must be taken to bring about that result. First, the social contract needs to be much clearer to people and must recognize the deficiencies of the past thirty years. This means looking very carefully at the distinction between a subsidized system and a true social insurance system. If under the current arrangements we were to try to turn Medicare into a true social insurance system paid for by working people through payroll taxes, we would need staggering increases in taxes. Alternatively, we could give up on any kind of payroll payment and no longer consider Medicare a social insurance program.

The federal government could simply pay for it out of general revenue without regard to any kind of control on costs. But this solution would create another staggering problem.

The right approach would be to redefine the contract by explicitly stating that Medicare should be partly a social insurance program, which guarantees people specific benefits, and partly a true means-tested subsidy program. This means we might want to consider not doing away with the distinction between part A and part B, as some people suggest. To do so would add to the problems of making any change and confuse the public even further about what kind of program Medicare really is. As an alternative, part A could be turned into a true, fully funded social insurance program. It could be made more comprehensive in the services it provides, but the extent of public financial support could be made leaner through higher deductibles, higher copayments, and so forth. At the same time, part B could be turned into a true means-tested program assigned to give people financial help if they need it to deal with the out-of-pocket expenses associated with a redefined and restructured part A.

In other words, through part A, an elderly person in America would have much more comprehensive benefits with higher deductibles and copayments. But through part B, a poorer elderly person would be heavily supported to pay for the out-of-pocket costs that he or she could incur. Wealthy people would get very little, if anything, in part B support. It seems to me that this proposal would lead to a public recognition that the current system is not equitable.

A second broad change that needs to be made is to alter the locus of control of the system's finances. Right now, central control means that Washington determines what payments should be made. Washington also determines what is good value for the money. But we should move toward allowing the elderly to take the financial value of their Medicare benefits and obtain a plan or coverage in some other way than through the traditional program or an HMO. This would constitute an important step in recognizing that it is the enrollees themselves who should be the arbiters of value. They should have the right to get the benefits that they need rather than those determined by Congress and the lobbyists. Taking this step would give incentives to providers to satisfy the beneficiaries rather than the latest rule from HCFA.

The National Academy of Social Insurance is currently engaged in this kind of rethinking, exploring these and other directions for change. There are many possible models to look at, and they are being examined in the various study groups.

One system that I have found very attractive is the Federal Employees Health Benefits Program. Whether one agrees with the FEHBP or not, it certainly suggests a very different structure for the way government could function: a revised Medicare system. The FEHBP model, like others we are looking at, would encourage the government to increase and improve the kind of information it provides to people, focusing much more on making options available. Instead of trying to micromanage pricing throughout the entire industry, an FEHBP-type Medicare would require the government to focus on allowing new services and options, providing better information, and carefully structuring a market in which to make decisions.

We may be at a stage in the debate over the future of Medicare where we can actually begin to have some thoughtful discussion about what kinds of changes can work and what they would mean. Americans need to have that if we are going to have a system that is modern and can actually fulfill the promised social contract.

Pundits, People, and Medicare Reform
Theda Skocpol

THE 1995–96 ELECTION CYCLE brought to national attention Medicare and its problems and revealed the chasm that separates elite and popular opinion about this crucial part of modern U.S. social provision. Pundits and people are not on the same wavelength, which could have dire consequences for the future of American democracy as well as for the shape and extent of the nation's commitment to decent health care for the elderly.

Contrary to the near consensus that grips Washington policy analysts, most Americans are not ready to have experts and politicians whom they profoundly distrust fundamentally restructure a cherished health security program on which they or their loved ones greatly depend. Most Americans do not want to give up a national commitment to fund a consistent set of health services with maximum choice of providers in favor of a leap into a world of more paperwork, more bureaucracy, increasing complexity and unpredictable costs for individuals, and much more anxiety for the elderly and their relatives. The pundits are ready to move from defined benefits to fixed and shrinking public contributions, but most of the people do not want to go along.

Bill Clinton trounced Bob Dole with nearly half the popular vote in 1996 while congressional Democrats also gained significant ground. The turnaround for Democrats was striking in that they had been left for dead after the Republican triumphs two years earlier. In large part, Democrats did well in 1996 because less economically privileged voters came back to the polls, looking to the president and other Democrats to defend "M2E2," that is Medicare, Medicaid, federal commitments to education, and national environmental regulations.[1] President Clinton may have pronounced big government dead in January 1996, but he rode America's biggest and best-loved public programs—Medicare above all—to his second-term victory. An immediate postelection poll found continuing majority support for universal health coverage and concluded that most of the American public "is focused on protecting Medicare from cuts, not on entitlement reform."[2]

Voters hardly had time to get home from the polls before editorialists and advocacy groups declared that the election was an endorsement for a "dynamic center" determined to undertake far-reaching entitlement reforms.[3] President Clinton was urged to be "courageous," to "rise above partisanship" by appointing a bipartisan commission led by experts to fundamentally restructure Social Security and Medicare. Clinton, the pundits declared, should avoid short-term fixes and instead undertake major restructurings, even more breathtaking in scope and departure from the status quo than his failed health reform effort of 1993–94.

Medicare is the prime object of structural reformist zeal. Crisis fever is harder to whip up about Social Security because its trust fund is, after all, currently in surplus; Social Security's problems will grow gradually only after 2012, and immediate modest adjustments could fend off the projected trouble. But Medicare part A has been declared near bankruptcy, meaning that some serious decisions about benefits or finances or both *do* need to be made very soon. Immediate difficulties in the program open the door wide for those who want the president and Congress also to address the projected rapid increases in Medicare spending that will accompany the aging of the baby boom generation. Since its inception as a program that catered to doctors and private insurance companies, Medicare has become part of the overall rapid increase in U.S. health spending; and it sticks out as a huge part of federal spending during an era of budget-balancing politics. In short, all sorts of crises and problematic trends converge to make demands for an immediate drastic Medicare overhaul plausible in elite circles.

Without going into the details of clashing plans for structural reform, it is clear that responsible experts and pundits (translation: conservatives and centrists, not "irresponsible" liberals) are focusing on plans to transform Medicare from a promise of predictable payment for a defined package of health services for each elderly person into a shrinking public contribution to part of the variable amounts individuals would need to pay for decent health coverage. There are also schemes for (more or less forcibly) injecting new kinds of so-called choices into each individual's situation: not just the choice of service providers (fee for service or an HMO) that already exists in Medicare, but also choices about how to spend a fixed voucher on one of hundreds of private insurance plans or perhaps even a choice between medical savings accounts and payments toward more complete coverage. The existing system of fairly open personal flexibility to connect to many doctors would be compromised or abolished in the schemes for structural reform that are currently fashionable.

Much of this book focuses on the details of alternative reform schemes, with arguments about the advantages and dangers of each. I will not burden readers with my opinions on every alternative. But I cannot resist saying that given the realities of U.S. politics and public administration, all the schemes for defined contribution reforms are likely to make inequalities of income worse and hamper the elderly's access to decent care. No matter how well designed on paper, all the schemes would end up allowing the better-off elderly and the momentarily healthier to separate themselves from increasingly inadequate provisions for the less-well-off and the sicker. The contemplated structural reforms in Medicare would promote what Robert Reich calls the "secession of the affluent" from shared public social provision. And there will be gender as well as class effects, because women tend to live longer. Even a well-off woman like me does not look forward to living to be a post-eighty-five-year-old subject to any of the plans for structural reform that are being bruited about. As the cartoon goes:

> Doctor to older patient: "I've got good news and bad news!"
> Patient: "What's the good news?"
> Doctor: "You're going to outlive Medicare!"
> Patient: "What's the bad news?"
> Doctor: "You're going to outlive Medicare!"[4]

Joking aside, my message is directed at all those clashing experts, everyone vying for a place on that Commission to End Medicare As We Know It. My message is, look before you leap. Trained (in most cases) as economists, health care experts are accustomed to arguing in terms of static technical design and rational claims about cost efficiency. But historically grounded moral understandings are much more important for other citizens. And institutional realities are much more relevant for predicting what will actually occur as plans meet politics, as proposals are eviscerated and reworked amidst congressional and interest-group maneuvers over reforming Medicare. Remember Ira Magaziner and his friends? They did not pay much attention to history, institutions, and predictable political processes when they drew up their ideal health care plan for the Clinton administration to lay before Congress. We all know what happened next.[5]

Consider the big picture of historically evolved public understandings about Medicare. Today Medicare has become a potential albatross for Social Security because Medicare's problems could end up dragging a much healthier Social Security system into a donnybrook over radical restructuring. But a little over thirty years ago, Medicare complemented a popular Social Security system. Medicare delivered much needed additional protections to retirees eligible for Social Security. More important, Social Security's main institutional feature—payroll tax financing and benefits delivered to former workers and their families without demeaning or intrusive means tests—provided a solid basis on which to build Medicare. Although Medicare was certainly more institutionally complex, reform advocates in the 1960s could argue that the program would work like Social Security. Most Americans heard that message, and liked it very much.[6]

From early in our nation's history, successful American social policies have shared certain basic features.[7] From public schools and Civil War benefits in the nineteenth century, through early twentieth-century programs for mothers and children, and on to Social Security, the GI bill, and Medicare, effective and politically popular U.S. social programs have embodied a recognizable moral rationale and encompassed broad constituencies. The best have promised supports for individuals in return for service to the larger community. And they have delivered benefits without means tests to individuals and families across lines of class, race, and place. Social Security and Medicare are both very much part of this tradition, offering substantial and honorable help to retired people who are understood to have contributed to the nation through lifetimes of work.

We need to realize that the social transaction here is much more than an individualistic investment of payroll taxes to buy pensions or services in the future. People believe that there is a morally grounded contract between families and the nation; they see eventual retirement benefits as something they earn through work, not just by virtue of making tax payments. Professional and managerial elites may have lost sight of popular moral understandings in recent years because most highly educated and powerful people do not look forward to retirement at all. But the bulk of American working people are not doing thrilling or self-fulfilling jobs. They are more likely to see their lives as a moral story with deserved rewards coming at the end.[8] People work hard, often in jobs that are neither well paid nor very secure, and they raise their children and cooperate with their neighbors. At the end of a lifetime of such socially responsible contributions lies a secure and dignified retirement, primarily anchored for most people in Social Security and Medicare.

As a poster in the 1930s put it, "Old Age Should Be the Harvest of a Fruitful Life," and most Americans still fervently believe this.[9] Perhaps all the more so today, in the wake of two decades of hard times for less privileged workers and families.[10] When people hear elites telling them that their hard-earned retirement protections may not be there, they profoundly resent and fear the message. Ordinary Americans feel betrayed by the thought that the federal government and the nation's leaders may break the social contract they have tried to live by and want to grow old by.

For more than a decade now, antigovernment conservatives have been pursuing a grand strategy to undermine Americans' faith in Social Security and Medicare, carrying out plans such as the one Stuart Butler and Peter Germanis outlined in the early 1980s article, "Achieving a Leninist Strategy."[11] This remarkable piece outlined tactics for undermining Americans' faith in public social insurance and preparing the ground for eventual individualistic and market-oriented privatization. Of course, there have been many parts to the overall assault that opponents of social insurance have mounted. One key part has been an effort to shake the faith of young people, especially affluent young people, that systems such as Medicare and Social Security are sound enough to be there for them in the future. Conservatives have talked incessantly about generational warfare, deploying economic projections and statistics sorted out by age cohorts. Conservatives in American politics are very good at getting their polemic messages broadly disseminated, so the generational assaults on Social Security and Medicare have spread much further than just to the readers of highbrow publications.

Efforts to undermine popular faith in social insurance have made some headway. Today, younger Americans are no longer sure that those protections will exist when they get old. But in another sense, generational warfare arguments have not worked well. Younger Americans remain just as supportive of generous social provision for the elderly as do the elderly themselves, indeed sometimes more so.[12] In real life, people are connected to one another as parents and children, grandparents and grandchildren.[13] Folks just do not think like "generational accounting" economists. Most American adults, especially adult women, report being in weekly or daily touch with their mothers.[14] Particularly among women, America's generations are not really socioculturally separated, let alone at war.

There is a perfectly understandable social dynamic behind the growing gender gap in American politics, especially about attitudes toward social programs such as Medicare. When an elderly woman starts worrying about "the government messing with her Medicare," the first person to hear about it is her daughter. And her daughter is very likely to listen closely, because she knows very well that if anything happens to the personal expense or quality of her mother's health care, it will not be Pete Peterson or Newt Gingrich who will have to take "more personal responsibility." She knows that *she* is the one who will have to do more to help her mother, perhaps taking money from a hard-pressed family budget or sparing precious hours amidst the pressures of her overcrowded days. After two hours getting everyone out the door in the morning, followed by eight hours at the office and several hours of housework and helping the children with their homework at night, our putative adult woman knows she can then look forward to talking with her mother about how to keep her beloved doctor or pay extra money to the right specialist. After a decade or so of doing all this, that same woman could look forward to a retirement full of hassles with whatever the Washington elites have dreamed up for her, too, instead of Medicare. She could anticipate worrying about which HMO to join, or wondering whether her voucher will pay for decent health care. Revisions of popular health programs like Medicare (and Medicaid) are, in short, not just issues for the elderly. They are family issues. Consequently, women of all ages will be paying close attention and worrying a lot about who is planning what for Medicare.

To get back to the big picture, there are good moral and social reasons why millions of Americans say that they are not very enthusiastic about big structural changes in Medicare. For all of its shortcomings people have come to trust and rely on Medicare as we know it. They like its predictable benefits and the choice of health care providers it allows. They do not see the sharp generational trade-offs that the privatizers posit. Nor do they care for the argument—now routine at places like the Brookings Institution—that elderly Americans have to be "brought into the same system" of health care delivery and financing as everyone else. Working-aged Americans of modest means know that many of them do not have health coverage or else have to pay more and more for increasingly niggardly and bureaucratically inflexible forms of care. Most people want better than that for their parents—and for themselves, too, when they make it to the promised land of retirement.

Experts, of course, believe that most Americans are childish about trade-offs, that they refuse to acknowledge national budget problems and do not want to pay taxes for a cherished program that is doomed by demography and medical technology. Maybe there is some truth in such views of the great unwashed. But it is also true that Americans have been fairly consistent, and not so irrational, in what they tell pollsters and their elected leaders.[15] Most Americans want the federal budget balanced but would prefer do it slowly if that is necessary to sustain Medicare. Most people argue for making cuts in payments to doctors and hospitals first. And most would consider raising taxes and premiums on very well off employees and beneficiaries. Americans have also made it clear that they would like to see cutbacks in government programs besides Medicare and Social Security.

Pundits routinely editorialize that America cannot abide an expanding proportion of its public expenditures devoted to the elderly (the implication is that old people are a waste, not a good investment). But average citizens apparently do not see things this way. Most seem willing to have more spent on the elderly as the country grays. And why is it so unthinkable that the United States might spend a growing proportion of its tax resources on our parents and grandparents (rather than, say, on corporate subsidies and B-1 bombers)? Understandably, congressional representatives and institutional elites want substantial tax monies channeled into manipulable programs rather than automatic entitlements. Meanwhile, though, most Americans might be very happy with a federal government that concentrates on well-understood social insurance programs that deliver a modicum of security with dignity to millions of families.

In the final analysis, maybe American elites just do not want to hear what a majority of their fellow citizens are saying, particularly about programs such as Medicare and Social Security.[16] Elites think they know what is best and are determined to forge ahead with structural reforms that may end up hurting and disillusioning millions of their fellow citizens. At a time when citizen distrust of the federal government is at an all-time high, policy experts, editorialists, and other pundits are urging the president and Congress to undertake radical transformations in Medicare, changes very much at odds with historically evolved moral understandings and different from the incremental steps that most voters have said they prefer.

With his eye on the editorial pages and his ear to the think-tank ground, President Clinton may soon take the plunge into commission-mandated structural reform. Maybe Congress will even manage to process recommended structural changes in Medicare, writing lots of subsidies for the health services and insurance industries into the details of the bills as they pass through committees. I hope not. Given today's bitter partisan divisions, I even tend to doubt it. (Sometimes gridlock is a good thing.) But all of this could happen, because the pundit consensus is so strong and elected politicians have so many incentives to slash the federal budget and avoid taxes while devising new subsidies for businesses.

But if top-down attempts at structural transformations of Medicare are made during the next several years, whatever finally spews forth from the congressional process is not likely to be good for average and less privileged Americans. Structural transformations proposed of by a commission and disposed of by Congress as we know it could be even worse for American democracy than for people's health care. Citizens who already believe there is little to like and trust about Washington may end up with their worst fears confirmed. This seems almost certain to be the result if experts and pundits insist on going forward with radical proposals for Medicare restructuring that head in directions most of the American people do not want to go.

So I say to all of the experts, for the sake of American democracy (not to mention for the good of old ladies, past and future), think carefully about institutional legacies, social morality, and political realities. Do not concentrate just on ideal plans and the technical details of reform proposals. Keep the health of American democracy in mind as you proceed, lest you leap too rashly into the brave new world of radically restructuring a program that most of your fellow citizens view as a keystone of the nation's social contract and a cherished support for their own life stories. Find gradual ways to adjust our shared and dignified Medicare program for the future. And if you must bring all Americans into the same system of health care and insurance, consider improving and universalizing coverage for working-aged families rather than reducing coverage for our retired grandparents.

Notes

1. Ruy Teixeira, "Who Rejoined the Democrats? Understanding the 1996 Election Results," Economic Policy Institute, Washington, November 1996.

2. "The Popular Mandate of 1996: The Voter Concerns That Decided the Election and That Will Shape the Future Agenda," Greenberg Research and CAF, Washington, November 12, 1996.

3. Details in Harold Meyerson, "Dead Center," *American Prospect,* no. 30 (January-February 1997), pp. 60–67.

4. This cartoon appears in Marilyn Moon, *Medicare Now and in the Future,* 2d ed. (Washington: Urban Institute Press, 1996), p. xvii.

5. See Theda Skocpol, *Boomerang: Clinton's Health Security Effort and the Turn against Government in U.S. Politics* (Norton, 1996).

6. Theodore R. Marmor, *The Politics of Medicare* (Chicago: Aldine, 1973); and Lawrence R. Jacobs, *The Health of Nations: Public Opinion and the Making of American and British Health Policy* (Cornell University Press, 1993), chap. 9.

7. For background, see Theda Skocpol, *Protecting Soldiers and Mothers: The Political Origins of Social Policy in the United States* (Harvard University Press, 1992); and Skocpol, *Social Policies in the United States: Future Possibilities in Historical Perspective* (Princeton University Press, 1995).

8. See the splendid research on the views of non-college-educated working people in Stanley B. Greenberg, *The Economy Project* (Washington: Greenberg Research, 1996).

9. The poster is cited in the *New York Times,* January 19, 1997, p. C1.

10. Sheldon Danziger and Peter Gottschalk, *America Unequal* (Harvard University Press, 1995).

11. Stuart Butler and Peter Germanis, "Achieving a Leninist Strategy," *Cato Journal,* vol. 3 (Fall 1983), pp. 547–61.

12. This finding appears again and again in opinion studies, including Fay Lomax Cook and Edith J. Barrett, *Support for the American Welfare State* (Columbia University Press, 1992).

13. Eric R. Kingson, Barbara A. Hirshorn, and John M. Cornman, *Ties That Bind: The Interdependence of Generations* (Cabin John, Md.: Seven Locks Press, 1986); and Vern L. Bengston and Robert A. Harootyan, *Intergenerational Linkages: Hidden Connections in American Society* (Springer Publishing, 1994).

14. Leora Lawton, Merril Silverstein, and Vern L. Bengston, "Solidarity between Generations in Families," in Bengston and Harootyan, *Intergenerational Linkages,* pp. 26–27.

15. In addition to "Popular Mandate of 1996," see Robert J. Blendon and others, "The Public's View of the Future of Medicare," *Journal of the American Medical Association,* vol. 274 (November 1995), pp. 1645–48.

16. The thesis that elites are not listening is elaborated and documented in Lawrence R. Jacobs and Robert Y. Shapiro, "The Politicization of Public Opinion," prepared for a forthcoming Brookings Institution–Russell Sage Foundation book edited by Margaret Weir.

Reflections on How Medicare Came About
Robert M. Ball

TO HELP READERS understand how this rather strange collection of legal provisions and administrative choices called Medicare came about requires me to try to recapture the times and the goals of those of us who put it together and, in my case, had the responsibility for administering it during its first seven years.[1]

Much can be explained by our reliance on the guiding hand of pragmatism, what we could get Congress to agree to—what could pass—and in administration what would work. As critics might say, our decisions were frequently the triumph of opportunism over principle. And there is truth in this observation, although on some points there was a stubborn defense of principle that at times seemed to threaten the very operation of the program. For example, we took the view that for hospitals, principally southern hospitals, simply to submit plans for desegregation would not be enough to qualify them for the Medicare program, although "plans" had been considered enough in the case of schools. Instead, just months before Medicare was to start paying for hospital services

Some of this material appeared first in "What Medicare Architects Had in Mind," *Health Affairs* (Winter 1995), p. 62.

and while hundreds of hospitals were not yet certified, the program had a thousand inspectors in the field, visiting hospitals to make sure that blacks and whites were being assigned to semiprivate rooms without regard to race. And remember, these were older people who had lived their lifetimes in rigid segregation. The *New York Times* suggested that the Johnson administration ought to make up its mind. Did it want to supply medical care services in the South or did it want hospital integration? The administration, it was argued, clearly could not have both. But in fact we did get both, just about everywhere.

There were a few holdouts, particularly in a chain of religious hospitals in the South. But to an extent pragmatism came to the program's aid here too. It paid for "emergency services" in unapproved hospitals if they were substantially closer to the patient at the time of the emergency than any other hospital. (And for a time, we were not too strict about the definition of an emergency.) No one died from lack of care because of the insistence on integration, or at least no one made that case. Perhaps here is a principle of successful public administration: Go as far as you can in the right direction from the beginning without causing a stalemate, but be prepared to tighten up later. Reimburse HMOs 95 percent of the cost of providing services on a fee-for-service basis, for example, but if with experience that proves to be too much, turn the screws a bit.

Although integrating hospitals principally illustrates devotion to principle, there was, as I have said, pragmatism too. Medicare legislation had marched up the Hill and back again several times before it passed. Votes were always close. The American Medical Association (AMA) was strongly opposed to the idea and had at least the superficial support of all parts of the medical enterprise, except the nurses, and the strong support of the insurance industry and most of the business community. When at last the legislation was in the Senate under circumstances in which passage seemed very likely—Lyndon Johnson had just been elected overwhelmingly to a new term—the application of the recently passed civil rights law to Medicare's hospitals was on the minds of most southern senators. They, and the administration, needed at all costs to avoid an explicit vote on the matter. So the only legislative history that we had to rely on for the drive against segregation was a colloquy on the Senate floor when Senator Abraham Ribicoff replied to a question that "Yes, title VI would, of course, apply." That was it. No debate, no newspaper story, nothing.

Pragmatism appeared in the shape of the program itself. Why, with no experience with a federal health insurance program, did the United States choose to start a program with the elderly, from any rational viewpoint the most unlikely initial group? The administration did not know how to run a health insurance program, so why did it decide to begin with the most difficult possible group? The elderly were by far the most costly group: admissions would be more frequent and stays would be longer than those of other age groups, the patients would have multiple illnesses, and after expensive treatment, they would, nevertheless, frequently die. Even when cured they were not a very good investment in terms of years of life ahead.

As a society if America was going to start with a given age group, it would seem to have made much more sense to start with children or perhaps mothers and children. They did not need expensive care very often, and the investment would make a difference for a lifetime ahead. So why not children? Why the elderly? Only one reason. Politically, the administration had the best chance with them. It is important at this stage of the story to remember that those who advocated Medicare wanted something more. The AMA was right. This was to be the entering wedge for a universal health plan. Those of us who were active at the time are still astounded that more than thirty years later only the disabled have been added to the program. We had hoped that long before now the feasibility and desirability of a universal system would have been demonstrated and it would be in operation.

Medicare came about because the advocates of universal health insurance were discouraged. The idea of a universal program had never made much progress in the United States. Ironically, national health insurance was advocated in 1916 by the leaders of the AMA, who were favorably impressed by the systems that had been established in Germany (1883), Britain (1911), and later in several other countries. Equally ironic was that much of the American labor movement in 1916 was opposed. Samuel Gompers, president of the American Federation of Labor, preferred collective bargaining to political solutions and feared that if workers began leaning on government, they might feel less need for unions.

These positions were soon reversed. By 1920 the AMA was firmly established in opposition to government health insurance. The unions, however, eventually went all out in favor of a government plan and indeed provided the backbone of its support. These two powerful groups became the main antagonists, first over national health insurance and then over the much more modest recommendations for Medicare.

President Franklin Roosevelt did not support national health insurance at the time of the 1934 recommendations of the Committee on Economic Security, and it was not included with the recommendations that formed the basis for the Social Security Act in 1935. He feared, probably correctly, that because health insurance had such strong opposition from physicians and others, if it were included in his program for economic security, he might lose the entire program. In later years he often commented favorably on universal health coverage, but he never offered or endorsed a national health insurance plan. He called for social insurance from the cradle to the grave, and in his 1944 State of the Union message, looking to the nations postwar needs and goals, he proposed an Economic Bill of Rights that included the "right to adequate medical care and the opportunity to achieve and enjoy good health." But occasional rhetorical sorties aside, he was content to let the Social Security Board push for national health insurance without adding his personal endorsement.

President Harry Truman specifically advocated a national health insurance plan. His power to get any domestic legislation passed, however, was weak, both while he was filling out Roosevelt's fourth term and after he had surprised everyone but himself by getting elected on his own in 1948. Facing Republicans in control of both houses of Congress, he had no chance of getting universal compulsory health insurance enacted, a situation that everyone but the AMA seemed to understand.

The AMA's opposition approached hysteria. For the first time, members were assessed special dues, which were used to fight health insurance. The organization created a $3.5 million war chest—very big money for the time—with which it conducted a campaign of vituperation against the advocates of national health insurance. It also exerted strict discipline over the few of its members who took an "unethical" position favoring the government program. This was a warm-up for later campaigns against Medicare.

Even before the AMA launched its attack, however, the Truman administration had given up on universal health insurance and was casting about for something less ambitious that might have a better chance. That is how Medicare was born—as a fallback. It was publicly advocated for the first time by a government spokesman when Oscar Ewing, head of the Federal Security Agency (now, after several reincarnations, the Department of Health and Human Services), unveiled it on February 27, 1952. The idea was to cover all Social Security beneficiaries: the elderly, widows, and orphans (persons with disabilities were not yet under Social Security.) Social Security was part of the Federal Security Agency, and we had worked up the plan for Ewing.

Initially, it went nowhere. President Truman never specifically endorsed the shift from support of universal health insurance to the limited Medicare program, but even if he had, he would not have been able to get Congress to consider it. He was within months of the end of his term. And Adlai Stevenson was soon to be overwhelmingly defeated for the presidency by Dwight D. Eisenhower.

The design of Medicare, which was taking shape in an unsympathetic political climate, was based entirely on a strategy of acceptability: What sort of program would be most difficult for opponents to attack and most likely to pick up critical support? Later modification to include just the elderly rather than all

Social Security beneficiaries and to cover them only for hospitalization had the same motivation. By the time John F. Kennedy campaigned on the issue in 1960, we had decided that even trying to provide coverage for inpatient surgery was a mistake. If physician services were left out entirely, we reasoned, the AMAs opposition would have less standing. By that time it was clear that the elderly had the most political appeal and potentially the most muscle. We wanted to get something going, and this seemed a politically plausible first step.

The elderly were an appealing group to cover first in part because they were so ill suited for coverage under voluntary private insurance. They used on average more than twice as many hospital days as younger people but had only about half as much income. Private insurers, who set premiums to cover current costs, had to charge them much more, and the elderly could not afford the charges. Group health insurance, then as today, was mostly for the employed and was just not available to the retired elderly. The result of all this was that somewhat less than half of the elderly had any kind of health insurance, and what they had was almost always inadequate, often paying only so much per day for hospitalizations of limited duration. So the need was not hard to prove, nor was it difficult to prove that voluntary individual insurance was not only not meeting the need, but that it really could not meet the need.

Our principles were pragmatic and goals were limited. We did not propose a program to reform the health care delivery system. We proposed assuring the same level of care for the elderly as was then enjoyed by paying and insured patients; otherwise, we did not intend to disrupt the status quo. Had we advocated anything else, it never would have received serious consideration. Thus the bill we wrote followed the principles of reimbursement that hospitals all over the country had worked out with the Blue Cross system. Government would be unobtrusive. Hospitals would be allowed to nominate an intermediary to do the actual bill payments and to be the contact point with hospitals. The carrot was that hospital bills that had previously gone unpaid because many of the elderly had no money would now be paid.

What the hospitals worked out with Blue Cross was retroactive cost reimbursement. Hospitals had an even better deal with the commercial insurance companies, which based their reimbursement on hospital charges that were ordinarily higher than costs. But at that time we had no plans for prospective payment or even prospective budgeting. By and large, our stance was not to rock the boat and to pay full costs, not intervening very much in how hospitals, at least the better ones, conducted their business.

We intended to bring the elderly, and under Medicaid the poor, the same standard of treatment as paying patients received. At that time amenities for the poor were very few, and the aged, who were mostly poor, were usually treated in hospital wards where their care was often left to interns and medical students. Indeed, one of organized medicine's objections to Medicare and Medicaid was that these programs would close off their main sources of teaching material. (Of course, that did not come to pass. After the Medicare legislation became law, it soon became evident that elderly patients in the program would happily cooperate with student caregivers under proper supervision.)

We believed that to make all of this happen, Medicare had to pay its own way and pay fully. We opposed shifting costs to other payers, and we avoided discounts beyond what the program's contractors might have secured for their own insured population. We pursued a careful, minute accounting for the costs of treatment for the elderly because the rule was to pay for them but for no one else. The program would not pay a share of a hospital's bad debts because it paid fully for its patients, but it would pay a share of teaching costs because everyone ultimately benefited from that. The program would allow a somewhat higher reimbursement rate for nursing the elderly on the theory that it took longer, but it insisted on lower per diem costs because of the longer stays of the elderly and the concentration of hospital costs in the first few days after admission.

One early frustration was the chaotic state of accounting in many if not most hospitals. They shared an unbusinesslike approach to management that was common at the time to many church-run and other nonprofit organizations. Nevertheless, we continued to believe that it was possible to set up systems that would produce good data on what it cost to take care of just the elderly.

As policymakers we did not try for more than we could accomplish. The program accepted the quality standard for hospitals as certified by the private Joint Commission on the Accreditation of Hospitals, as long as the hospital also had a utilization review committee and met the civil rights standard. We set up somewhat less stringent quality standards for other hospitals, mostly smaller ones, and contracted with state public health agencies for their inspection. This limited approach brought most hospitals into the program and gradually improved their quality. But we bent where we had to. For example, one of the requirements was that there be a trained nurse on duty at all times, and a little hospital in Johnson City, Texas, did not have one for some shifts. However, with Lyndon Johnson president, I could not conceive of not certifying the one hospital in Johnson City, so we stretched the requirement. We held that if a physician was on duty when there was no nurse, we would assume that the physician could perform the same duties as a nurse. That is not really true, but we stretched it.

It was important that the program start up smoothly. We worked with the hospitals and physicians and considered all shades of opinion in getting advice before we issued rules. At one time, nine informal working groups were discussing the interpretation of various provisions of the program. Each group had representatives of just about all the forces in American medicine. Many of these people would not have come into the same room together before the Medicare legislation passed. The groups were made up of fifteen or twenty people: experts from the universities, representatives from the AMA, specialty medical organizations, group practice prepayment plans (which were then anathema to organized medicine), and labor unions and consumer groups, all working with the government and doing their best to come forward with the most desirable interpretations of this new law. They did not always try for agreement, but each group gave us their best advice after discussing the matter with each other. And I really mean that. To a remarkable degree, opponents as well as supporters tried hard to be helpful.

It is a long way from legislation to a going program. We consulted very widely, and in setting up the regulations worked finally with a legislatively required advisory body that was also broadly representative of diverse interests and opinions. Although we could obviously not decide in the end in favor of all the varying positions, just about everybody came through the process feeling they had had their day in court. Thus, actual administration of the program began with widespread support among the hospitals, physicians, and the public.

Establishing the program went off, really, without a hitch, although there were some hectic moments just before the deadline for beginning to provide services. A couple of weeks, or maybe somewhat more, before the program was to go into effect, for some reason the president got nervous. When the president is nervous, the cabinet officer under him gets nervous. That made me nervous because I was just one step below that and in charge.

The president was worried that people who were eligible had been saving up for years all their handicaps and illnesses—everything that was wrong with them—and on the day the program opened there were going to be lines around the block at every hospital because just about everyone older than 65 was going to be seeking services. But a 20 percent increase in the use of hospital beds by the elderly would have amounted to only a 5 percent increase in the total number of people in the hospitals. And the program was to begin in July, when hospital occupancy is lowest. So until the president stirred things up, we felt pretty comfortable. An increase of 20 percent for the elderly seemed an adequate allowance.

Nationally, we believed, there were plenty of hospital beds. But it is true that the best hospitals frequently are near their capacities even in July. So, we got out the maps. There was a pin on the map representing every major hospital in the country. Helicopters were standing by to move people to where there were vacancies. Public health hospitals, veterans hospitals, and army hospitals all across the country were alerted to be ready to handle emergency cases. And then absolutely nothing happened. There was no line anywhere. Medicare had a very smooth start.

The principle of our mostly accepting the current situation and gradually tightening up later is also illustrated in the initiation of Medicare part B, covering physician services. For part B there was no civil rights or utilization review requirement. The program was explicitly based on a private insurance plan, an Aetna plan for federal workers under the Federal Employees Health Benefits Program. It was to be voluntary: not paid-up insurance but insurance financed by a current premium with half paid by the elderly who elected coverage and half by the federal government.

Part B had been added to the administration's hospital insurance plan at the last moment by Wilbur Mills, chairman of the House Ways and Means Committee, who wanted part of the plan to follow the principles advocated by some of the congressional Republicans. The government subsidy, now controversial, was an unavoidable result of making part B voluntary. Without it, rates based on the average cost of all of the elderly would have been unattractive to the younger group of elderly persons, but if the rates were varied by age, the premiums would have been prohibitive for those older than 80.

We had spent many years perfecting the legislation covering hospitals, but we had only one weekend in which to try to adapt the private Aetna plan to a government-run plan. There were no quality standards in the Aetna plan and no cost controls other than a vague stipulation that services had to be "medically required." Reimbursement was to be a "reasonable" charge determined by the customary charges of the particular physician and the prevailing charges in the locality for similar services. We had considerable concern about such a plan but decided that it was better than not covering physician services at all and that this was our only chance. So the administration supported it. We also had a naive faith that when we had more experience with the program, we could get reasonable changes made in the law.

With a government program, sooner or later, public policy concerns such as cost and quality move front and center. These concerns caused the program to become a leader in the health insurance field. After-the-fact reimbursement for hospital costs clearly was a flawed policy, and within a couple of years other government officials and I were calling for some form of prospective payment. When Medicare finally adopted the diagnosis-related group (DRG) system in 1983, it was an important advance for all who reimbursed for hospital care. The principle of setting in advance a rate for a given diagnostic group gave hospitals a huge incentive to keep costs down as compared with the previous system of reimbursing them case by case for whatever "reasonable costs" were received. This change, applied to all age levels by many plans, made the lengths of stay in U.S. hospitals the shortest in the world.

Similarly, we knew from the beginning that we needed some kind of fee schedule in part B, but we had to struggle with the term "reasonable," defined as "customary and prevailing," all through the early years. When Medicare finally adopted the resource-based relative value scale (RBRVS) in 1992, it was again pioneering a technique that helped other insurers. After Medicare adopted physician reimbursement standards based on the resources required to deliver the service and related the relative cost of one service to another, the method was widely adopted. The unit underlying the comparison of one service to another could be set generally at any level desired, but the relationship among services could stay the same and the level of the unit negotiated. It is doubtful that this method would have been feasible before Medicare did the necessary research and adopted the system. Other contributions to health insurance were the program's insistence on more careful administration by contractors than they were used to and better accounting by hospitals.

But to return to the early steps of implementing the program, we were greatly aided by the tremendous build-up of excitement among elderly people and their sons and daughters. After the long fight, there was great enthusiasm. I remember talking to maybe 15,000 people in Detroit, and you could feel the excitement in that group of older people who were being told for the first time about the start-up of Medicare.

Part B was voluntary, and we had to sign people up for it. We sent out punch card applications to all the addresses that we had for people 65 and older. We had, of course, addresses for Social Security beneficiaries, people in private retirement plans, welfare beneficiaries, and anybody who had paid income tax. We sent applications out to almost everybody—hospital and nursing home patients too—then followed with other efforts to emphasize the need to sign up by a specified date: the sides of post office delivery trucks carried the deadline for signing up. Forest rangers looked for hermits in the woods. Everybody participated.

The program was immensely popular. One of the punch card applications came back from a man who was afraid that we might misunderstand his intentions. You could check yes or no on the application, but he wanted to be sure and had cut the no right out of the card. It did not work very well in the punch card equipment, but we managed.

As I said, there was no intention of reforming the nation's health care system. The intention was to put Medicare patients in an equal position with those already covered under private insurance or those who could pay their own way. In fact, the law forbade us to interfere in any way with the practice of medicine or the administration of hospitals. But it became clear that the original direction in the law had to be interpreted liberally. There was no way the program could be administered without some interference with the practice of medicine and the operation of hospitals. But the language in the law shows the extreme of the hands-off policy the program started with.

Medicare has done well what it was designed to do. Because of the program, hundreds of millions of older people and their children have been better off. Not only has the cost of medical bills been made bearable, but lives have been saved and the quality of life of the elderly has been greatly improved. Medicare has made available modern medical techniques—cataract removal, artificial hip transplants, cardiac bypasses—that otherwise might have been affordable only for the affluent. Medicare also has undoubtedly contributed to longevity: the United States (with Japan) leads the world in the expected remaining length of life for those who have reached age 65. In its present form, however, Medicare is clearly not prepared to cope with the huge increase in the number of beneficiaries that will take place beginning about 2010. To keep the program solvent and viable, changes will have to be made.

It is as true now as it was thirty years ago that the Medicare program is needed to give the elderly the same health care under the same conditions as is available to insured younger patients. Now, as then, most group insurance is furnished through employment, and individual insurance is simply too expensive for an age group (and those with disabilities who are also now included in the program) that needs much more health care and, on average, has lower incomes than do younger employed persons. For elderly persons and for the family members who otherwise would be saddled with their medical bills, Medicare continues to be—often literally—a lifesaver.

But it is a lifesaver itself in need of saving. Once a leader in providing health care, the program has fallen behind. First of all, Medicare's benefit package is considerably less comprehensive than packages offered by the better employer plans. In any long-range reform, the package should be improved, particularly by including a stop-loss provision to protect beneficiaries and their families against catastrophic costs and by adding drug coverage and more prevention services. Medicare also needs to take the lead once again in developing important cost-reduction techniques that can be followed in private plans, as it did with the invention of DRGs and the RBRVS.

I have one other thought. I do not know exactly what the next steps in cost control should be, but I find very promising the proposals Robert Reischauer and others have been working on that would set the value of a government-paid-for voucher at the average offer of bids to supply the Medicare package of services in a given geographical area. And I want to confess a major mistake we made. If there is a way to correct this mistake, it might make a difference. We had no idea that the Medicare cost-sharing provisions—the copayments and the deductible—would be canceled out by the growth of a medigap industry. We thought that the bills Medicare left uncovered were mostly too small to justify the administrative costs of supplementary insurance programs. Maybe they are, but a major industry of Medicare supplementation has developed nevertheless, and Medicare is paying a heavy price as private insurance rests on top of the basic Medicare coverage. The result is that neither the patient nor the physician on behalf of the patient has an incentive to think twice about the cost of a procedure. Somehow, we must get private insurers to share the costs they have created for Medicare by nullifying the copayments and deductibles, and somehow we must get the patients and physicians to agree that costs make a difference. With all its problems, managed care does help keep physicians aware of costs. In addition, are there well-constructed experiments to be performed on applying the hospital DRG-type approach to other services? How can we put back together some of the services that have been unbundled?

It is clear, I think, from the Medicare experience that in such a program everything depends on the human factor, on how patients, physicians, hospital administrators, insurers, and others behave. The program is not a mechanical model but a system that has all the messiness that arises when human beings are called on to run complicated, interrelated institutions that depend on human behavior. We should not be discouraged about further extensions of health insurance, but neither should we expect a smooth-running, purring machine. As Mark Twain said, "Man was made at the end of the week when God was tired."

Notes

1. Some of the details in the following discussion are indebted to Peter A. Corning, *The Evolution of Medicare from Idea to Law,* research report 29 (Office of Research and Statistics, Social Security Administration, 1969); Richard Harris, *A Sacred Trust* (New American Library, 1966); and Social Security Administration, bound volumes of the Social Security Act and its amendments.

Social Insurance Commentary
E. J. Dionne

SOCIAL INSURANCE is, to my mind, one of the most brilliant creations of a century of democratic (small "d") politics. It is an idea rooted in socialist, and arguably biblical, thought that saved capitalism. Social insurance arises from the understanding that competitive market economies do not distribute their fruits equally and that competitive economies sometimes break down. Competition has benefits and costs, and both are shared unequally.

Social insurance was a wise admission on the part of supporters of competitive economies that citizens would take the risk such economies require only if they were provided with a degree of security, especially against old age, unemployment, the sudden death of a spouse, and the vicissitudes of health. Risk is tolerable, even desirable, as long as every one of life's risks does not become an all-or-nothing game. This is especially true when one's family, not simply one's self, is put at risk. The power of the social insurance idea rests on a respect for individualism, not on a utopian and mistaken view of what radical individualism can accomplish.

In 1910 in *Social Insurance,* Henry Rogers Seeger, a Columbia University economist, wrote,

> Up to a certain point, it is moral and commendable for each to look after his own interests and the interest of those dependent upon him. It is a mistake to think that self interest in this sense is synonymous with selfishness. Adam Smith's assertion that "it is usually by pursuing our interests with due consideration to the interest of others that we contribute most to the common well being," is true of the ordinary man in the ordinary situation. But along with our individual interests, which can best be cared for by individual enterprise, industry, and forethought, there are other interests that call for a collective and cooperative action.

Seeger then described risks that we now have forms of social insurance for: industrial accidents, illness, premature death, unemployment, and the like. He concluded, "By . . . the means of cooperative action and the creation of social insurance, and by these means only, in my opinion, can we hope to raise the whole mass of wage earners to higher standards of efficiency and earnings and to more intelligent appreciation of all of life's possibilities." He turned out to be right. That is why we embarked on a system of social insurance.

Franklin D. Roosevelt said it even better. In a 1938 radio address on the third anniversary of the Social Security Act, he observed that the first in

American history to seek governmental protection were not the poor and lowly but the rich and strong. They sought protective laws to give security to property owners, industrialists, merchants, and bankers. He did not blame the wealthy for seeking these protections. Instead, he saw that workers, too, sought protections as they became more articulate through organization.

> Strength or skill of arm or brain did not guarantee a man a job. It does not guarantee him a roof. It did not guarantee him the ability to provide for those dependent upon him or to take care of himself when he was too old to work. . . . Long before the economic blight of the Depression descended on the nation, millions of our people were living in wastelands of want and fear. Men and women too old and infirm to work either depended on those who had but little to share or spent their remaining years within the walls of a poorhouse. . . . Because it has become increasingly difficult for individuals to build their own security single handed, government must now step in and help them lay the foundation stones just as government in the past has helped lay the foundations of business and industry. We must face the fact that in this country we have a rich man's security and a poor man's security and that the government owes equal obligations to both. National security is not a half-and-half matter. It is all or none.

The United States has been remarkably successful because it followed the path laid down by Seeger and Roosevelt. Other industrial economies did the same. In many cases they did more than we did in the sphere of social insurance. We have established throughout the industrial democracies what Walter Russell Meade has called "the social democratic bargain," a marriage between market economies preached by capitalists and worker protections preached by socialists. Most economic decisions remain in private hands, but national governments use the tools at their disposal, notably taxing and spending. You are not supposed to talk about these anymore. But it was spending to take the edge off economic downturns that hastened the return to prosperity.

Labor laws guaranteed workers the right to organize, which boosted their share of economic largess. Government helped citizens of modest means secure housing, educate their children, and have a decent retirement. That social democratic bargain has been a good deal. It was possible because market economies delivered the goods and national governments had the power to tax, spend, and regulate pretty much as they and their electorates chose.

I would argue that the political unhappiness we are experiencing now in the United States and in many countries of Western Europe is not primarily the result of scandal; it is not primarily the result of negative advertising; and it is not the product of politicians being mean to one another. Politicians have long been mean to one another. Instead, it is the result of the weakening of the social democratic bargain and of the social insurance state.

This bargain is under siege from many directions. The global economy puts new competitive pressures on both businesses and governments to trim benefits that had once been taken for granted. In the welfare states of western Europe, this pressure is largely on public benefits. In the United States, we have an intensive system of private benefits in the form of company-provided health insurance and pensions. As we debate our public social insurance benefits, these basic private social benefits are being eroded. The proportion of workers without health insurance is growing. And the proportion of workers with pension plans involving substantial assured contributions from their employers is shrinking.

A second factor weakening the social democratic bargain is the decrease in the proportion of workers who are unionized. This is especially pronounced here and in Great Britain. A third factor is aging populations, accompanied by rising health care costs, which are putting great pressures on social insurance programs for health care in every country in the West. Finally, a technological economy that puts a high premium on skills and education seems to be widening economic inequalities. This produces a paradox. Growing inequalities create new dissatisfactions with government and taxation, while at the same time putting more pressure on government to rectify the imbalances.

In the most pessimistic light, the social insurance state faces a profound political contradiction. On the one hand, we have steadily increasing demands on government precisely because the social democratic bargain is breaking down. On the other hand, we have increasing mistrust of government, which makes it difficult to expand the social insurance state where necessary, particularly in providing health care. I am an optimist, so I do not accept this pessimistic view. I believe that the idea of social insurance is becoming more popular again precisely because the underlying reasons for its existence are becoming more explicit.

The basic idea behind social security, the need for collective provision against certain forms of insecurity, remains deeply and broadly popular despite the rise of the ideology of privatization. Advocates of privatization keep running into the stubborn fact that most Americans broadly like Social Security because it works and because it accords with their values.

The original idea of the Social Security Act could have been proposed by new Democrats no less than old Democrats, and a lot of Republicans. If there was ever a program designed to help those who "work hard and play by the rules," to use the president's phrase, this is it. If there was ever a program designed to offer a "hand up, not a handout," surely Social Security and other provisions of the social insurance state meet that criterion.

Some believe that the strongest danger facing America is financial insolvency in these programs. Others talk about a low savings rate. Still others emphasize the dangers of big government. But I believe the biggest danger is that we will forget why we have social insurance, and why its preservation is necessary not only to a civilized society but also to the very market economy that has provided us with so much wealth.

The programs of the social insurance state, especially Medicare and Social Security, loom very large on the balance sheets of government. As the baby boomers march inexorably toward old age and retirement, the costs will loom larger still. Nevertheless, fixing the social insurance state is very possible and within our reach. Saving it is absolutely necessary. Social insurance is the basic insurance policy Americans have for social stability, a modicum of social justice, and a society in which risks are taken freely and energetically because there is some protection against catastrophe and social breakdown.

Few business people I know would cut their expenses by canceling their fire insurance. Social insurance is the cost of doing business for a society that seeks to remain dynamic and inventive as well as just and fair. We need to rediscover the power of this idea and its value to us all.

3

Financing Medicare

O PTIONS for strengthening the Medicare program to with-
stand severe fiscal challenges in the next century range
from short-term fixes to long-term changes, as reflected in the papers in this
chapter.

Preparing for the Retirement of the Baby Boomers
Joseph R. Antos

THE MEDICARE PROGRAM finances the health care of 38
million elderly and disabled Americans and will spend more than $200 billion
in 1997. It is the second largest entitlement program; only Social Security is
larger. Still, the growth of Medicare spending has long been far faster than
spending in other major federal programs or the growth of the economy itself.
This trend is projected to continue unless America makes substantial changes
in policy.

Slowing the acceleration in Medicare spending has been a longstanding
focus of policymakers, and major reforms of the program have been proposed
in recent years. Concerns over the program's financing have been heightened
by the projected depletion in 2001 of the Hospital Insurance trust fund. But
current financing problems will be dwarfed by the crisis that could occur as the
baby boom generation reaches age 65.

The views expressed here are those of the author and do not necessarily represent the
position of the Congressional Budget Office.

Table 3-1. *Medicare Outlays, by Category, Projected for Fiscal Years 1997, 2002, 2007*

Billions of dollars unless otherwise specified

| | Outlays | | | Average annual rate of growth, 1997–2007 |
Category	1997	2002	2007	(percent)
Hospital Insurance	137	202	290	7.7
Supplementary Medical Insurance	75	116	179	9.1
Gross outlays	212	317	469	8.3
Premium receipts	−20	−26	−32	4.8
Net outlays	192	292	436	8.6
Gross domestic product	7,829	9,870	12,379	4.7

Source: Congressional Budget Office.

The United States is now experiencing historically low growth in Medicare enrollments as the baby bust generation, born during the Depression and war years of the 1930s and 1940s, reaches age 65. After 2010, however, the first wave of the baby boomers will reach 65, and Medicare enrollments will grow at exceptionally rapid rates for two decades. Demand for services will increase dramatically as succeeding baby boom cohorts enter the program through 2030.

We are thus in the calm before the storm, at least in relative terms. Policy actions taken during the next few years will shape the future of Medicare. Deciding what those actions should be has already proven contentious. But there is no question that action must be taken.

Near-Term Outlook

In its January 1997 projections of Medicare spending, the Congressional Budget Office estimates that the program will spend $60 billion less between 1998 and 2002 than had been projected in April 1996. Nonetheless, gross outlays will reach $317 billion by 2002 and $469 billion by 2007 (table 3-1). From 1997 to 2007 Medicare spending will grow 8.3 percent a year, considerably faster than the 4.7 percent average annual growth rate projected for the GDP.

Payments to hospitals account for most of the reduction in baseline spending for Hospital Insurance, or part A. The level of hospital spending in 1996 was somewhat lower than had been anticipated, causing the CBO to revise spending downward over the period projected. Medicare payments to providers of

Table 3-2. *Medicare Benefits, by Type of Service, Projected for Fiscal Years 1997, 2002, 2007*

Billions of dollars unless otherwise specified

	Outlays			Average annual rate of growth, 1997–2007
Type of service	1997	2002	2007	(percent)
Fee-for-service				
Hospital Insurance				
Inpatient hospital	87	105	125	3.7
Skilled nursing facility	13	19	27	7.6
Home health care	19	30	43	8.6
Hospice	2	3	4	5.7
Subtotal	121	156	198	5.1
Supplementary Medical Insurance				
Physician[a]	31	35	39	2.5
Outpatient hospital and other services[b]	18	27	38	7.8
Laboratory services, durable medical equipment, and other services[c]	13	21	34	10.0
Subtotal	62	83	111	6.1
All fee-for-service benefits	182	239	310	5.4
Health maintenance organizations	26	73	153	19.6
All Medicare benefits	208	312	463	8.3

Source: Congressional Budget Office.

[a]Includes payments by carriers to physicians and nonphysicians under the physician fee schedule.

[b]Includes outpatient hospital services, laboratory services in hospital outpatient departments, hospital-provided ambulance services, and other services paid by intermediaries.

[c]Includes independent and physician in-office laboratory services, durable medical equipment, ambulance services paid by carriers, and other services paid by carriers.

postacute care, especially skilled nursing facility (SNF) services and home health care, will continue to rise rapidly (table 3-2). Thus patterns of future growth in part A spending remain similar to past trends.

A more significant slowing of spending growth under baseline assumptions is projected for Supplementary Medical Insurance (SMI), or part B. In line with recent trends the CBO has reduced the projected growth in the volume of physicians' services per enrollee. The recent decrease in use of services may be related to the use of volume performance standards, which limit payment updates if the volume of services exceeds certain targets. However, spending for other SMI services, particularly outpatient services, is projected to increase at rapid rates over the next ten years.

Perhaps the most significant change in the CBO's projections is the significant upward revision of enrollments in Medicare health maintenance organizations in the next decade. By 2007 a third of all Medicare beneficiaries are projected to be in HMOs, up from about 12 percent in 1997. That projection reflects two assumptions. First, an increasing proportion of people becoming eligible for Medicare upon turning 65 will already be HMO members, making the program's HMO sector more familiar. Second, HMO enrollment will become more attractive as premiums for private medigap coverage rise, reflecting the upward spiral of costs in the fee-for-service sector.

The CBO report is good news for policymakers. Slower growth in Medicare spending implies that achieving a balanced budget in 2002 will likely require smaller spending reductions than had been projected. Moreover, the improved outlook for managed care is a promising development for the Medicare market. But that good news is modest. The underlying forces driving the rising cost of the program remain largely unchanged.

Sources of Spending Growth

High rates of growth in Medicare spending reflect the rapid rise in medical costs per beneficiary. These costs are projected to grow by 6.9 percent a year in the next decade, and much of that growth will be due to increases in the volume and intensity of services provided through the program.

Incentives built into traditional Medicare are driving the rapid growth in spending. Despite recent growth in enrollments in Medicare HMOs, most beneficiaries remain in fee-for-service Medicare, which provides limited financial incentives to encourage prudent use of services. Cost-sharing requirements are fairly weak, and most beneficiaries have supplemental coverage that covers the copayments. Providers have little incentive to limit the number or cost of services they provide because they know that insurance is picking up all or most of the bill. Moreover, the Medicare program does not realize savings possible from managed care because federal payments to HMOs are linked to costs in the fee-for-service sector.

The significance of payment incentives in fostering spending growth is underscored by considering how the prospective payment system (PPS) for hospital services has affected the actions of hospitals and other providers. Under PPS, hospitals are given fixed payments based on the diagnosis of their patients. This fixed payment provides an incentive to hospitals to reduce their costs by discharging patients sooner into post–acute care services.

Payment incentives combined with actions that liberalized Medicare's coverage of home health and skilled nursing facility services increased both the demand for and supply of post–acute care services. Home health care and SNF will account for 25 percent of spending in 1997 under part A. In the next decade Medicare's payments to fee-for-service providers of these services are projected to grow 7.6 and 8.6 percent a year, respectively—much faster than the 3.7 percent annual growth in hospital payments projected for the same time period. By 2007, home health care and SNF services will have grown to about 35 percent of part A spending.

This rapid growth is contributing to the depletion of the Hospital Insurance trust fund, projected by the Medicare trustees to occur under current law in 2001. It is not surprising, then, that attention has focused on shifting some of home health spending from part A to part B as a way of extending the solvency of the fund. Such shifting would not by itself help slow the growth of Medicare spending. But it could be a useful step if it leads to agreement on additional policies to slow spending. There is, however, a risk that extending the trust fund depletion date in this manner could delay the difficult policy decisions that are needed to ensure Medicare's long-term viability.

Long-Term Outlook

Medicare spending is already growing faster than the resources available to pay for the program. Over the longer term the situation is likely to deteriorate. A 1997 CBO analysis shows that as the baby boom generation reaches retirement age, federal spending for entitlement programs—particularly Social Security, Medicare, and Medicaid—will increase dramatically.[1] In addition, continued expansion in the volume and intensity of services provided through Medicare and Medicaid is expected to put upward pressure on federal spending for each beneficiary enrolled in the programs. If no policy actions are taken to relieve the budgetary pressure, deficits will mount and seriously erode the nation's future economic growth.

Medicare enrollment will rise rapidly after 2010 as the baby boomers become eligible for the program. The Medicare trustees project that enrollment will grow by 2.4 percent a year between 2010 and 2030, up from the 1.4 percent average annual growth projected through 2007. By 2030, Medicare enrollment will have doubled, to 75 million people. The enrollment increase will be accompanied by a slowing growth rate of the working-age population. The number of workers will drop from 3.8 for every Medicare beneficiary in 1997 to 2.2 by 2030. Consequently, demographic trends will drive up the demand for services after 2010 at the same time that the work force that provides the bulk of Medicare's financing will be growing relatively slowly. In addition, the cost per beneficiary could continue to spiral upward, placing an enormous burden on the federal budget and the economy. Even under the Medicare trustees' assumption that growth in spending will gradually slow to be more in line with growth in national income per capita, however, the CBO projects that Medicare spending will overtake spending for Social Security within thirty years.

Clearly, staying on Medicare's current spending path is not sustainable over the long term. Although Americans might decide to devote a larger share of the budget and of national income to the program in the near term, no program can indefinitely grow faster than the economy.

Policy Options

Short of a major program restructuring, policy options for treating Medicare's financial ills would retain both a traditional fee-for-service sector and risk-based plans. Consequently, the traditional fee-for-service sector, with its open-ended claim on federal payments, would continue to drive the growth of Medicare spending.

A more ambitious option would provide a fixed payment for every beneficiary, in effect converting the entire program into a defined contribution plan. Under the option, beneficiaries could enroll in any health plan, including fee-for-service plans. Those who choose lower-cost plans might pay no more than they do now, but each would be liable for the full additional cost of selecting a plan that is more expensive than Medicare's payment. Those enrolling in fee-for-service plans might be required to pay such a surcharge under a defined contribution program.

A defined contribution program that eliminated the special status of Medicare's fee-for-service sector would be practical only if beneficiaries had more than one health plan from which to choose. New methods would be needed to determine the federal payment to health plans because the payment would no longer depend on the amount of service provided to each enrollee. Payments would have to be adjusted both to ensure that health plans had a financial incentive to enroll people who were less healthy and to avoid overpaying plans that attracted a mix of patients that was less costly than average. Oversight might also be needed to ensure that each health plan met an acceptable level of quality and services. The federal government's experience in running a successful health insurance program for its employees based on the principles of a defined contribution plan could be useful in establishing the mechanics of such a system for Medicare.

Whether a defined contribution option can slow the growth of Medicare spending to sustainable long-term rates and provide adequate health coverage for a growing number of beneficiaries depends on how well competition among health plans fosters efficiency. A restructuring of the program that is poorly designed could fail to meet the policy goals. Nonetheless, a market-based strategy may be the most promising way to resolve the problem of financing Medicare in the long term.

Although a complete restructuring of Medicare could require years of development, practical steps to begin could be adopted now. Policies that foster program restructuring and cost containment could also contribute to the immediate goals of reducing the deficit and improving the solvency of the Hospital Insurance trust fund. Several broad approaches have been discussed, including

—slowing the growth in spending per enrollee by reducing rates paid to providers or increasing the cost-sharing amount that beneficiaries must pay;

—raising the age of Medicare eligibility; and

—increasing Medicare revenues through higher premiums or higher payroll taxes.

Slowing the Growth of Provider Payments

Medicare payments to fee-for-service providers are adjusted annually to reflect inflation or cost increases. But Congress has frequently enacted policies that adjust payment rates by less than the increases in the relevant indexes of inflation. Such policies induce providers to offer more services, however, and may not effectively curb the growth in expenditures, which represent price times volume of services. Nonetheless, these policies are virtually certain to be part of any budget proposal.

Introducing payment systems in fee-for-service Medicare that limit spending, rather than prices, could be a more effective strategy for the long term. Options might include prospective payment or bundling, which pays a fixed amount for a specified set of related services; volume performance standards, which reduce annual updates to payment rates if the growth in total payments for particular services exceeds the standard; and competitive bidding, which replaces administered prices with payment rates based on market conditions. These options would, however, require detailed development before Medicare could adopt them.

Medicare savings could also be achieved if the method used to pay HMOs were modified. Risk-based HMOs are paid a fixed amount per beneficiary that is tied to costs in the fee-for-service sector. These organizations thus have an incentive to enroll relatively healthy beneficiaries, who use fewer services. Because the current payment formula does not fully account for this "favorable selection" of enrollees,

Medicare pays a little more for typical enrollees in risk-based HMOs than the enrollees would have cost in the fee-for-service sector.

Even if adjustments for favorable selection remained crude, payment levels could be set to lower overall Medicare spending. The simplest option would change the payment rate from 95 percent of fee-for-service costs to some lower percentage. Alternatively, the payment update could be set equal to the growth rate in some appropriate index, such as the overall economy, rather than growth in fee-for-service costs. Greater program savings could, however, reduce the attractiveness of risk-based plans to beneficiaries because the plans would be less likely to offer the array of additional benefits that most now offer. Some plans might be discouraged from participating in the risk-based Medicare sector at all. Consequently, options that could encourage enrollment in risk-based plans, even as the plans became less generous, should be considered.

Increasing Beneficiary Cost-Sharing Requirements

Medicare requires beneficiaries to pay deductibles and coinsurance when they use covered services. Raising these requirements would provide savings to the program. In principle, increasing what beneficiaries must pay when they receive services also provides an incentive to limit their use. But most beneficiaries have supplemental coverage through private medigap insurance, health plans for retirees, or Medicaid. These plans typically pay for Medicare's cost-sharing requirements, dampening the incentives to limit use of services.

One way to restore the incentives would be to allow private supplemental coverage to provide only an annual cap, such as $1,000, on enrollees' liabilities for cost sharing. This would require beneficiaries to pay deductibles and coinsurance up to that amount each year, but would provide a limit on out-of-pocket costs that is not currently available under Medicare.

Raising the Age of Eligibility

The age of eligibility for Medicare could be gradually increased from 65 to 67 between 2003 and 2025 to be consistent with currently scheduled increases in the normal retirement age for Social Security benefits. This would reduce Medicare enrollment about 9 percent by 2025, when the policy would be fully phased in. Spending would fall about 5 percent over this period—less than the decline in enrollment—because those who are 65 to 66 years old are typically the least costly enrollees.

Even increasing the age of eligibility beyond 67 would have a limited effect on Medicare spending in the long term. The policy would do little to reduce total health care costs and nothing to increase the efficiency of the health care system. It could also shift some costs now paid by Medicare to private employers, who might face several additional years of expenses for people retiring early. Moreover, it may be desirable to provide significant advance notice to people and employers of any change in the age of eligibility, which could alter the timing of retirement for some individuals.

Increasing Medicare Revenues

Raising the premiums paid by current Medicare beneficiaries or the payroll taxes paid by current workers would also help improve Medicare financing and contribute to reducing the federal deficit. But increased revenues would do nothing to slow the growth in spending that threatens the program's long-term stability.

Conclusion

There is reason for optimism that the policy process will soon culminate in an agreement that can improve Medicare's financial outlook, at least for the next few years. The CBO's 1997 projections of Medicare spending trends certainly suggest that near-term financing problems may be less challenging than they have appeared. Moreover, the United States is now experiencing slow growth in Medicare enrollment and a sizable working-age population. The relatively small cohort of Depression-era babies retiring during the next decade, coupled with the large number of baby boomers who are in their prime earning years, provides very favorable circumstances for financing the program. There may not be a better opportunity to begin the difficult process of restructuring Medicare for the long term.

Notes

1. Congressional Budget Office, *Long-Term Budgetary Pressures and Policy Options* (1997).

Comment by Charles Kahn III

THERE IS A GAP in perceptions between certain health care elites and the public regarding Medicare. The 1996 election clearly shows this. Whereas many in Washington consider Medicare in fiscal crisis, the polls showed that the public was satisfied with the status quo for the program. Politicians who challenge this conclusion do so at their peril.

Nevertheless, as an analyst, I believe the fiscal status quo for Medicare cannot be sustained in the coming decades, and that to maintain current benefits and financing would require more spending than we as a society are going to be willing to spend. If you accept this assumption, Medicare spending will have to be tempered.

I say tempered because the basic agreement on Medicare between our government and its citizenry will not be broken. There will be a Medicare program, and it will not look that much different from what we have today. Still, however, affording such a program is another matter. Particularly with the advent of baby boomers' retirement or a few years later, it is unlikely the taxpayers will be willing to pay the tab for Medicare as we know it.

In a first step, as the responsible steward of the Medicare program, Congress should consider, as it has been considering, whether expenditures can be reduced in a reasonable way, that is with no loss of benefits, no loss of quality. Because volume times price equals expenditures, program administrators have done about all they can with price administration strategies to reduce costs. That is not to say there is no room to manuever. Obviously, the president's $100 billion of reductions in the growth of Medicare will be primarily maneuvering, and I assume Congress will take that amount or something close to it and put in some of its own ideas. But in terms of the long range, it is unlikely that fiddling will help very much to keep the promise that was made to keep the program affordable. Clearly, it is not possible to do much to affect expenditures, at least in terms of increasing volume, by playing with prices. The diagnosis-related groups (DRGs) have affected both the share of clients and hospital costs; but the balloon of increased expenses pops out in other places, such as home health care and skilled nursing facilities.

So from a strategic standpoint it makes sense to talk about restructuring and capitation as a possible alternative, but we must proceed in this direction while still preserving quality and the basic benefit structure.

This leads to my last point: another political reality of the last election and the president's veto of the 1995 Republican budget bill, which included a major reworking of Medicare, is that this Congress, and probably those in the near future, will not impose new taxes. Taxes will not be raised to fund this entitlement. But at the same time, the president has been successful, and his party has been successful, at preventing serious consideration to changing the structure of beneficiary liability, whether increasing premiums for the wealthier elderly, or sharing costs with beneficiaries, or moving to a fixed contribution. These changes will not occur anytime soon. It is a political equivalent to what the Democrats did to the Republicans back in the early 1980s regarding Social Security. The Democrats have blocked any policy to ask the beneficiaries to pay more by labeling any initiative to do so as destructive of the very fabric of Medicare. That is a shame, but it is a reality.

The attitude of the members of Congress whom I work for is that if the president wants to propose increasing Medicare premiums, they will talk about it. If he wants to talk about income relating to the program, they will talk about that too, but he must talk about it first. And clearly, the budget the president presents for Medicare that is likely to be discussed will not include such alternatives. So, in the near future we are left with short-term fixes that do not deal with the dynamic problem Joseph Antos described.

I will end with this. At a minimum policymakers should not accept in these short-term fixes any tricks; and the shift of part of the home health care benefit from part A to part B, which has been discussed and is included in the measures that the president is likely to send to Congress, is a trick that helps the near-term financing of part A but moves the long-term Medicare crisis off only a few years. This is disadvantageous. We need the pressure of having this checkbook of part A, rather than moving some of those expenditures off budget as in part B, which is going to get paid because the government pays its bills.

Shifting the Medicare fiscal crisis to the future by sleight of hand is problematic because making fundamental changes in the program to solve the longer-term financing problems is going to be easier the sooner they are made. If Congress continues making short-term fixes to triage long-term problems, it will harm the very people Medicare is meant to protect.

Comment by Judith Feder

I WANT to address what is potentially wrong or right as policymakers consider the financing problems that face the Medicare program. There are two prominent risks. The first is the temptation to be led by numbers and to treat Medicare financing issues as overwhelmingly a budgetary problem. There is no question that it is a budgetary problem, but it is much more than that. Medicare and the way we address it is a matter of how Americans as a society want to deal with ensuring affordable access to health care for the nation's elderly and some of its disabled population. The second danger is social engineering. Incrementalism is a good thing, and in dealing with a rapidly changing health care system and the risks we are aware of in those changes, we must be cautious in making changes in a program so valuable, important, and effective.

Let me begin by focusing on what we should not do. From the budgetary perspective, it is extremely tempting simply to fix or limit federal liabilities for Medicare. Capping the Medicare program ought to be off the table. To cap the levels of federal spending would be to move Medicare from a defined benefit to a defined contribution. That action would not address the program's financing problems. It would simply mean that the federal government is washing its hands of them.

I know that David Kendall does not advocate an arbitrary cap. He is discussing a way to set a premium. However, capitations or fixed payments slip very easily into fixed amounts that apply regardless of elderly people's ability to buy adequate benefits with the amounts they receive. We have to be very careful of shifting liabilities instead of addressing problems.

With regard to social engineering, policymakers must be very sensitive to the difficulties posed by a competitive insurance marketplace. Medicare has had the advantage of insuring all the elderly in a single pool. With Medicaid's help, it avoided segregating lower-income beneficiaries from those with higher incomes, and it did not separate the healthy from the sick. Any time we move toward choices, we raise the risk that a competitive insurance market will splinter beneficiaries and undermine the appropriate spreading of risk. Policymakers must be very careful that they do not move the Medicare program in the direction of the private insurance market for the under-65 population, particularly the individual insurance market.

As a society we can pursue choice in better or worse ways. What kind of a marketplace we structure, how we set up mechanisms to enable people to make choices, how we hold plans accountable, how we provide information, and what kinds of plans people can choose will determine how much we are inviting risk selection. Included here are medical savings accounts and balance billing. Some arrangements can make risk-selection problems worse and can manage choice well or poorly. But, coming back to my social engineering comment, good arrangements are difficult to operate as well as design. To adopt what on paper seems a well-designed system but one that cannot work in practice would be a big mistake.

Now, what should we do? It is critical that we begin to address the financing problems. The right way to begin is by making Medicare as efficient as it can be to avoid unnecessary growth in the size of the financing problem.

Most observers agree on the mechanisms that should be used to reduce current spending. Although there is also disagreement, the parties are moving in a common direction. We ought to take advantage of the slowdown in cost growth in the private sector to slow growth in Medicare payments to hospitals and physicians. We ought to address the inefficiencies in current payment mechanisms for home health care and skilled nursing facilities, but without undoing the benefits they provide. We should avoid overpayment in managed care. And at a reasonable pace we should be moving toward making choices work effectively, perhaps broadening the range of choices, improving the program's ability to monitor care, and informing consumers about their choices.

Joseph Antos ended his remarks by noting the importance of incentives. I would urge policymakers to review the incentives in the current system. People's financial liabilities under Medicare continue to grow without structural changes. Part B deductibles have not increased with inflation, but the part A deductible is huge. Under current law a typical elderly person pays about 20 percent of his or her income on health care costs. These payments create incentives for people to buy systems of care in which they have confidence. We ought to promote more choice only to the extent that we have confidence we are preserving the program and its protections.

Taking these actions to slow cost growth carefully puts society in a position to address the broader financial question: "How are those costs to be distributed across generations?" To date, we have not been ready to address that question in a constructive way. Our job is to be ready to do so when the time for that discussion comes.

Comment by David B. Kendall

MEDICARE AS IT STANDS now is unsustainable. The program's share of the economy is projected to triple by 2030, assuming that current benefit levels are sustained. Congress could, of course, increase taxes to cover the costs of these benefits. But that would be a tax on work, which would make the situation worse by slowing economic growth. Higher payroll taxes would make it harder for the economy to assume the burdens of social programs. And there are significant moral hurdles in raising payroll taxes. How can we ask low-income workers, who often do not have health care coverage themselves, to pay higher taxes to support health care for wealthy retirees? How can we ask generation X to bear the full burden of the baby boomers' benefits when, in fact, the baby boomers have already put the burden of a huge public debt on generation X?

Joseph Antos has outlined what could be called three radical reforms: restructuring Medicare, increasing the program's cost-sharing requirements, and pushing back the age of eligibility. I would argue that parts of each of these proposals are consistent with the original intent of the program, and taken together they would be more consistent with its origins than are the existing laws and regulations.

Let us start with one of the premises of Medicare: that it should have a geographically uniform and constant set of benefits. Today, there is no uniformity and consistency. If a person lives in southern California or Florida, Medicare will pay for dental benefits or for a health club membership if the beneficiary joins an HMO. If a person happens to live in rural Ohio, as my grandmother did, he or she gets nothing approaching such benefits.

Medicare benefits are not constant over time because of inflation. For example, the lack of inflation adjustments to Medicare's deductibles in the part B premium have increased the generosity of the benefits. The part B deductible would have to be more than doubled to compensate for the effects of inflation in the past thirty years. The original part B premium was a 50 percent of total part B costs. Today, it is only 25 percent.

Similarly, increasing lifespans have made Medicare benefits more generous because the benefits are not adjusted for life expectancy. The life expectancy of 65-year-olds has increased by 2.5 years since Medicare's inception, but the age of eligibility has not changed.

Another premise behind Medicare is that the program's health care delivery system should be consistent with that in the rest of the marketplace, as it was when it was enacted. When the law was passed, fee-for-service health care was the dominant form of coverage. Today, less than 30 percent of insured workers have fee-for-service coverage, but 89 percent of Medicare beneficiaries still have this more expensive form of care.

A third premise behind Medicare is that rich and poor should have equal access to care. Originally this was not quite true: low-income elderly persons did not have access to reliable care because of high deductibles and copayments. So Medicaid supplemental benefits were created to offset the inequity. But the benefit design for upper-income retirees was never reconsidered. A $100 deductible for elderly Americans of modest means would curb some unnecessary care, but for wealthy Americans it is more like an excuse to spend $100 so that Medicare will pay for future health care. As health care economist Mark Pauly has said, to make health care consumption equal among different income levels, the level of insurance coverage needs to be unequal.

So, how can we return to the founding principles of Medicare?

To make benefits constant, they simply need to be updated to reflect three decades of inflation and indexed to inflation and to increases in the lifespan. To make benefits geographically uniform, there are two choices. The existing HMO program could be limited so that the benefits do not exceed current Medicare program benefits. This is essentially what the Clinton administration is doing by proposing to reduce Medicare payments to managed care plans from 95 percent of the fee-for-service cost to 90 percent. The action would surely curtail the extra benefits offered under an HMO program.

But that fix is inconsistent with the idea of updating Medicare's delivery system to be consistent with today's managed care system. So instead, the Medicare subsidy should be tied to a competitively priced package of uniform benefits. This would also be consistent with what is happening in the private sector. Instead of paying for all benefits, large employers today are offering employees a choice of plans and a defined financial contribution that guarantees a basic level of coverage and gives employees the responsibility for paying more if they choose a more expensive plan. Essentially, a managed care plan is guaranteed, but a fee-for-service plan is still an option if an individual wants to pay the higher price.

Medicare should go one step further, however. Rather than guaranteeing a managed care package, the program could guarantee standards of quality of care as well as a subsidy tied to a market price. In other words, let us set measures for performance on quality as well as costs and then let the competition begin; whether it is fee-for-service or managed care that wins the battle, the winner will set the standard.

Finally, to create equal access to health care for the poor as well as the rich, upper-income Americans should receive a subsidy worth no more than the cost of a catastrophic policy, and Medicaid supplemental benefits for low-income elderly should be protected. Such a program might even be expanded to help address cost differentials among income classes that would occur because of the new pricing schemes in Medicare. For example, a $20 difference per month in premiums between managed care and fee-for-service for a low-income retiree might inhibit choice. The difference could be narrowed by increasing the subsidy to low-income retirees. In short, there may be some simple ways of making the system work for lower-income beneficiaries.

If reforming Medicare is a simple matter of updating the original ideas of the program, why have we strayed so far from its original path and why do our political leaders seem so incapable of presenting and resolving the choices that have to be made?

Medicare was enacted, of course, in the spirit of mutual responsibility. As a society we did not want to see older Americans die because they were too poor to get treatment for an illness, and we did not want them to be denied modern medicine. But in the intervening thirty years the politics of entitlements has taken hold. Political pressure has so expanded benefits that future Medicare beneficiaries will be entitled to more than they contributed in taxes. This imbalance can work as long as the economy expands faster than the burdens that society places on it. But the coming retirement of the baby boomers will force society to admit that this is a kind of Ponzi scheme and will fundamentally reshape the political forces that govern both Social Security and Medicare.

We have to return to the principle of mutual responsibility and imagine a new role for government that is consistent with the age in which we live. Instead of bureaucracies that, as Stuart Butler says, centralize decisionmaking, the government should give citizens the means to solve their problems and set their own priorities. Modernizing Medicare to empower consumers and patients with choice, information, and responsibility is the right platform for reform.

If I have not convinced fellow progressives that this is the right path to take, let me make one final observation. As it stands now, Medicare is a major political obstacle to providing health care coverage for the uninsured. As long as the program remains an open-ended entitlement with runaway costs, its reputation will blacken all other attempts to expand coverage. For example, the Daschle-Gephardt bill to cover children is the most fiscally conservative measure that the Democratic leadership has ever introduced. Yet some critics have already dismissed it as the creation of another budget-busting entitlement.

We need to modernize Medicare, if for no other reason than to prove that the simple humanitarian deed of taking care of each other's health care needs does not have to be a fiscal and political nightmare. To date, all we have proved is that no good deed goes unpunished.

4

Building a Sound
Infrastructure for Choice

THE PAPERS in this chapter describe ways to structure choice for Medicare beneficiaries: ways of addressing the special needs of those with chronic illness and disability, features of competitive pricing proposals, the role of public and private purchasing alliances, and specialty or population carve-outs for certain conditions.

The Medicare Beneficiary as Consumer
Stan Jones

AFTER YEARS of regarding Medicare as their only choice for health insurance, and perhaps being somewhat taken for granted by the program, beneficiaries in many parts of the country find they have a choice. Indeed, they find themselves being sought by alternative health plans that offer excellent benefits and premiums designed to appeal to them. In 1996 an average of 80,000 beneficiaries a month left traditional Medicare for such plans, a rate that the Health Care Financing Administration says will result in one-third of the beneficiaries being in such private plans by 2007.[1] It is safe to say that many private insurers have hopes of capturing even more of this new market.

This evolving marketplace confronts beneficiaries with very important changes in what they can expect from their Medicare plan, health care providers, and the federal government. To choose well, that is, to choose in their own best interest, beneficiaries must unlearn old attitudes and learn new skills more appropriate to shopping in a competitive marketplace. If the marketplace is to produce health care for beneficiaries at acceptable prices and quality, they must learn these skills and drive the market in these directions by their choices.

To get a realistic sense of the high stakes for beneficiaries in their choice of a health plan and the challenge that such a choice poses, this discussion invites the policy-oriented reader to look at the changes from the beneficiary's point of view. It shows how they must reorient their understanding of Medicare and learn how to choose well among health plans and providers to suit the realities of the emerging program. I focus particularly on what the changes mean from the perspective of the millions of chronically ill Medicare beneficiaries. Based on this assessment of the stakes and challenge, I urge that government or private agencies should use for beneficiaries at least the best practices large employers use to help their employees choose, as well as providing more adventurous experiments and pilot efforts.

Changes in Health Plans

Beneficiaries have been assured of receiving basic Medicare coverage without having to make a serious choice (although some choose to decline part B coverage). Their choice has been focused on Medicare supplemental (medigap) policies marketed to them by private plans. The potential for both gain and loss has been less than it has in the new Medicare marketplace, where private plans offer choices of the basic coverage plus supplemental coverage that vary in important respects from traditional fee-for-service Medicare plus supplemental. Plans vary in how they select and pay their providers, how accessible care is to the various areas served, how they define "necessary" and "appropriate" health care, and how they handle emergency and out-of-area care. Beneficiaries or their children or caregivers must now assume responsibility for finding the best deal in basic health coverage amidst this variety. And they are faced with adopting a skeptical or buyer beware attitude appropriate to any market in which competitive vendors are aggressively selling to them. They must learn to read the fine print and allow for the oversell every consumer should expect in the marketplace.

Health plans compete to develop and market attractive premiums and benefits. This competition includes valuable additional benefits such as lower cost-sharing and prescription drug coverage, and prices that may vary as much as $1,000 a year or more from the cost of traditional Medicare plus supplemental coverage. In fact, the variation in benefits and costs among plans and traditional Medicare can be even greater, especially for those who depend on high volumes of a specific service, such as home health services, on the necessity for which there may be professional disagreement. Although all plans must cover basic part A and part B benefits, within these coverage definitions plans can vary their own definitions of what constitutes appropriate care so as not to pay for services that the beneficiaries have enjoyed in traditional Medicare or in another plan. Alternatively, plans can pay for services under parts A and B for which traditional Medicare has refused to pay. The beneficiary is faced with understanding and comparing plan marketing materials accurately enough to make an informed choice among them.

To keep premiums competitive, health care plans generally limit their choice of physicians, hospitals, laboratories, pharmacies, and other providers to those that will accept their clinical culture or their payment arrangements, discounted fees, reporting, and utilization review process. Some allow use of nonparticipating providers, but at a higher level of cost-sharing, not unlike Medicare, which allows use of providers who decline to accept assignment. All insurers, including the traditional Medicare program, attempt to limit referrals to and use of high-cost services from providers such as specialists, hospitals, emergency rooms, nursing homes, and home health care. Private health plans have stronger means and incentives than traditional Medicare for limiting use of such services and providers and seem more effective at limiting use. Beneficiaries are faced with determining whether a plan with an attractive premium and acceptable coverage includes their customary providers, whether it defines patterns of care so as to give them access to the specialists and other services they customarily use, and whether their place of residence or travel patterns are consistent with providers' locations. From the beneficiaries' perspective the choice is complex and involves substantial clinical risks, and reliable information is hard to obtain.

Beneficiaries have been trained to rely on their political representatives and advocates to keep Medicare attractive and affordable. They are now being asked to make their influence felt in a marketplace by their purchasing decisions. What plans they favor and how much they are willing to pay will gradually determine the market standard for what is covered, what constitutes appropriate care, and how plans structure care. That is to say, how well beneficiaries choose among plans will not only determine what they individually get from their Medicare coverage, but their collective choices will determine the range of what is budgeted by health plans for care of the elderly in the future. Health plans, in effect, are the agents that accomplish this budgeting when they set premiums and offer competitive benefits and definitions of necessary and appropriate care to compete for market share and operating margins.

They also have an opportunity to budget to achieve greater collective good for their enrollees (as well as market share and profit) through trade-offs between the amount of services provided all their enrollees and specific services to individuals with particular needs. For example, a plan might elect not to do further expensive tests or referrals for diagnostic purposes, even though it would marginally improve the accuracy of the diagnosis, so that it can devote more revenues to preventive services for enrollees or for profits or salaries. The legal status and limits of this private budgeting (it could be called allocation of resources or even rationing) activity are still unclear, given the uncertain benefit of many clinical procedures and the variations in their use. A critical question is whether this private budgeting can be held effectively accountable by beneficiaries' purchasing decisions, or whether an element of public or political budgeting is required if U.S. health care is to reach a balance that serves both the individual and society in an acceptable way.

Changes Beneficiaries Face from Providers

Under Medicare's traditional fee-for-service system most patients have become accustomed to coordinating their own care. They try to keep track of what providers they have seen for what services, and they have wide discretion to seek at Medicare's expense any of a wide variety of covered services they believe they need.

Health plans attempt to manage this coordination more efficiently, usually through a primary care physician who exercises control over what services are provided, or at least what services are paid for by the plan. For beneficiaries there is the potential for improved quality of care in such management, especially if they have complex health care needs. The drawback is that they may find that plans sometimes do not refer them to specialists or give tests or services that under fee-for-service Medicare they have come to believe are good for them. And because the plans' financial best interest may be served by fewer referrals and services, beneficiaries have reason to be skeptical about such refusals. They therefore need to choose a plan and a primary care provider whom they trust with this level of control over their health and costs.

Under traditional Medicare the most important step beneficiaries take in determining what kind of services and care they receive is choosing their physicians and the style of practice and philosophy they bring. The choice has relatively little to do with the Medicare insurer. But health care plans become more closely involved than traditional Medicare with physicians' clinical practices and use incentives to influence physicians' practice styles to conform to plan review protocols and guidelines. These guidelines may be based on statistical or actuarial studies, the advice of panels of experts, the plans' own clinical or claims experience and judgment, the collective good of their enrollees versus the good of individuals, desire to keep premiums low to increase market share or keep claims low to increase margins, and how well premium revenues are doing relative to claims. Indeed, beneficiaries must expect that to some extent the guidelines can and will reflect all of these.

Beneficiaries are faced with taking these hard-to-discover clinical practices into account when they choose a doctor. Their choice is also a choice of plan philosophy and vice versa.

Under the fee-for-service system the provider's financial self-interest is in some ways aligned with that of the beneficiaries. Both have an interest in getting Medicare to pay for all the care, referrals, tests, and services that the physician and patient agree are needed. This is consistent with trusting that the physician will not skimp on care, although it does raise questions about whether the practitioner may be recommending too much care.

Effective health care plans enlist the providers in the plans' effort to constrain use of high-cost services and referrals. This may be done by incentive payments, bonuses, payment of global fees or capitation amounts, or by dropping providers who seem to use excess services. Plans can also contain costs by educating their providers and cultivating a conservative clinical culture. Providers may feel their contractual arrangement, employment, or implicit partnership with a plan is threatened if they object to its refusal to cover a service to a patient, inform the patient that there is a clinical option the plan does not cover, or advise a patient to join another plan. This perception may be reinforced through so-called anticriticism clauses in the contract between plan and provider.

Beneficiaries with complex needs have grown accustomed to asking and trusting completely their physicians' best judgment about what course of care is most promising for their condition and even what health plan (or traditional Medicare) best covers it. However, in health plans there may be incentives for physician's to offer less than their best professional opinion about what would be in a patient's best interest. Beneficiaries must take these providers' incentives into account when they discuss referral and treatment options with physicians.

Changes in Government Incentives

It is not clear that beneficiaries have thought of Medicare as a health care plan or an insurance plan per se. It has been the government program that pays their medical bills. Today government has taken on three roles: it manages a health care plan for beneficiaries (traditional Medicare) as in the past; it certifies and offers alternative private health care plans to beneficiaries; and it administers a process that allows beneficiaries to choose among these options.

Beneficiaries must learn to consider their former sole benefactor, traditional Medicare, as one choice among many. They must see the government as offering a choice of plans that compete with traditional Medicare. And they must consider government as like many large self-insured employers in being a source of help to them in choosing well among traditional Medicare and these plans.

In the past, government has exercised direct control over the one program available to beneficiaries, and beneficiaries have lobbied government to make their one choice a good deal. In the new model, government has less direct control over health care plans and their practices. It must certify that plans meet various basic standards, including limits on plan variations, as a condition for selling to beneficiaries. But plans have latitude beyond these standards. And standards can only go so far in disciplining a market. The ultimate discipline is in the choice of traditional Medicare or one or another health plan by the purchaser. The government is presently not acting as a wholesale purchaser on behalf of beneficiaries, as do many leading private employers. In fact, it seems to be headed in the direction of certifying a widening variety of health care plans. The current trend leaves the primary burden of purchasing with the beneficiaries, who must look out for themselves by choosing plans whose practices seem most likely to produce satisfaction.

The government has viewed its constituency as beneficiaries entitled to payment for covered health services. It now must view them more broadly as entitled to a choice in their own best interest between various private plans and a government-offered traditional Medicare program.

From the perspective of the managers of the traditional program, beneficiaries begin to look like customers shopping for their best. For traditional Medicare to choose to compete for customers would be a great advantage to beneficiaries. However, this also suggests they may not trust traditional Medicare to encourage or inform them as much as it might about other plans that could be better for their individual needs. Perhaps these competitive concerns account for governments' slowness to provide beneficiaries the basic information—lists of participating alternative plans and basic information on them, for example—that private programs and such public programs as the Federal Employees Health Benefits Program make available to their employees.

Changes as They Apply to the Chronically Ill

Chronically ill beneficiaries face a special challenge from these changes in health care plan, provider, and government incentives. Most important, capitated health plans have strong incentives to avoid enrollees who are likely to cost them more than they will be paid in premiums. And to the extent providers are paid by plans to encourage less use of services, they too have incentives to avoid high-cost patients.

Chronically ill beneficiaries must learn to aggressively seek out and choose health plans and health care that are in their best interest in a system where they are often not wanted and where plans avoid (demarket) them by not signing up their favorite providers, making referrals to specialists hard to get, restricting services enrollees believe they need, and above all by giving them no marketing information on whether the plan is good for people with their condition.

Chronically ill people can be expected to put energy and time into choosing their providers because a lot is at stake for them both clinically and financially. They have been accustomed under traditional Medicare to having the program pay for whatever provider they choose, with the caveat that they may have to pay a higher percentage of a nonparticipating physician's bill. They must now learn to live with a system in which they may have to research and choose new providers or remain in traditional Medicare and lose the added benefits and lower costs available from private plans.

The unwillingness of chronically ill beneficiaries to change providers is sometimes cited as a just reason to let them pay more. But it is very difficult to find information that helps identify physicians who will be skilled in meeting complex needs and that beneficiaries will believe can be trusted to manage their care, especially when the plans and physicians involved are not actively seeking their business. The high-stakes and difficult task of changing physicians seems likely to lock chronically ill beneficiaries into traditional Medicare or the plan their physicians are presently in and to whose practices they have grown accustomed.

Because health care plans and their providers have the latitude to change the patterns of the care they give to Medicare beneficiaries based on their definitions of necessary and appropriate care, it is difficult for beneficiaries to know before joining a plan whether specific services they enjoyed under traditional Medicare or another plan will continue to be available or paid for in a new plan. The plan makes this determination only after enrollment when a beneficiary consults one of its clinicians. Chronically ill beneficiaries can discover after joining a plan that it will not provide or pay for expensive services or referrals that they have previously been told are needed or are justified for quality of life by what they believe to be competent physicians. The chronically ill badly need to trust their specialists to discuss their clinical options candidly with them and offer their best opinion, before enrollment, about how different plans are likely to provide or pay for the types of services the beneficiaries are getting or are likely to need. Without this candid advice, and sometimes even with it, chronically ill beneficiaries are faced with buying a pig in a poke.

In American medicine, chronically ill patients are often told not to give up hope. Clinical care is constantly being improved. Patients have become used to this prospect and sometimes have overreacted by asking their providers to try every procedure or test reviewed in the popular press. Yet the chronically ill have reason to be fearful of the competitive health plan marketplace. Whether plans budget their premium revenues to achieve better market shares and operating margins and to remain within their budgets to maximize the collective good, it is possible that healthier (and perhaps short-sighted or uninformed) beneficiaries may choose among plans in such a way that the market standard for coverage and care falls short of the specific needs of the chronically ill. This may create a marketplace in which there are weak incentives at best for plans to invest to do better for the chronically ill. How much investment in improving clinical care for high-cost patients is likely in a system that has incentives to avoid them? The chronically ill need special help in forcing the system to respond to their needs.

The Beneficiary as Consumer

It is difficult to quantify the extent of the challenge to beneficiaries posed by the emerging Medicare marketplace. They must learn to deal skeptically with people they have generally trusted and to seek out and make sense of complex information about plans and providers. Their physicians are likely to face pressures and have financial incentives to behave differently from the ways they have in the past, and the health plan salespeople may be getting a $500 commission for each enrollment. For many people, a crucial choice can hinge on relatively technical information about practice protocols and provider incentives.

Medicare beneficiaries are likely to face a wider range and larger number of choices than almost any employee group. At the same time, they may be less well equipped to research and make the choices because of frailty in mind or body (almost 4 million beneficiaries are older than 85, and well over 4 million more are disabled).[2]

Helping Beneficiaries Become Consumers

Given the extent of the challenge and the disadvantages many frail and chronically ill elderly people face in this enterprise, a case can be made for providing assistance to them that is at least comparable to that provided by many employers and for extraordinary and venturesome pilot efforts by the government and private organizations to give them a fighting chance as consumers.

First, the government must find ways to pay a fair premium to health care plans (and to the traditional Medicare program) for beneficiaries with high-cost chronic conditions. It is not reasonable to expect chronically ill beneficiaries to fare well as consumers if they are facing a sophisticated and technical system that has strong financial incentives to avoid them and to avoid investments that might attract them. Given the high incidence of chronic illness among Medicare beneficiaries, the highest priority should be given to using existing technology and developing additional or alternative ways to pay providers and health plans so as to create a market with incentives to invest in and market to the chronically ill.

Research on risk-adjusting premiums has extended far beyond the averaged adjusted per capita costs (AAPCC) method and needs to be used by Medicare as a way of adjusting payments to plans and also of holding traditional Medicare accountable on a fairer basis for its per capita costs.

In addition, because risk adjustors can be gamed and are in fact largely untested under market conditions, and because the chronically ill are such an important cost and quality concern for Medicare, the federal government should open new and venturesome lines of research, demonstration, and pilot activity on adjustors. For example, the Health Care Financing Administration might solicit proposals from providers and health plans for new ideas of how to provide care for chronically ill people in innovative ways at fair market prices. The federal government might accept bids for comprehensive care or subsets of care (so-called carve-outs) to beneficiaries identified by diagnosis, functional status, or other criteria. One promising beneficiary group is composed of those ill with a condition that is likely to be terminal and a primary factor in their care as well as in the quality of the remainder of their lives (virtually all Medicare beneficiaries die while members of traditional Medicare or one of its certified plans). These pilot projects might involve global fees, capitation, or a mix of these and fee for service appropriate to the insurance risks involved. This and other lines of research face complex problems, but so do risk adjustors; and the need for a solution (or many small solutions) to the problem is crucial to providing adequate care to Medicares chronically ill.

The beneficiary as consumer needs help from a "purchasing agent." This is particularly true for the chronically ill. The purchasing agent would review and offer a consumer a choice of the health care plans that are the best deals in the area according to the agent's published criteria. In many large public and private organizations, the personnel department serves this function, presenting a limited number of plan choices to employees.

The government's ability to perform as purchasing agent is hampered by its enormous size as a buyer and by the inflexibility of its rule-setting and contracting process. However, it might conduct pilot projects or evaluate venturesome efforts by private agents who might contract with it to perform the function of agent or who might contract with beneficiaries to perform the function on their behalf. For example, private organizations that represent groups of Medicare beneficiaries with chronic conditions might evaluate and negotiate arrangements with providers and plans and then offer them to their members. This would, of course, require a means of fair pricing to overcome risk selection. The goal of the government should be to set standards for purchasing agents to ensure their objectivity.

In the absence of purchasing agents, the extent and importance of the choice faced by beneficiaries and their compromised ability to choose argues for setting higher basic standards for Medicare plans. At present, the government's relaxation of the 50/50 rule and minimum enrollment requirements for health care plans under Medicare constitute a trend toward lower standards. Standards for beneficiaries' health care plans should be higher even than those of some employer programs such as the Federal Employees Health Benefits Program. In this program all plans that meet the minimum standards are theoretically admitted, and federal retirees eligible for Medicare often purchase high-option coverage that yields extremely little additional benefit over standard options at a very high additional premium.

Additional Proposed Standards

The Health Care Financing Administration already enforces such standards and is developing more. Further standards might reasonably be argued.

—There should be clinical parameters or limits of some sort on budgeting and utilization review of health care plans. Specifically, limits are needed on how differently Medicare and other plans can define appropriate services and referrals in sensitive areas of Medicare part A and part B benefits. There should also be requirements that health plans make available and justify their criteria of appropriateness and their practice and review guidelines. The justification should be based on clinical evidence or credible judgment, including budgeting decisions regarding how services are allocated between the collective good and the individual good of their enrollees. One goal would be to assure beneficiaries that variations in traditional Medicare and plan service or payment practices reflect credible clinical or public health opinion in our society (and legal system), not just a plan's desire to increase its market share or operating margin. A second goal would be to limit plans' freedom to redistribute resources between collective and individual good or to hold plans accountable for these judgments not only to the marketplace but to the political process. A third goal would be to reduce the harm beneficiaries might do to themselves if they select a plan without knowing much about it.

—There need to be requirements that health care plans, traditional Medicare, and supplemental insurers contract with providers in ways that encourage them to share relevant clinical information and possible treatment choices with their patients and, to the extent their professional judgment warrants it, to be advocates for the patients with the insurers. The goal would be to allow the plan to pay for services based on its appropriateness criteria to the extent the criteria are within the limits discussed earlier, but prohibit the plan from applying the criteria to what the provider can freely describe, recommend, or even provide as a service to beneficiaries outside of plan coverage. The best practices of health care plans in these matters might be reviewed for possible adoption for all Medicare plans.

—There should be limits on financial incentives for providers to cut back on providing expensive services to patients in Medicare, Medicare supplemental, and health plan contracts. For many physicians the current limit that incentives account for no more than 25 percent of income allows the purchase of a new Mercedes or sailboat to hinge on reducing services. In addition, government might set guidelines for how plans and providers must describe these financial incentives to encourage a proper skepticism in beneficiaries when they choose plans and providers.

—There should be standards for basic types of specialists and services needed for specific chronic conditions of high prevalence among Medicare beneficiaries. There could also be requirements that health plans and providers must advertise or make easily available information on their capacity to treat specific chronic conditions. The National Committee on Quality Assurance has begun important work toward this end. The standards might be further developed in collaboration with consumer advocacy organizations, which might in turn analyze the performance of Medicare and health care plans in these respects and publish the analyses. The goal is to get otherwise unadvertised information to chronically ill beneficiaries so they can choose in their own best interest.

—There should be some standardization in coverage and standard definitions of terms used to describe coverage in traditional Medicare, supplemental policies, and health plans. For example, if a plan claims to offer prescription drug coverage, it should describe succinctly whether it restricts coverage to a formulary, what portion of the prescription cost it pays, and from whom drugs must be obtained. For some coverages, and prescription drug coverage may be one of them, confusion is so easy that the benefit should be standardized. Out-of-area and emergency coverage requirements are also among these. Consider that several years ago CalPERS, the California Public Employees Personal Employee Retirement System, standardized its requirements for the coverage that plans must offer because health administrators were convinced the coverages offered were too complex for meaningful comparison by employees and that this situation watered down price competition.

—The marketing practices used by plans must be limited. This includes continuing the ban on door-to-door marketing and, in deference to the frailty of the beneficiary population, adding a ban on outgoing (plan-initiated) telephone marketing. Also, the commissions paid to brokers for selling to a Medicare beneficiary could be limited. Alternatively, agents could be required to inform beneficiaries immediately of the amount of commission they would receive in the sale, again as a way to encourage appropriate skepticism.

—Plans should be rated good or fair based on the value they represent. Traditional Medicare, supplemental, and health plans can be compared and ranked by the premium of the plan relative to the actuarial value of the benefits it offers. The day may come when quality can also be quantified to some extent and added to the ranking. The government, a purchasing agent for government, or private organizations such as employer or consumer organizations might publish the figures. Some private organizations already publish the figures in some markets, such as the Federal Employees Health Benefits Program, and show that plans vary greatly in their ratios of premiums to benefits. Beneficiaries could still choose a plan with a low ratio of benefits to price if they perceive that the plan is of a higher quality than others. Or in lieu of a rating one could argue that a plan that charges more than, for example, 1.5 times the average premium for a benefit unit in a geographic area is not likely to be a good buy. Government or a private purchasing agents might go a step further and limit participation to those plans that achieve at least a certain basic level of benefits to premium.

Providing Information and Education

Another way government and private plans could help beneficiaries choose well is to provide education, trustworthy information, and careful management of the process of choosing. The best practices of large employers in these regards, including the Federal Employee Health Benefits Program, make governments efforts to inform Medicare beneficiaries look primitive. Various remedies should be undertaken.

—The federal government should conduct a massive and continuing retraining and education program on what Medicare is, what health care plans are, what the consumer has to gain and to lose in choosing traditional Medicare or a health plan, and the kinds of consumer attitudes and skills needed to weigh choices. During open season it should educate consumers about the information that is available to help them evaluate the choices. This campaign might be launched in some future year in anticipation of starting open seasons and could be funded with a one-time appropriation. It might be conducted in collaboration with voluntary organizations involved with the elderly and chronically ill.

—Beneficiaries need to be provided with trustworthy, objective, comparative information when choosing plans and providers. The best practices of large private employers indicate the type of information that should be provided. Traditional Medicare, supplemental coverage, and health plans should give prices, benefits, participating providers, referral guidelines and practices, geographic locations, provider payment policies and incentives, payment review guidelines for prescribed sentinel conditions and illnesses, and out-of-area and emergency coverages.

—Objective government or independent private agents should provide a number of information services. Given conflicts in the Health Care Financing Administration's multiple accountabilites, it would be useful to establish a government entity independent of traditional Medicare to oversee this function. Because funds for these types of information, counseling, and grievance resolution activities have traditionally been hard to get from Congress, the activities might be funded from a levy on health plan premiums and traditional Medicare's per capita costs. The assumption is that helping beneficiaries choose well is critical to the long-term cost control in the program.

The information services should take on three major responsibilities. First, they should provide current comparative information on traditional Medicare and health plans that is developed by independent parties. The infomation should include performance indicators, outcome and satisfaction measures, satisfaction and quality indicators for specific chronic conditions, ratios of premiums to benefit values, and estimates of the out-of-pocket costs for caring for sample conditions.

Second, the services should make available comparative information on area physicians and other providers that would allow beneficiaries to evaluate the desirability of giving up their current providers for new ones. The information should include the chronic conditions or illnesses in which the providers specialize, their training and experience, whether their practice is open to new patients, their financial arrangements with health plans, their clinical philosophy for conditions and illnesses in which they specialize, and satisfaction and outcome indicators. The goal here is to reduce the risks of changing providers to a reasonable level so that health plans can continue to restrict physician panels without excluding large numbers of chronically ill subscribers. If this type of difficult-to-acquire and controversial information cannot be provided, the political and perhaps unavoidable alternative will be to require all plans to offer point-of-service choice of providers at a reasonable additional cost, as some legislative proposals have suggested.

Third, the services should provide counseling to beneficiaries attempting to choose so that they do not surrender or compromise their own or their spouse's or dependents' Medicaid or retiree benefits. The current advisory services offered by Medicare are available in only some areas. Comparable services should be available nationwide to help beneficiaries evaluate the treatment they are getting from providers and plans when they have questions or doubts and function as advocates for them the way large companies' benefits staffs function for employees.

Fee-for-Service as a Choice

The government should equip the traditional Medicare program to try to remain a competitive option for Medicare beneficiaries. Many features of the competitive Medicare plan market suggest there is likely to be substantial risk selection against Medicare. In addition, private plans have the freedom to offer additional benefits and cover Medicare's cost-sharing much less expensively than Medicare plus Medicare supplemental can. Managed care plans also offer better coordinated care to beneficiaries through their various provider panel arrangements and contracts. If traditional Medicare is not given the means to compete with these plans in price and coverage, it is likely to continue to lose enrollees, and to lose the healthier enrollees first, raising the per capita cost of the program. Given the magnitude of educating beneficiaries to be savvy health care consumers and the risk that they will not succeed in choosing in their own best interest, it would seem prudent to maintain for the foreseeable future Medicare's viability as a choice.

Notes

1. Health Care Financing Administration, *Profiles of Medicare* (Department of Health and Human Services, 1996), p. 96.
2. Ibid., pp. 16, 18.

Structuring Choice under Medicare
Roger Feldman and Bryan Dowd

GREAT CONTROVERSY surrounded the passage of the original Medicare legislation in 1965. President Johnson's initial proposal was restricted to hospital coverage for the elderly. In an attempt to weaken the opposition from the American Medical Association, which charged that Medicare would lead to socialized medicine, strategists for the bill had opposed including coverage of physicians' services.[1] Ultimately, Medicare emerged as a multilayered program. The original proposal for compulsory hospital insurance under Social Security became part A. The second layer consisted of government-subsidized voluntary insurance under part B to cover physicians' bills.

To lessen the opposition from powerful hospital and physicians' associations, several features were included in Medicare that mirrored the prevailing financial arrangements of American medical care. Hospitals were reimbursed for Medicare's share of their reasonable costs. On the doctors' side, fee-for-service reimbursement for physicians was preserved, with payment based on a method borrowed from Blue Shield plans: reimbursement at "usual, customary, and reasonable" fees. Thus physicians as a group were allowed to determine their own payment levels.

Medicare also enshrined the principle that patients had the right to choose any provider who was willing to supply services to the program.[2] Freedom of choice was so important that at the request of Blue Cross almost all states passed laws prohibiting a health insurance company from negotiating with specific providers for lower charges and then directing patients to those providers. This same principle was further institutionalized in Medicare.

Having adopted provider-determined reimbursement and freedom of choice, Medicare's costs expanded rapidly, far outpacing original projections.[3] As concern over costs grew, almost all proposals to resolve the problem were regulatory. The one exception was President Nixon's 1971 proposal to encourage the formation of health maintenance organizations as a national strategy to

This report was prepared under a contract from the National Academy of Social Insurance as part of its initiative, Restructuring Medicare for the Long Term. We wish to acknowledge contributions from Robert Coulam of Abt Associates. We also benefited from the support of the Health Care Financing Administration under contract 500-92-0014 (Medicare Competitive Pricing Demonstration, Project Officer Ronald W. Deacon). The opinions expressed here do not represent official HCFA policy.

contain the costs. He recommended that the federal government facilitate the development of HMOs in all states by contracting with them to provide services to Medicare beneficiaries. In the ensuing congressional hearings the experience of these plans, particularly the Kaiser HMOs, was cited as promising relief. By paying physicians fixed, capitated amounts and owning their own hospitals, Kaiser groups were able to control costs significantly. As usual, the American Medical Association strongly objected to the movement toward HMOs, claiming the concept needed further testing.

In 1972 Congress added section 1876 to Title 18 of the Social Security Act, authorizing capitation payments for HMOs based on either cost or risk. Section 1876 established a precedent for a limited group of providers to receive a capitation payment for the Medicare benefit, with the right to retain some of the savings resulting from their efficiencies. During the years that followed, the Health Care Financing Administration (HCFA) developed several demonstration projects to test alternative forms of risk contracting for HMOs.

The 1982 Tax Equity and Fiscal Responsibility Act authorized enrollment of Medicare beneficiaries in HMOs and other competitive medical plans. HMOs contracting with Medicare were paid 95 percent of the estimated cost of serving similar beneficiaries who elected to remain in the fee-for-service (FFS) sector. This payment rate was named the adjusted average per capita cost (AAPCC). HMOs were not allowed to give direct premium rebates, even if they could provide benefits for less than the government payment. The refusal to allow premium rebates further entrenched a third idea in Medicare: hostility to financial incentives and other market signals as a means to encourage enrollees to choose different health plans, including fee-for-service Medicare.

In the many congressional hearings on the role of HMOs in the Medicare program, two themes stand out: ensuring fairness in access to health care and improving the efficiency of the market.[4] Fairness in access was emphasized by representatives from the prepaid plans. From the health care plans' perspective, fairness meant that all health plans (not just FFS plans) should have an equal opportunity to enroll Medicare beneficiaries. Fairness was also characterized as giving Medicare beneficiaries the same access to prepaid health plans enjoyed by employed people.[5] In areas where HMOs were available, it was argued that beneficiaries should be able to join them. Other meanings of fairness, which we describe in the following section, were not evident at this time.

It was hoped that allowing HMOs into the Medicare market would improve efficiency in two ways. First, replacing fee-for-service reimbursement with capitation would give providers an incentive to keep their enrollees healthy. Second, it was hoped that HMOs would promote a more competitive health care delivery system, with long-term savings for the government and more coverage for beneficiaries.[6]

The introduction of prepaid health plans into the Medicare program raised a number of questions. How should the plans be paid? What prices should beneficiaries face in making their choices among health plans? How much management of the Medicare market was required, and who should do it? Unfortunately, it was not widely recognized that these operational matters could affect the ability of the program to meet its goals of fairness and efficiency. Despite advice to the contrary, Congress prescribed a heavily regulated administrative pricing system in which the government rather than a competitive market determined the payments to HMOs.

Because of this choice of payment methods, it has been hard for risk plans to compete with fee-for-service Medicare.[7] Basing the government's contribution on fee-for-service costs and prohibiting premium rebates forces the HMOs in high-AAPCC areas to compete by offering more benefits instead of lower premiums. This form of competition has its limits. In an effort to avoid returning money to Medicare, HMOs may offer benefits that are of little value to consumers. This may be the reason that enrollment in Medicare risk plans has not grown at rates matching those in the private sector.[8] Moreover, evidence suggests that better-than-average risks have enrolled in HMOs. Payment based on 95 percent of the average risk therefore may increase rather than decrease costs to the Health Care Financing Administration.[9]

Early indications of a desire to reform the HMO payment system appeared in 1985 when a White House working group, chaired by presidential advisor William L. Roper, recommended several testable ways to bring more competition and cost efficiency into Medicare. One was contracting with a single entity, on the basis of competitive bids, to provide services for all beneficiaries in the demonstration area.[10] Another was to offer all beneficiaries in the area the choice of several plans through the use of vouchers. Neither proposal was tried at the time.[11]

Virtually everyone now agrees that the current method of paying Medicare HMOs is seriously flawed. The AAPCC may not accurately reflect fee-for-service costs that would have been incurred by HMO enrollees, and payments vary widely among nearby geographic areas. And within the same area, payments may differ significantly from one year to the next. There is far less agreement on what should be used in its place. Congressional Republicans recently proposed that the government contribution to Medicare be specified in statute, with per capita growth rates determined by explicit decisions of political leaders.[12] Although the government contribution under that proposal would be the same for both fee-for-service and HMOs, the Republicans' plan still represents administered pricing rather than the competitive bidding that is typical of premium setting in the private sector.

What Is Wrong with Medicare?

Before proceeding with our analysis of options to fix Medicare (in particular, before analyzing competitive pricing), it is important to explain what is wrong with the program. We see two problems: it is unfair and it is inefficient.

During the congressional hearings on Medicare HMOs, fairness was narrowly interpreted in terms of health plans' access to Medicare beneficiaries and beneficiaries' access to health plans. There is also a much broader sense in which the program is unfair: Medicare takes hundreds of billions of dollars from working Americans and uses the money to subsidize the costs of current beneficiaries. The program has no plausible plan for ensuring that current taxpayers will receive benefits when they become eligible for Medicare.

In our book *Competitive Pricing for Medicare* we deliberately avoided discussing fairness: "This is not a book about fiscal responsibility or fairness. It is about *efficiency*. One of the greatest contributions of economists to the field of policy analysis is the clear distinction between issues of fairness and those of efficiency."[13] Although still recognizing the distinction, we believe that economists can also contribute to discussions of fairness.

We consider two types of fairness: fairness within a generation and across generations. Medicare is fair within a generation if it meets the tests of horizontal and vertical equity. *Horizontal equity* requires that all people in a cohort with similar abilities to pay should be treated equally. *Vertical equity* means that people of differing abilities to pay should be treated differently. As applied to Medicare, these principles imply that people with less income should enjoy proportionately more benefits from Medicare, or pay proportionately lower taxes, than those with more income.

The government's share of Medicare expenses is funded from three sources: the Medicare payroll tax, general tax revenue, and part B premiums. Working Americans begin contributing to the program as soon as they begin paying personal income and social security taxes. The 1997 Medicare tax rate was 2.9 percent. Unlike the Social Security tax base, which ends at $62,700, all eligible wages are subject to the Medicare tax. It is thus proportionate to income. Personal income taxes, which fund much of the program's costs, are progressive because the percentage of income taken for taxes increases with income. Part B premiums do not vary with respect to income, but they fund a relatively small proportion of total part B costs (25 percent in 1997).

Except for the fact that nonwage income escapes the Medicare payroll tax, two people with equal income will pay equal Medicare taxes. Thus broadly speaking, the current Medicare financing arrangements are horizontally fair. In terms of vertical equity, however, Medicare is not fair. Although part B (less the beneficiary premium) is progressive because it is financed from general tax revenues, the Medicare payroll tax is proportionate to income. This violates the principle that people with less income should pay proportionately lower taxes than those with more income.[14]

There is no reason to suppose that Medicare benefits are horizontally unfair. Vertically, the program may favor the wealthy, because they live longer than the less wealthy and tend to spend more money on medical care.[15] These problems, however, do not seem intentional. The relatively greater benefits enjoyed by those who live longer can be justified on the grounds that the program is intended to protect people from the possibility that they will live to very old ages and incur large medical bills.

A significant problem with Medicare is that the program is unfair across generations. This can be understood with the help of two concepts: present value and the zero-sum constraint. Present value expresses a stream of payments over time by what they would be worth if they were all paid out at a given date as one sum.[16] The zero-sum constraint says that future generations must pay with interest for purchases that past and present generations did not pay for. It can be expressed by the following accounting identity:

PV of current generation's taxes + PV of future generations' taxes – PV of current generation's expenses – PV of future generations' expenses + PV of Medicare deficit = 0

Present value and the zero-sum constraint represent a method for determining whether current Medicare policy is sustainable. This is done by fixing one or more of the terms in the constraint at prespecified values and calculating what must happen to the other terms in order to satisfy the constraint. For example, suppose that current Medicare policy is carved in stone for the generation that retired in 1994. This group will receive, on average, $5.19 in part A benefits for every dollar they and their employers paid into the program and the interest on those payments.[17] Therefore, to satisfy the zero-sum constraint, the present value of future generations' benefits must be less than the present value of their taxes or the program must a run permanent deficit or both.

Now set the permanent deficit at zero and freeze Medicare's current benefits in place.[18] The taxes on future generations needed to support this program would increase from 2.53 percent of GDP in 1994 to 8.63 percent in 2065, according to the Medicare trustees' reports.[19] The Medicare tax would rise from 3.16 percent to 10.11 percent of the wage base. Although taxes at these levels would fix Medicare's financial problems, they are not in the realm of political reality. All possible fixes for Medicare are likely to involve at least some reduction in benefits for future generations. The question is: what type of cut would be perceived as least unfair to future generations?

Several types of empirical evidence suggest that eliminating the beneficiary's right to enroll in a fee-for-service delivery system at no cost beyond the part B premium would be the fairest way to reduce Medicare benefits. First, the federal government already has decided to allow HMOs to market to Medicare beneficiaries. Thus the principle of offering plans that limit access to some medical care providers is well established in Medicare. Second, the experience of the private sector suggests that the working population (who will be future Medicare beneficiaries) does not demand freedom of choice at no out-of-pocket cost as an entitlement.

Third, a more subtle argument suggests that eliminating the entitlement to fee-for-service delivery would reduce a regressive benefit of the Medicare program. Evidence from the employed sector points to the fact that demand for expensive (unmanaged) health care plans is related to the employee's income.[20] Medicare pays the full cost of unmanaged fee-for-service. Thus, the current Medicare program provides an unequal subsidy for the wealthy. Converting the Medicare entitlement from fee-for-service medicine to a basic benefit package obtained from the most efficient health plan would curtail this subsidy.

In contrast, across-the-board cuts in other Medicare benefits (for example, by increasing the hospital deductible) would fall equally on all beneficiaries, regardless of their income. Cuts of this type could be criticized as vertically unfair. Continued reductions in payments to fee-for-service providers are another option for controlling Medicare costs, but it is unlikely that reductions can continue without at some point affecting provider participation in the program.

In summary, Medicare is not fair across generations. Some combination of cuts in future benefits and future tax increases will be needed to guarantee the long-run solvency of the program. Unlike defined-contribution proposals, which set the beneficiary's entitlement at a dollar value without regard to what that amount of money can purchase, eliminating the entitlement to fee-for-service medicine would preserve the beneficiary's right to have a basic level of coverage.

In addition to being unfair, Medicare is inefficient. In our previous study, we identified two primary sources of inefficiency in the program. The first involves the price that the government pays for Medicare benefits. When the government adds another benefit to Medicare, it pays the inflated price of that benefit in the inefficient fee-for-service sector. Economic theory predicts that any buyer, facing an inefficiently high price, will buy too few services. As applied to Medicare, this theory predicts that the government will buy too few Medicare benefits.

There is ample evidence to support the claim that HMOs are more efficient than the fee-for-service sector. In carefully controlled studies, including a randomized trial, hospitalization rates, length of stay, and use of costly procedures have been lower in HMOs.[21] Additional evidence is the ability of many HMOs to provide the current Medicare benefit package plus supplementary benefits at no charge to beneficiaries. In 1996, some 63 percent of all Medicare risk plans were charging no supplementary premiums.[22] Favorable selection within the AAPCC payment categories could account for some of the excess revenue but probably not all of it. For example, the *Los Angeles Times* reported that one HMO offered free drug benefits that cost as much as $2,500 per year per beneficiary.[23]

Unfortunately, estimates of the government's demand for Medicare benefits are not available. Therefore, we do not know how many benefits have been left out of the Medicare entitlement because of the inefficiently high cost of fee-for-service. However, indirect evidence suggests that at least some benefits (such as expanded long-term care) would be added to the entitlement if they could be purchased for a reasonable cost.[24]

The second source of inefficiency in Medicare is that beneficiaries face distorted prices when they choose health care plans. This problem is the direct result of the Medicare HMO payment policy. Beneficiaries are entitled to the full cost of basic coverage (less the part B premium) if they choose FFS coverage; if they choose an HMO, the government pays 95 percent of that estimated cost. Because HMOs can produce basic benefits for less than that payment, competition among them would force them to convert the "overpayment" into additional benefits that consumers want or into direct cash rebates if consumers would rather have the money. However, HMOs are not allowed to give cash rebates. There are even limits to the types of additional services they can offer. Until recently, for example, Medicare HMOs could not use their surplus funds to offer a point-of-service option that would pay a portion of the cost of services obtained from providers outside the HMO's own provider network. Advocates of medical savings accounts for Medicare also believe that if beneficiaries were given the cash equivalent of their Medicare endowment, they would choose to spend it in ways that are not available under the current program.

Because they cannot give cash rebates, HMOs in high AAPCC areas will spend their surplus revenue on additional benefits. They will even provide benefits such as health club memberships or free transportation to the doctor's office that cost more to produce than they are worth to beneficiaries. We refer to those benefits that Medicare beneficiaries would not choose to purchase with their own money as *inefficient benefits*. In fact, beneficiaries would not even purchase inefficient benefits if they were spending someone else's money, if they had the option of taking the cash instead.[25] Inefficient benefits will not be offered by HMOs in areas where beneficiaries' payments do not cover the cost of all efficient benefits, and would not be offered if HMOs were allowed to give cash rebates.

Our previous analysis also identified other problems with Medicare. For example, Medicare beneficiaries often lack even basic comparative information on the health care plans available in their market area, much less the comprehensive information on health plan quality and satisfaction that many employers have made available to their employees. The result is that beneficiaries make poorly informed choices, including the purchase of duplicate coverage. A complete description of these problems can be found in *Competitive Pricing for Medicare*.

Competitive Pricing as a Solution to Medicare's Problems

The beauty of competitive pricing proposals is that they use the proven efficiency of HMOs to determine the right price for basic Medicare benefits. The government, facing the right price of Medicare benefits, would be able to buy more Medicare benefits; Medicare beneficiaries, facing the right price of more expensive health plans, would have an incentive to make efficient choices. In all likelihood, some consumers would want to purchase additional benefits and amenities (including unmanaged care), but their choices would be efficient because they would be spending their own money for those amenities.

In our recommended version of competitive pricing, the government would specify a basic benefit package (possibly the current package), take bids on this package, and set its contribution equal to the lowest-priced plan in the market area. The government contribution would apply to fee-for-service Medicare as well as HMOs. Beneficiaries could purchase additional benefits and other amenities with their own money, ensuring that all efficient benefits would be purchased if they happened to be left out of the basic package. We recommended converting medigap insurers into full-fledged risk plans that would submit bids with other health plans and would be responsible for all Medicare benefits.

We also called for open enrollment periods with limited plan switching between open enrollment periods. That proposal was modeled on the current practice of large employers who offer multiple health plans. Virtually without exception, employees in those firms can freely change health plans during the open enrollment period without facing medical underwriting, regardless of their health status.

Much of the current Medicare program would remain unchanged under our competitive pricing proposal. Traditional fee-for-service Medicare would continue to be offered in all markets. The Health Care Financing Administration would continue to sponsor Medicare, with responsibility for determining the conditions of market entry and monitoring health plan performance. But the agency would take a more active role in distributing information on health plans to beneficiaries in each market area before the open enrollment period.

Why Further Analysis of Competitive Pricing Is Needed

Competitive pricing proposals, including our own, are heavily influenced by the experience of large employers, who use similar competitive pricing systems to manage their health insurance programs.[26] But there are important distinctions between the health benefit plans of large employers and the Medicare program, indicating a need for further analysis of competitive pricing in Medicare.

One aspect of employment-based insurance that distinguishes it from Medicare is the employee's trade-off between wages and more generous fringe benefits, including health insurance. The cost of employment-based health insurance is paid by employees, either directly through out-of-pocket premiums or indirectly through lower money wages.[27] Because the ultimate users of the health insurance product are the ones who pay for it, they have incentives to monitor the quantity and quality of insurance benefits that are supplied.

In contrast, the demand for Medicare benefits is a political decision made by the voters, only some of whom are Medicare beneficiaries. It is quite possible that the political demand for benefits does not coincide with the ultimate users' demand. Thus, it is important for the government to monitor the quantity and quality of benefits that are supplied. Merely specifying a package of basic benefits may not be sufficient to do this. For example, HMOs will have an incentive to submit bids on a package that includes more than the basic benefits if extra benefits attract customers and if the exact makeup of the package is difficult to monitor. Can a bidding system be designed to stop this form of benefit creep should it occur?

We also did not fully appreciate the role of employer-sponsored health insurance for retirees. Many employers offer health benefits that supplement Medicare, and an increasing number of retiree programs include HMOs. This raises the possibility that HMOs might submit high bids to the HCFA but then discount those bids to employers. In other words, HMOs might submit bids that they never intend to collect. How should the HCFA respond to opportunistic premium discounts by HMOs?

Numerous other details of a more technical nature need to be worked out in any competitive bidding system for Medicare. These include:

—On what basis should health plans be allowed to participate in Medicare?

—Should Medicare have a limited open enrollment period?

—How should the government's contribution to premiums be determined?

—Should government and beneficiary contributions be adjusted for risk?

—At what level should the competitive pricing system be administered, and should the HCFA be the only administrator of Medicare?

Monitoring the Products on Which Bids Are Submitted

Our competitive pricing proposal called for health care plans to submit bids on the current package of basic benefits, with the government's contribution based on the lowest bid submitted by a qualified plan. Plans also could submit bids on any packages of supplementary benefits they wanted to sell. Further analysis suggests that this proposal may be flawed. The problem is that health plans may submit bids for basic benefits that include the cost of popular supplementary benefits, that is, they may submit bids that are higher than the cost of basic benefits so as to induce a government contribution to fund below-cost supplementary benefits. This strategy might cause the government to contribute to the cost of supplementary benefits that it does not want to buy. Other proposals to induce HMOs to reveal the cost of basic benefits should be considered.

The Problem Illustrated

The following example illustrates the problem of getting plans to submit bids on basic Medicare benefits.[28] We make four assumptions regarding the cost of basic Medicare benefits and the extent and cost of supplementary benefits in fee-for-service Medicare and HMOs. Given these assumptions, we explore the pricing practices of Medicare HMOs under both the current AAPCC payment system and a competitive pricing system. The assumptions are:

—The cost of basic fee-for-service Medicare benefits (including the "spill-over" cost induced by fee-for-service medigap supplements) is $4,000 a year.

—HMOs produce *basic* Medicare benefits for $3,000.

—HMOs and fee-for-service are equally efficient at producing *supplementary* benefits.

—All consumers want to purchase a supplementary policy that costs $600 a year.

First, consider the HMOs' pricing problem under the current payment system. The HMO receives $4,000 from the government.[29] This payment exceeds its total cost of basic plus supplementary benefits by $400. Both HCFA regulations and marketplace competition will force the HMO to return the difference to the beneficiary. Since the HCFA will not allow the HMO to do this through a part B premium rebate, the HMO has to add more optional benefits that cost $400. Suppose that those benefits are worth $200 to beneficiaries (who wanted only $600 of supplementary benefits).[30] Thus, under the current payment system, the HMO "gives away" supplementary benefits that are worth $800 to beneficiaries. The fee-for-service system also receives $4,000 from the government. Fee-for-service beneficiaries must pay $600 for their medigap policy. From the beneficiary's perspective, the relative price of choosing the fee-for-service sector over the HMO is equal to the medigap premium plus the forgone value of the HMO's optional services, or $800.

Now, consider a competitive pricing system in which HCFA bases its contribution to premiums on the lowest submitted bid. The government's contribution is invariant with respect to the beneficiary's choice of health plan, including the fee-for-service sector. We also assume that all HMOs in the market are equally efficient, and thus we can concentrate on the bid from a typical HMO. Initially, we assume that there is only one HMO in the market.

The optimal outcome under such a system (from the HCFA's perspective) is for the HMO to bid its true cost of basic benefits: $3,000. It drops the $400 of optional services that consumers did not want to purchase at their cost, and charges $600 for the standard supplementary policy. Beneficiaries choosing fee-for-service Medicare must pay $1,000 out of pocket for basic coverage plus $600 for supplementary benefits. The difference in the out-of-pocket cost between the two sectors is $1,000.

Compared with the current strategy of offering $400 of inefficient supplementary benefits, this "optimal" pricing strategy allows the HMO to increase the attractiveness of its product in relation to fee-for-service Medicare ($1,000 versus $800). Thus, the optimal pricing strategy would replace the current strategy. However, the HMO has another pricing strategy that may be better from its perspective than the optimal one from the HCFA's perspective: it

Table 4-1. *Comparison of Fee-for-Service and HMO Pricing Strategies*
Dollars

Category	Fee-for-service sector	Ideal HMO bid	HMO bid with efficient supplements
Cost of basic benefits	4,000	3,000	3,000
Cost of supplementary benefits	600	600	600
Bid for basic benefits	4,000	3,000	3,600
Bid for supplementary benefits	600	600	0
Government contribution to premiums	3,000[a] 3,600[b]	3,000	3,600
Beneficiaries' out-of-pocket cost for basic benefits	1,000[a] 400[b]	0	0
Beneficiaries' out-of-pocket cost for supplementary benefits	600[a] 600[b]	600	0
Beneficiaries' total out-of-pocket costs	1,600[a] 1,000[b]	600	0
Fee-for-service minus HMO total out-of-pocket cost	1,000[a] 1,000[b]	. . .	. . .

[a]Ideal HMO bid.
[b]HMO bid includes efficient supplementary benefits.

could include the cost of efficient supplementary benefits (those that benefici-aries value at least as much as they cost the HMO to provide) in its bid for basic coverage. In table 4-1 we assume that HMOs are asked to submit prices for both basic benefits and their proposed supplementary benefits. Would the HMO include the cost of efficient supplementary benefits in its bid for basic benefits?

The ideal HMO bid creates a $1,000 difference in out-of-pocket cost be-tween fee-for-service coverage and the HMO. The strategy of including effi-cient supplementary benefits in the bid for basic coverage produces the same out-of-pocket difference. Thus, the HMO does not change the attractiveness of its "product" by bidding $3,600 for basic benefits and nothing for supplemen-tary benefits. Under the assumptions of our model, therefore, competitive pricing may or may not produce the ideal bid.

Would this uncertainty be resolved if there were two equally efficient HMOs? The answer is easily no. Whichever strategy the first HMO chooses, the second will be indifferent between submitting an ideal bid and a bid for basic benefits that includes efficient supplementary benefits. In fact, all bids that total $3,600 for basic and efficient supplementary benefits will be equally attractive to consumers, and therefore we cannot predict the bidding strategies that will be chosen by equally efficient HMOs.

This would also be the case if the second HMO could produce basic benefits at lower cost ($2,500, for example) than the first HMO. The more efficient HMO would reduce its total bid by the amount of the efficiency difference, but it would be indifferent concerning the division of its bid into separate components for basic and efficient supplementary benefits. Likewise, the uncertainty is not resolved if we assume that HMOs can produce efficient supplementary benefits at lower cost ($450, for example) than fee-for-service. This new assumption would simply widen the out-of-pocket difference between sectors to $1,150 under both pricing strategies.

The only tie-breaker that we have discovered is the possibility that not all beneficiaries demand $600 of supplementary benefits. Suppose, for example, that some beneficiaries would not purchase any supplementary benefits if they had to spend their own money. In that case HMOs have an incentive to exclude the cost of supplementary benefits from their bids.[31] Relying on this argument may be overly optimistic, however, because the demand for supplementary Medicare benefits is widespread.

Possible Solutions to the Problem

To increase the likelihood that HMOs will submit bids for basic benefits that reflect their costs, it may be necessary to impose further incentives on the bidding process. The first is a penalty for high bidders. The extreme sanction against bidding high would be exclusion from the Medicare program. Exclusion would increase an HMO's incentive to submit a low bid, but it would decrease beneficiaries' access to HMOs. The second incentive would be a reward for bidding low. For example, the HCFA might pay an additional $10 a month per beneficiary to the HMO submitting the lowest price for basic benefits. Notice that this incentive differs from a policy of setting the government's contribution to premiums $10 above the lowest bid for basic benefits. The latter policy would affect the revenue of all HMOs, while the former would affect only the revenue of the lowest priced plan.

We are not confident that the HCFA can ever discover an HMO's true cost of basic benefits through the use of accounting methods such as the adjusted community rate methodology. If costs could be discovered through this method, there would be no need for competitive pricing. However, there may be a limited role for cost accounting in a competitive pricing system. In the extreme case an HMO that offers generous supplementary benefits at no out-of-pocket premium is definitely shifting the cost of those benefits onto its bid for basic benefits. The HCFA might require that such HMOs justify their bids, with a presumption that generous supplementary benefits should cost *something* to provide.

Another strategy might be to examine the types of supplementary benefits that are offered, and the premiums for these packages, in low-AAPCC markets. HMOs in such markets should offer efficient supplementary benefits at premiums that approximate their costs.[32]

HMOs could also be required to sell supplementary policies separately. Suppose that the demand for supplementary benefits is widespread. This rules out the tie-breaker that we have discussed, but it raises another intriguing possibility for separating the bids on basic and efficient supplementary benefits: require that all supplementary policies be sold separately to anyone who wants to buy them. Under this requirement, beneficiaries who want to purchase an HMO supplement to basic fee-for-service Medicare could do so. If the HMO was unwise and continued to give away the supplement (as in the third column of table 4-1), it would surely lose money.

For this strategy to be realistic, two other conditions must be met. First, supplementary policies sold by different insurers must have the same effect on the cost of any insurer's basic policies. Otherwise, health plans would have to submit different bids for their basic policy, depending on who was supplementing it. Second, the supplementary policies must be standardized (as they are in this example) so that they can be attached to any basic plan. It is not clear whether these conditions can be met.

The Role of Employers in a Competitive Pricing System

The employer group market is a growing share of the total Medicare HMO market. Anecdotal information suggests that it is the largest share in some areas. Exclusion of this significant market segment from a competitive pricing system would substantially lessen the potential efficiency gains from competitive pricing. However, inclusion of employer-sponsored Medicare plans might cause significant problems for the HCFA. Two such problems deserve particular emphasis: What should the HCFA do if an employer subsidizes the HMO premium? What should the HCFA do if a health plan agrees to waive its out-of-pocket premiums?

Employer Subsidy of the HMO Premium

Suppose the employer decides to pay the retiree's share of the HMO premium for HMOs that require an out-of-pocket premium contribution. What attitude should the HCFA take toward this behavior by employers?

Competitive pricing works best when beneficiaries face the full marginal cost of choosing more expensive health plans. Therefore, we do not favor an employer subsidy for the out-of-pocket premium of any plan, including fee-for-service, for active employees or retirees. This policy reduces the financial penalty for choosing costly, inefficient plans and therefore artificially inflates the market share of those plans. However, if an employer remains committed to subsidizing inefficient health plans, we do not see much that the HCFA can or should do about it.

HMO Premium Discounting

Suppose the employer and the HMO negotiate an arrangement in which the HMO agrees to waive the out-of-pocket premium. What attitude should the HCFA take toward premium discounting? Premium discounting could arise for four reasons: favorable risk selection, real efficiencies, monopsony power, and opportunistic behavior by the HMO. The appropriate response to premium discounts may depend on how they arise.

FAVORABLE RISK SELECTION. The retirees of certain firms who enroll in Medicare HMOs may be healthier or sicker than the average Medicare HMO enrollee. In this case the HCFA's payment to the HMO would differ from the HMO's costs, after adjusting for other risk factors. An accurate risk-adjustment formula would have to include "retiree of firm X" as another risk factor. However, this level of refinement is probably impossible to achieve in practice and might not be desirable. Devising a risk adjustor based on fee-for-service Medicare costs in firm X would be especially difficult because such costs depend in part on the provisions of the firm's current fee-for-service supplementary coverage. Firms with more generous fee-for-service supplements would receive larger "risk" adjustments under this scheme, which is not a desirable outcome from the HCFA's perspective.

REAL EFFICIENCIES. Firms may reduce the cost of providing the Medicare entitlement through investing in activities that go under the broad heading of "sponsorship." These activities include providing information on health plans and organizing annual open enrollment periods. Some of the activities may duplicate those conducted by the HCFA or its agents in the competitive pricing system. Although firms may cut back their investment in sponsorship when it can be obtained at no cost from the HCFA, in most cases they will continue to provide some sponsoring activities as long as there is a return on this investment. This return could take the form of negotiated premium discounts from the HMO. Alternatively, the HCFA could reduce its payment to the HMO and forward the money to the firm. A final policy option would be for the agency to pay the firm without reducing its contribution to the HMO. The last strategy, while providing optimal incentives for the firm to engage in sponsorship, would allow the HMO to keep its windfall profit.

Implementing any policy in which the HCFA pays the firm for sponsorship activities would be difficult because it requires an assessment of the savings from firm sponsorship. These savings would be extremely difficult to measure with available data sources, even as the cost of lost sponsorship may be the least worrisome of the costs of competitive pricing. Arguably, the HCFA should take the lead in reforming Medicare and should not let private efforts that remedy the agency's own sponsorship difficulties stand in the way of something more important: competitive pricing.

MONOPSONY DISCOUNTS.   Discounts may arise because a firm is a monopsonist (a buyer with a significant amount of purchasing power) in the market for Medicare supplementary benefits. Provided that the supply side of the market is competitive, monopsony is inefficient because it results in too little insurance being purchased. The case in which the supply side is not competitive is more difficult to analyze. However, we doubt whether monopsony is a significant problem in the Medicare supplement market. No buyer, not even a large firm, is likely to purchase a significant fraction of all the Medicare supplementary insurance sold in most local markets.[33]

OPPORTUNISTIC DISCOUNTS.   The last reason discounts may arise is that the HMO never intended to collect the full amount of the premium. This possibility is very troubling. By submitting a high bid, the HMO may be able to influence the HCFA's premium contribution (this is especially likely if all HMOs expect that their competitors will do the same thing). An HMO that requires an out-of-pocket premium contribution because of its high bid can then offer a discount to employer-sponsored retiree plans. If these plans represent a substantial share of the market, the opportunities for discounting may be widespread. This would reduce the cost of submitting high bids and might substantially undermine the incentives in the bidding system. We are not certain that the HCFA has the authority to prevent HMOs from discounting their premiums. Nonetheless, if that authority does exist, the agency should seriously consider requiring HMOs to sell each benefit package at one price to all buyers.[34]

Technical Problems in Competitive Pricing

All forms of competitive pricing involve at least a modest amount of organization of the demand side of the market for health plans (for example, specifying the product on which prices are submitted). An important dimension of demand-side organization is determining who should be allowed to participate. Options range from a very restrictive winner-take-all system to a very open program in which every qualified plan is offered. In between are several semirestrictive options: the Federal Employees Health Benefits Plan (FEHBP) is open to any HMO; the state of Minnesota allows only some HMOs to be offered; and the Buyers Health Care Action Group (BHCAG) in Minneapolis will offer any plan that meets the terms of a request for proposals, but the RFP specifies that participating providers cannot belong to more than one plan.

The argument in favor of offering all health plans available in the market area is based primarily on two beliefs: that the best judge of a health plan's value is a well-informed consumer and that open participation maximizes the competitive pressure on plans in the market and avoids the possibility that the government could become an accomplice (either knowing or unknowing) in restricting market entry. As long as consumers have good information on the premium, coverage, quality of care, and other relevant characteristics of each health plan in the market area, all plans should be offered and consumers should judge value for themselves.

Additional reasons not to restrict the number of winning health plans are:

—alternatives are available in the market should a health plan experience problems with financial solvency;

—adequate capacity is provided;

—participation by health plans is encouraged; and

—it is easier to identify a poorly performing plan if there are more opportunities for comparisons of performance.

Although we believe that well-informed consumers are the best judges of health plan value, several arguments in favor of limiting the number of health plans must be considered. Aside from savings in administrative costs (about which there is not much evidence), there are two primary reasons to restrict the number of qualified health plans. First, restricting the number would add a second layer of competition to the market. Heightened competitive pressure would be brought to bear on the plans if, in addition to bidding for enrollees, they had to bid for entry to Medicare. When the health plans know that the price and benefit package they submit will be used to select winning bidders, they may submit more competitive prices. Second, limiting the number of participating plans might reduce the problem of biased selection because there would be less opportunity for plans to compete by designing special benefit packages that attract low-risk beneficiaries.

We will illustrate the argument for limiting the number of health plans with the experience of two programs: the state of Minnesota's Group Insurance Program for state employees and the Buyers Health Care Action Group in Minneapolis–St. Paul. The experience of the Federal Employees Health Benefits Program (FEHBP) will be examined as a possible illustration of biased selection in a system that allows unrestricted HMO participation.

State of Minnesota

If heightened competition is the rationale for limiting the number of qualified Medicare plans, the criteria for selecting plans may differ dramatically from those used to determine whether the plan simply meets a minimum quality standard. Minnesota follows a policy of offering all licensed staff and group-model HMOs to state employees. The state believes that staff and group-model HMOs offer products that are unique in that physicians predominantly see patients belonging to that health plan. Independent practice association (IPA) plans with broad provider networks are more likely to be very close substitutes from the consumer's perspective, and offering several such plans simply increases administrative costs and dilutes the state's bargaining power without increasing consumer choice.

Minnesota's resistance to offering identical IPA plans with broad provider networks is understandable. The issue is complicated, however. If consumers can keep the same physician and coverage when switching health plans, they are likely to give greater weight to the out-of-pocket premium when they shop for a plan. This creates a strong incentive for health plans with broad provider networks to reduce their costs and thus their premiums. In fact, one could argue that price competition is more intense among plans with broad provider networks than among staff and group HMOs. The fact that consumers in these HMOs must change physicians when they change health plans actually may give some monopoly pricing power to the HMOs.

There might be some benefits to offering more than one plan of the same type.[35] A study of health plan choices of the Twin Cities employed population found that consumers were most sensitive to out-of-pocket premium differences among health plans of the same type (for example, staff and group-model HMOs in one category versus IPAs and fee-for-service plans in the other category). This study focused only on shopping by employees among the plans that they were offered, however, not on shopping by the employers.

Whether competition for consumers among similar plans produces lower premiums than competition for entry to a firm is a unresolved question. The issue is complex, and the arguments about optimal management of a set of plans are largely speculative. If Medicare decides to limit access to its program even among qualified plans, monitoring and nurturing the competitive market becomes much more important. Medicare must ensure that exclusion of a qualified health plan does not drive the plan out of existence if its presence as a potential competitor is considered beneficial to the market.

Buyers Health Care Action Group

The Buyers Health Care Action Group, a coalition of approximately two dozen of the largest employers in Minnesota, has taken a somewhat different strategy by requiring that bidders have provider networks that do not overlap. BHCAG was formed in 1992 and is known for its past efforts to implement a value-based purchasing strategy with an emphasis on quality management.[36] Starting in 1993 BHCAG contracted with a single health care organization that was capable of responding to its demands. This situation was recently altered in a dramatic fashion. Hoping to develop a consumer-driven health care environment, the group implemented contracts in 1997 with fifteen nonoverlapping care systems that met performance standards and were willing to provide better information to consumers. Most employers contribute a fixed amount to any of the care systems chosen by their employees. To preserve their protection under the Employee Retirement Income Security Act (ERISA), the employers will retain financial risk for the new program.

The new initiative is the result of evolution in the thinking of BHCAG members based on their previous efforts. In particular, the group was concerned that it was difficult to hold providers accountable given the overlapping provider networks in most Twin Cities health plans and that there was a lack of progress in creating better-informed, active consumers.[37] In addition, BHCAG was concerned that its previous sole-source contract had stimulated consolidation among Twin Cities health plans, reducing the choices available to consumers and increasing the market power of the remaining plans. BHCAG is determined that the new approach will increase, rather than decrease, the amount of consumer choice.

Federal Employees Health Benefits Program

The third argument for limiting the number of qualified plans is that this would reduce the problem of biased selection. Biased selection occurs when some health plans (typically those that offer more generous benefits) attract the sickest employees in a group. Prices for more generous plans will thus be higher than would be justified based on benefit differences alone. According to a recent report by the Congressional Budget Office, "Those patterns isolate sick people in selected plans that then experience increases in cost and risk financial instability."[38] In the extreme case, a plan that attracts high risks may experience progressively poorer risks and higher premiums until it is forced to leave the program.

The Federal Employees Health Benefits Program provides health insurance for more than 4 million active federal employees and annuitants, as well as their 4.6 million dependents and survivors, at an annual cost to the government of about $11 billion.[39] Participants in the FEHBP can choose among many health plans that offer varying levels of benefits and premiums.[40] Biased selection should flourish in this type of environment, and two actuarial studies have found evidence of some selection in the FEHBP. However, those studies do not make a compelling case that the plan suffers from severe selection problems.

Analyzing data from 1981 to 1984, the first study found that adverse selection had increased the cost of high-option FEHBP plans offered by Blue Cross and Aetna.[41] Analyzing data from 1982 to 1985, the second study reported that unfavorable selection appeared to deteriorate over time.[42] Citing "significant structural defects" in the program, Aetna withdrew its indemnity plan from FEHBP in 1990.[43] But the study that found adverse selection against Blue Cross and Aetna from 1981 to 1984 concluded that "comprehensive plans *as a class* have not been selected against (yet)." And the second study found that favorable selection tended to deteriorate over time, suggesting that favored plans may not be able to maintain their selection advantages over the long run.

Furthermore, both studies of biased selection in the FEHBP had a serious methodological flaw: the only variable used to standardize the benefits offered by each plan was its coinsurance rate. Oddly, the authors reported that Blue Cross's high-option plan had the same coinsurance rate as its low-option plan (one expects high-option plans to have lower coinsurance rates), resulting in similar actuarial values for the two plans. Standardization for other benefits, which were omitted from the analysis, would have increased the actuarial value of high-option coverage and thus would have reduced the reported extent of adverse selection.

According to some observers, the selection problems experienced by some high-option plans in the FEHBP could be corrected easily. Much of the adverse selection occurs because retirees younger than the age of Medicare eligibility tend to congregate in a few indemnity plans. Walton Francis, a leading expert on FEHBP, has recommended that the government make an added premium contribution for this high-risk group.[44] The retirees would carry that contribution with them as they changed plans, thereby "holding harmless" any plan that experiences adverse selection.

Another perspective was offered by Peter Welch, who argued that biased selection is inherent in situations in which employees can choose among several conventional carriers.[45] All it takes for consumers to switch conventional carriers is some paperwork. In contrast, switching among HMOs, or between fee-for-service coverage and HMOs, more often involves changing one's physician. Welch believes that the "obvious" solution is for FEHBP to offer just one conventional plan in each area. In fact, the FEHBP already comes close to this optimal solution. The government generally allows new HMOs to enter the program without any barrier.[46] In contrast, new fee-for-service competitors generally are prohibited (although a major fee-for-service expansion occurred in the middle 1980s, after Congress bowed to union pressure to admit new plans). Aetna's withdrawing from the program and the government's policy of not allowing new fee-for-service plans to enter have created a situation strikingly similar to Welch's recommendation. Therefore, it is not surprising that the FEHBP, like many other large employment-based health plans, can survive without experiencing severe selection problems.

Should Medicare Have a Limited Open Enrollment Period?

Annual open enrollment periods, with limited plan switching between those periods, are an almost universal feature of employment-based health insurance programs. The advantages of open enrollment to employees are obvious and numerous. First, open enrollment guarantees that all employees have access to every health plan, regardless of their health status or prior use of health care services. Second, during open enrollment, most large employers provide employees with information regarding total premiums, out-of-pocket premiums, and comparisons of benefits.[47] Some employers also conduct surveys of employee satisfaction with health plans and typically release this information during open enrollment. All of these activities improve the quality and timeliness of employees' information about the available health plans.

Finally, open enrollment with a lock-in mitigates biased selection. Between open enrollment periods, which are held once every year in most firms, employees cannot voluntarily change health plans. This requirement reduces the employee's incentive to enroll in a plan simply to obtain needed (and foreseen) services. If the employee has any doubts about the plan's ability to provide services after the foreseen episode of illness is over, he or she will be less likely to join a plan on the basis of anticipated use of services.

Because of these advantages, many large employers believe that open enrollment is crucial to the success of their health benefits programs. In *Competitive Pricing for Medicare* we recommended that Medicare should adopt open enrollment periods even if competitive pricing is not implemented. We argued that open enrollment would offer the same advantages for Medicare beneficiaries as it does for private employees: access to all health plans, good information, and a reduction in the problem of biased selection. However, many details of the Medicare open enrollment proposal need to be specified. Among these are:

—Is the schedule of events in open enrollment practical for Medicare?

—Should the length of the lock-in period be different from the one-year contract that is typical of employment-based health insurance?

—Should disenrollment occur without any preconditions or under conditions (for example, screening) set by health plans or the government?

—Should consumers have the option to select the open-enrollment program?

—Would risk adjustment eliminate the need for lock-ins?

IS THE SCHEDULE OF EVENTS IN OPEN ENROLLMENT PRACTICAL FOR MEDICARE?   The HCFA has believed that open enrollment would be difficult to implement in the Medicare program because the AAPCC payment rates must be announced early in the year in order to provide time for health plans to comment on changes in methodology or assumptions of the AAPCC. This would necessitate basing the rates used during open enrollment on estimates that may prove to be inaccurate.[48] However, this is a problem only because of the current regulatory pricing system, in which Medicare tells the health plans how much they will be paid. If the health plans told Medicare how much they were going to charge, the need for comments on methodology and assumptions would vanish.

Minnesota's experience suggests that all activities of open enrollment can take place with adequate lead time for the enrollment process to occur in the fall and the effective date of the new contract on January 1 of the following year. Collection of data on price, coverage, and other characteristics of competing health plans takes place in April or May. Two meetings are scheduled between the health plans and the state program administrators: the first concerns plans' proposed benefits packages and provider networks; the second, scheduled in late June, focuses on plans' proposed premium rates. Open enrollment is held during October. There is no reason why Medicare could not follow a similar schedule. If the sheer volume of Medicare enrollees posed a logistical problem for health plans, enrollment periods could be staggered by market area, or even county of residence.

Selection of market areas and service areas also needs to take place during the summer before open enrollment. A *market area* is the area over which beneficiaries can choose among a set of health plans at given premiums. A *service area* is the geographic area over which a health plan can sell its product. Retaining the county unit as the market area would have obvious advantages for Medicare because health plans are already familiar with this definition. And it would be advantageous for the HCFA because the premium of the fee-for-service sector is already calculated by county.

HOW LONG SHOULD THE LOCK-IN BE FOR MEDICARE?   Open enrollment is a clear example of the tension between two conflicting objectives: consumers want to be able to make instant changes among health plans, but they also want true insurance against risk. We do not believe both objectives can be satisfied without some trade-offs.

When consumers can move from one health plan (insurance contract) to another on short notice, they are likely to shop for health care services at the time services are needed. If shopping among health plans for short-term consumption of services is allowed to continue unchecked, the market for health insurance can deteriorate into a market for health care services. Although it may seem advantageous for consumers to be able to shop among different plans for the best physician to treat their cancer or the best coverage of services they need immediately, this freedom has the potential to destroy the market for health insurance. Health plans that attract sick people would have to raise their premiums to reflect the fact that new enrollees joined the plan to consume services immediately. Their premiums would reflect the cost of providing services to sick enrollees, not the cost of providing insurance to all enrollees, some of whom will become sick during the period of the insurance contract.

If health plans are restricted from charging different premiums to different individuals (for example, to new enrollees for a certain period of time), or using other screening devices such as medical underwriting or restrictions on preexisting conditions, premiums simply will rise for everyone in the plan. If premiums are not allowed to rise, plans will find some other way to segment the market, perhaps by offering different levels of coverage or of managed care. Taken to its extreme, the market for health insurance might subdivide into plans designed for healthy enrollees and plans designed for sick enrollees. Premiums for the healthy persons' plans would be extremely low and those for the sick persons' plans would be very high. The healthy persons' plans might compete to provide low premiums and limited services, and the sick persons' plans might compete to provide efficient treatment of sick enrollees. However, plans would not compete to provide high-quality, low-cost health insurance.

Risk-averse consumers will reject this market outcome because they want to purchase insurance against uncertain future health expenditures. These consumers will demand insurance products with enough restrictions to allow the market for insurance to survive. Consumer demand for restrictions that preserve the market for insurance is the reason for the current structure of the group health insurance market, with limited plan switching between open enrollment periods. To our knowledge, it is not possible to allow consumers to shop freely for services among different health plans and, in the long run, preserve a healthy market for true insurance. Thus a lock-in provision is advantageous because it helps ensure that consumers can choose health plans based on the desirability of the plan as an insurer rather than as a provider of services for immediate consumption. The main beneficiaries of a lock-in provision for Medicare would be the enrollees in health plans that experience adverse selection based on consumption of services immediately following enrollment. Those plans might include some HMOs (because of low coinsurance, deductibles, and supplementary premiums), or the fee-for-service sector (because of unrestricted access to specialists).

Some HMOs might object to a lock-in provision because they believe that high risks who are not satisfied with the services they are receiving will be most likely to leave for fee-for-service plans or another HMO. This might appear to be a safety valve that reduces pressure to change possibly unreasonable HMO practices. Although HMOs might benefit in the short run by losing high-risk members, disenrollment precipitated by the need to improve the quality of one's current health care might lead to the demise of the market for insurance. Any health plan whose disenrollees characteristically exhibit high levels of service use immediately following disenrollment poses a serious threat to the Medicare program and its beneficiaries, and the HCFA should terminate its contract. This rule applies equally to the fee-for-service sector, where steps should be taken immediately if HMOs are found to experience high costs for new enrollees switching from fee for service.

Annual open enrollment periods are virtually universal in employment-based insurance, although some employers are beginning to experiment with two-year periods between open enrollments. Large employers that organize open enrollment periods for their retirees seem to offer them annually, but that may occur out of habit rather than experimentation. We recommend annual open enrollment periods, but we suggest that the HCFA evaluate health plan selection carefully, including a requirement for plans to submit data on the use of sentinel medical procedures (major but postponable surgeries such as joint replacement) by new enrollees. The HCFA should also monitor the use of services by disenrollees from Medicare HMOs and compare their data to a sample of continuing fee-for-service enrollees to determine if beneficiaries who need services are choosing or leaving particular health plans.

Additional evidence on the persistence of high expenditure levels in Medicare also would be useful in setting the length of the lock-in period. To the extent that high use persists, the lock-in period needs to be extended because the time horizon for hit-and-run use of services is longer. Evidence from the employee group market suggests that high expenditure levels typically do not last for many years.[49] However, the situation might be different for Medicare, and evidence of persistent high use would suggest that a longer lock-in period is appropriate. The HCFA might also experiment with limitations on preexisting conditions for certain persistent conditions, although these are not found in employment-based health insurance.

SHOULD CONSUMERS CHOOSE THE OPEN ENROLLMENT PROGRAM? Most open enrollment programs feature automatic membership, that is, the consumer chooses health plans within the program but does not choose to join or not join the program itself. This is not always the case, however. Minnesota state retirees have a one-time opportunity to join the state's open enrollment program. To become eligible, they must have continuous health insurance coverage and must purchase an annuity of at least $10,000 cash value.[50] If they elect to do this, they have the right to switch among Medicare health plans (including a fee-for-service plan and several HMOs) offered by the state during annual open enrollment periods. Otherwise, they can participate in the individual market for retiree health insurance coverage and are subject to any preconditions legally imposed by the plans.

Although not specifically designed as such, the Minnesota program protects the participating plans against opportunistic shopping for health care services. Most retirees are probably healthy when they choose to participate in the program. Therefore, those who choose open enrollment probably represent a cross-section of all employees. Some of the participants will become ill, but this percentage is not expected to be higher than in the overall population. The key to protection is the one-time opportunity to choose the open enrollment process and not the $10,000 annuity, which is immaterial to the provision of protection. Without such a program, retirees might elect nonparticipating plans as long as they remained healthy, but switch to the state's plans after they became ill.[51] This would force the premiums for participating plans to increase.

WOULD RISK ADJUSTMENT ELIMINATE THE NEED FOR LOCK-INS?   Later we will analyze the use of adjustments to compensate plans that attract higher risks. Because such adjustments would pay for the costs of beneficiaries who enroll to use needed services, would they eliminate the need for lock-ins? We do not think so. Without lock-ins, the market for insurance (as opposed to reimbursement for foreseen use of services) would be damaged or destroyed. The health plan's premium might become a negotiated schedule of fees for services that beneficiaries expect to use when they enroll in the plan. But the premium would not represent a pool that protects every enrollee against risk. In fact, in the worst case there would be no protection against risk.

Setting the Government's Contribution to Premiums

The way the government sets its contribution to premiums can have a dramatic effect on the competitiveness of the Medicare market. The government's contribution can be set in two basic ways: by a Dutch auction or by picking a point on the distribution of bids.

In a Dutch auction, an auctioneer begins by announcing rates that are very attractive to sellers. Less attractive rates are announced and sellers begin to drop out of the auction. The process continues until only one seller remains. This seller is paid at the rate where the second-to-last seller dropped out. In Medicare the government could announce very high capitation rates, then reduce the rate until only one HMO agrees to serve Medicare beneficiaries at the announced rate. Alternatively, the government could reduce the rate until the desired balance between low payments, participation, and benefit levels is achieved.

If, for reasons suggested earlier, persuading HMOs to submit bids for basic benefits that exclude the cost of efficient supplements is an intractable task, a Dutch auction might allow the government to discover the HMOs' cost of basic benefits through a process of attrition. Final prices under the Dutch auction could be lower than prices attained under the second approach (taking bids and choosing a point on the bid distribution as the government's contribution). Because of the similarity of the Dutch auction to the second-lowest-bid method, we discuss it further later.

From the HCFA's perspective, an advantage of the Dutch auction is that the agency retains full control over the payment rate. In that sense the Dutch auction is closer to the current AAPCC payment system than any alternative that bases the government's contribution on the distribution of bids. A possible disadvantage of the Dutch auction for Medicare is its administrative complexity. Each time the HCFA announces a lower payment rate, the HMOs would have to calculate a new benefit and premium package. The number of steps needed to reach the lowest price may be cumbersome, raising the possibility that the HCFA would stop the auction when the payment rate was too high, thus allowing the plans to continue to offer "inefficient" supplementary benefits.

Alternatively, the government could ask HMOs to submit bids at which they are willing to provide a designated level of services. Those bids would be used to determine the government's contribution to premiums. The principal question becomes *how* this process will work—in effect, a question of what point on the distribution of bids the government should pick. There are five basic alternatives for making this choice.

LOWEST BID FROM A QUALIFIED PLAN. An obvious and appealing decision rule would be to choose the lowest bid to establish the government's contribution. This rule is simple to administer, easily understood, and unlike the other alternatives, it does not subsidize higher-cost plans.

But there are three potential problems with it. The first is not unique to the lowest-bid system but requires special attention in that system. All health plans, including the lowest bidder, would have to meet minimum-quality criteria. There are valid concerns that the government may not be able to monitor the quality of health plans sufficiently well to preclude the presence of unacceptably low-quality plans in the market. In addition to concerns over quality, there could be concerns over the legitimacy of the price submitted by the lowest bidder. Other health plans often complain that the lowest price will be a predatory bid submitted by a plan that is using its reserves to drive competitors out of the market.

We have discussed at length the problem of uncertain quality and objections to basing the government's contribution to premiums on the lowest bid.[52] We have suggested that any plan offering a questionable level of quality (though not questionable enough to exclude it from the market) should be placed on probation. Its premium should not be included in the computation of the lowest bid. The probationary plan should be given a fixed amount of time to prove that its price or quality is genuine. This would allow the government to set a payment level that permitted access to a plan of acceptable quality at minimum out-of-pocket cost to beneficiaries.

The problem of predatory pricing is both conceptually complex and, from a practical standpoint, very difficult to address. One response is to note that the practice is illegal. Unfortunately, it is often very difficult to prove that in a court of law. In fact, F. H. Easterbrook has suggested that courts not even hear predatory pricing suits until one firm has been driven from the market and the remaining firm has raised its price.[53] Although an after-the-fact trial might deter future potential offenders, the damage to the integrity of the competitive pricing process done in the interim could be substantial. Another response to predatory pricing concerns is to note that as long as the market is contestable, that is, as long as new firms can enter the market, the predatory plan can survive only by *not* earning abnormally high profits.

A related objection to the lowest bid is that it contains no information on the extent to which the plan has gained acceptance by beneficiaries. In the extreme case the government's contribution to premiums could be based on a plan that has no enrollees. Given some basic monitoring of health plan quality, the notion that the lowest-priced plan would be unpopular with beneficiaries runs counter to the best empirical evidence on the demand for health plans.[54] Consumers gravitate toward, not away from, health plans that cost less. But still, it is possible for the lowest-priced plan, in various unobserved ways, to be an inadequate product to offer consumers.

The last objection is that HMOs do not have an incentive to submit the lowest possible bids (that is, equal to their average costs) when their payment is equal to the lowest bid. This may seem somewhat paradoxical, but if the HMOs know they will be paid at the lowest bid, they have an incentive to guess that bid. For example, if an HMO with monthly costs of $300 per enrollee thinks that other HMOs may submit bids of $400 and $450, it may decide to bid $375. The potential reward for submitting the higher bid is a $75 profit; the potential penalty is that this HMO may not submit the lowest bid.

SECOND-LOWEST BID.   Under second-lowest-bid systems, the lowest bidder wins the right to supply the product, but it is paid an amount equal to the second-lowest bid. The winning bidder is not required to rebate the difference between its bid and the second-lowest bid to consumers. It may keep this difference as a reward for bidding low.

Of all the systems for purchasing Medicare benefits from a single winning health plan, paying the second-lowest bid provides the strongest incentives for plans to submit low bids. The rationale for this conclusion is simple: by bidding low, the plan maximizes its chance of winning the Medicare contract without incurring any penalty because its payment will be based on a bid submitted by another plan. Thus the plan will bid as low as possible. This result is identical to a Dutch auction, in which the government awards the contract to the last remaining bidder at a payment equal to the rate where the second-to-last plan dropped out.[55]

Despite this powerful advantage, the second-lowest-bid system has three disadvantages. First, and most important, the incentive to submit low bids may be reduced substantially when there are multiple winning bidders. This is almost certain to be the case in Medicare, where bids are not likely to be rejected unless the plan is found to have unacceptably low quality. When there are multiple winners in a second-lowest-bid system, each plan has an incentive to be the second-lowest bidder. This strategy increases the plan's expected revenue at no cost, because there is no risk of disqualification from submitting a high bid. Thus the most significant advantage of the second-lowest-bid system (and of the Dutch action) over paying the lowest bid would be reduced in bidding for Medicare contracts.

Second, paying the second-lowest bid may be substantially less successful in markets where there are structural differences in efficiency among types of suppliers. Suppose, for example, that bids submitted by staff-model HMOs typically are lower than bids submitted by IPAs. If there was only one staff-model HMO in a market, paying the IPA's bid would deny the staff-model HMO the price advantage represented by its greater efficiency.

Finally, like all other systems except paying the enrollment-weighted average premium, the second-lowest-bid system does not address the objection that health plan payment is unrelated to market acceptance, measured by enrollment.

A PERCENTILE OF THE BIDS.   Under the third alternative, the government chooses a percentile on the distribution of bids. This percentile can be announced beforehand or after the bids are received. Steps would have to be taken to avoid paying the low bid under some rules (for instance, paying the 25th percentile in a market with fewer than six bidders).

Suppose the government's contribution was set at the 50th percentile. The first question that must be resolved is how to pay plans bidding below the 50th percentile cutoff. One option is to pay plans their bid amount. The second option is to pay the 50th percentile amount to plans bidding below the cutoff.

If plans bidding below the 50th percentile are paid their bid amount, plans with costs below the 50th percentile would cut their own revenue by bidding low, without gaining the usual benefit of doing so, that is, distancing themselves from other plans' bids. Such low-cost plans would have a strong incentive to try to guess the 50th percentile and submit a bid at that level. As long as bids were randomly distributed around the "true" 50th percentile, paying plans that bid below the 50th percentile probably would not affect the government's costs very much. In other words, the government's cost would increase every time a plan whose costs were below the 50th percentile overestimated the 50th percentile (thereby raising the 50th percentile). However, the government's costs would be reduced for every bid below the 50th percentile.

If the government paid low bidders the 50th percentile, plans with costs below the 50th percentile would not have to worry about having their payments reduced by bidding their cost, but the government would not benefit from low bids, unless the 50th percentile itself was reduced—a possibility, in view of the discussion immediately above.

It is unclear which method is best for the government. However, we are somewhat more skeptical of paying plans the amount of their bid. Low-cost plans are probably very averse to submitting bids that cut their revenue with no consumer response to show for it, and thus they may tend to submit bids on the high side of the 50th percentile. That strategy will raise the 50th percentile and increase the government's costs. Therefore, we recommend paying the 50th percentile amount to health plans that are below the 50th percentile.[56]

Otherwise, the advantages and disadvantages of the percentile method are similar to those of the second-lowest bid. In our example, beneficiaries would "see" the additional cost of plans bidding above the 50th percentile as additional out-of-pocket premiums. The percentile method does not address the problem of price differences arising from different types of health plans such as staff-model HMOs versus IPAs. Also, the percentile method does not make the government's contribution to premiums a function of health plan enrollment.

A FIXED PERCENTAGE OF THE LOWEST BID.   The government could set its contribution to HMO premiums at a fixed percentage of the lowest bid. By a fixed percentage, we mean a multiple such as 1.10, or 10 percent higher than the lowest bid. There are precedents for this system in the employment-based sector. The state of Wisconsin sets the employer's contribution at 105 percent of the lowest bid. If a health plan's bid is less than the employer's contribution, there is no rebate to the employee. The state and several of the participating health plans have criticized the 105 percent rule. All parties believe that the rule reduces the incentive for a health plan to attract enrollees by offering a lower price.[57]

It is easy to see that if all health plans add 5 percent to what they believe to be the lowest price, this will result in higher bids than if health plans vied to *be* the lowest bidder. In the absence of cash rebates, the health plans' incentive under a "percentage of the lowest price" system is to bid the government's contribution to premiums, rather than their average cost. That incentive raises the lowest bid and thus the government's costs. Otherwise, the advantages and disadvantages are similar to the second-lowest-price and percentile systems.

ENROLLMENT-WEIGHTED AVERAGE PREMIUM.   The final alternative is to set the government's contribution at the weighted average of the bids submitted by all qualified health plans. The weights could be the plans' market shares (the proportion of beneficiaries in the market area choosing each plan). This payment system is similar to the "big six" method used to set the ceiling on the federal government's contribution in the Federal Employees Health Benefits Program.

The advantage of the enrollment-weighted average premium is that the government's premium contribution is sensitive to beneficiaries' enrollment decisions. That is also its greatest weakness. A plan with a dominant market share will have a strong influence on the government's contribution to premiums. Any ability of health plans to manipulate the government's contribution to premiums must be taken very seriously and avoided if possible.

Another disadvantage is the fact that market share weights must be based on the previous year's market shares, because the current year's shares will not be known until after the open enrollment period, and beneficiaries need to know their out-of-pocket cost for each health plan before open enrollment. In addition, it would not be possible to assign a weight to a plan that was offered for the first time.

The most important consideration in choosing the premium contribution method is that the government sets a defined contribution to premiums (one that does not vary with the plan chosen). The government can announce that the contribution will be based on the bids received. Among the alternatives, the level-dollar contribution based on the lowest bid has the advantages of simplicity and maximum correction of distorted prices from both the government's and the beneficiary's perspective.

Should Government and Beneficiary Contributions Be Adjusted for Risk?

Whenever multiple health plans are offered to a group of individuals, risks are unlikely to be distributed equally among the plans. Some plans will enjoy favorable selection—the enrollment of relatively low-risk individuals—and others will face adverse selection. Favorable or adverse selection, summarized by the term *biased selection,* can result from either biased enrollment or biased disenrollment. Health plans have expressed great interest in biased selection, and the subject has received a great deal of attention from health policy analysts. Numerous proposals have been made to adjust HMO payments for biased selection (beyond the present adjustments in the AAPCC). Other analysts are skeptical that a workable risk adjuster can be devised and have recommended abandoning full capitation in favor of a blend of capitation and fee-for-service payment.[58]

In our earlier analysis we took a different (and distinctly less popular) view: we suggested that biased selection was not a serious problem and that further adjustments for risk were likely to be counterproductive. This is despite the fact that HMOs enjoy favorable risk selection in the current Medicare program.

In the current administrative pricing system, the HCFA determines the payment level for each AAPCC risk cell. Health plans have a strong incentive to reduce their cost for beneficiaries in each cell below the payment rate. They can do that by increased efficiency or by attempting to enroll relatively healthy beneficiaries within the rate cells. In a competitive pricing system, however, health plans can set their premium at any level they choose. Competitive pressure from other plans gives them a strong incentive to submit a price equal to their average cost. The result is that plans with lower-cost enrollees will submit lower prices.

Analysts who recommend further adjustment of health plan prices for risk view the low submitted prices with skepticism: they believe them to be inefficient and unfair. Low prices would be inefficient if they reflected not only differences in health plan efficiency but differences in enrollee health risk. Ideally, each beneficiary should face prices that reflect only efficiency differences among plans. Any factor that alters the set of ideal prices, such as failure to adjust for the average risk of individuals choosing each plan, may result in too many people picking the low-priced plans. Low prices would be unfair if wealthier consumers tended to have better than average health risk. Then the benefits of low prices would be enjoyed primarily by the wealthy while the burden of high prices would fall primarily on poorer consumers.

We agree that unfavorable selection against fee-for-service occurs in the current Medicare program, but in our book we argued that market conditions will work against unfavorable selection in a competitive Medicare program. Our argument was based on the evolution of fee-for-service plans facing similar conditions in the health insurance market for those younger than 65. The characteristics of health plans are not fixed in concrete; they can adjust to market conditions. In the Twin Cities, unmanaged fee-for-service plans have become preferred provider organizations or gatekeeper plans (which require that a primary care physician preapprove visits to specialists) to compete with HMOs. Higher deductibles are another way that fee-for-service plans can manage risk selection against HMOs. It is important to remember that healthy people are attracted to the medical practice style found in managed care plans. In our experience, the threat of adverse selection has led many fee-for-service plans to take a greater interest in the management of medical care for their enrollees.[59]

We also suggest that the current payment system, without risk adjustment, is fairer to low-income beneficiaries than a risk-adjusted system. There is ample evidence (at least among the under-65 population) that health care spending is positively related to income.[60] Thus, if certain plans charge low premiums because they enroll low risks, those plans are more likely to serve low-income enrollees.

We concluded that biased selection, though potentially important, deserves less attention from policymakers than basic market reforms. Furthermore, failure to discover an optimal set of risk adjusters should not slow progress toward installation of a competitive pricing system for Medicare. In addition, we noted the following points that should receive careful consideration:

—A competitive pricing system featuring open enrollment periods with limited plan switching between open enrollment dates probably would do more to alleviate concern over biased selection than complex systems for risk-adjusting health plan payments.

—Risk adjustments are extremely rare among large employers, many of whom have offered multiple health plans for years.

—Risk adjustments, if miscalculated, could embody substantial, perverse incentives for health plan behavior. For example, if health status after enrollment were included in the payment formula, health plans would receive more money for enrollees who became sick after they enrolled. This could create a perverse incentive for inappropriate treatment.

—The positive relationship between managed care and favorable selection means that the threat of adverse selection provides an incentive for inefficient health plans to improve their management of care.

—The current administrative pricing system provides a strong incentive for health plans to gain favorable selection because they cannot adjust their revenue for the effects of unfavorable selection. That is not the case under competitive pricing.

Another point to be considered is whether biased selection among Medicare beneficiaries is different from what it is among the employees under managed competition conditions. It would be interesting to determine whether there are systematic differences in selection related to income and the presence of chronic conditions. Firms that use managed competition often have higher-income employees than the typical firm and incomes considerably higher than those of Medicare beneficiaries. Lack of selection problems among these large employers (on which we based our earlier conclusions) might not apply to Medicare.

A study by Bryan Dowd and colleagues may be useful in clarifying the type of selection that occurs in Medicare.[61] They studied selection in Minneapolis–St. Paul, which had a mature Medicare HMO market in 1988 with two IPAs and three network HMOs. The sharpest contrasts in beneficiary characteristics were not found between fee-for-service plans and the HMOs, but within the fee-for-service sector, where the oldest, poorest, and sickest beneficiaries were found in fee-for-service Medicare without a supplement. The authors' results suggested that some low-income beneficiaries might switch from basic fee-for-service to HMOs if the HMOs were less expensive. This could be accomplished in the current payment system, without risk adjustment, by allowing HMOs to give premium rebates to enrollees choosing basic coverage.

In an analysis of the Federal Employees Health Benefits Program, Stuart Butler and Robert Moffit reached conclusions that (we believe) are similar to ours.[62] They noted that the FEHBP permits plans to offer a wide range of benefits but requires them to charge the same premium to all enrollees. This would seem to be an invitation to severe selection problems, yet the program is remarkably stable. The authors attribute the stability to the fact that the FEHBP restricts plan switching except during the annual open enrollment period. This makes it difficult for enrollees to destabilize the system by transferring to generous plans just to cover predictable health care costs, while protecting the enrollees' access to all plans, regardless of health status, during open enrollment. They also emphasize that information on plan features and enrollee satisfaction is widely available from both private and public sources. Our proposal for competitive pricing likewise called for information on Medicare to be distributed before the open enrollment period.[63]

Unlike us, however, Butler and Moffit recommend risk adjustment for the demographic factors used by the current Medicare AAPCC: enrollees' age, sex, reason for eligibility, institutional status, and whether they have end-stage renal disease. Despite our concerns about risk adjustment, in the next section we discuss two options for instituting it in Medicare. In both options all beneficiaries pay the same premium regardless of their demographic rate cell. The difference is in how the HCFA's contribution is set: in the first option the agency pays a fixed contribution equal to the demographic factors times the cutoff price; in the second it pays the residual after the beneficiary premium is subtracted from the product of the demographic factor times the plan's bid. The systems lead to different, but subtle and surprisingly complicated results for beneficiaries, health plans, and the HCFA.

The simplest risk adjusters, which are already available, are the demographic cost factors from the current AAPCC. These factors are ratios representing the average fee-for-service Medicare expenditure for beneficiaries in a demographic cell in relation to a standard or 1.0 beneficiary.[64] There are separate cost factors for aged, disabled, and end-stage renal disease (ESRD) beneficiaries. A simple bidding system would have plans submit a bid for the 1.0 enrollee in each category. The HCFA would rank those bids and choose the winning bidders. It would be possible to have different HMOs being the winning bidder for aged and ESRD enrollees, for example.

But even this simple system raises complex issues. With any given cutoff price and set of bids, there are three questions to consider:

—Can HMOs predict their reimbursement levels and thus be sure to cover their costs, regardless of the cutoff price?

—Do all beneficiaries pay the same out-of-pocket premium, regardless of their demographic risk?

—Does the HCFA contribute a strict multiple of the cutoff price for any demographic cell?

If the answer to any two of these questions is yes, then the answer to the third must be no. That presents a potential confusion in how the plans will formulate bids and how the HCFA will explain the bidding process to the plans. The following examples illustrate the difficulties that would arise if the HCFA (in the interest of fairness) required that all beneficiaries pay the same premium, regardless of their demographic risk class.[65]

THE HCFA CONTRIBUTES A MULTIPLE OF THE CUTOFF PRICE.   In our first example, the HCFA's contributions are equal to the demographic factors times the cutoff price.[66] Under this system, plans cannot know their reimbursement unless they are at or below the cutoff price and they cannot know they will be at or below the cutoff until long after their bid is formulated.

The following numerical example will clarify this problem. Assume a cutoff price of $300 for the 1.0 enrollee. Plan A (a plan bidding above the cutoff price) bids $400. If we assume level-dollar out-of-pocket premiums for all beneficiaries, all plan A enrollees will pay $100, regardless of their demographic cell. For example, plan A enrollees in a cell with a demographic factor of 1.5 will pay $100. Assume that the cost weight for this cell, times plan A's bid, accurately reproduces plan A's cost of $600 for this cell.

If the HCFA's contribution is a strict multiple of the cutoff price, then the agency pays $1.5 \times \$300 = \$450$ for this beneficiary. The beneficiary pays the fixed premium of $100. And plan A gets paid $550, the sum of the HCFA contribution and the beneficiary premium. The problem with this example is that when plan A prepares its bid, it has no way of knowing that its reimbursement for this enrollee will be $550, rather than its cost of $600. The cutoff price will be known only after bids are submitted, too late to affect the formulation of bids.

With this formula, plan A may be reimbursed more than expected for demographic cells with weights less than 1.0, and the reimbursement increases as the cutoff point declines. Thus, a 0.8 enrollee in this example would result in

$340 total reimbursement for the plan ($100 out-of-pocket premium and $0.8 \times \$300 = \$240$ HCFA contribution). If the cutoff declined to $200, the HCFA's contribution for the 0.8 enrollee would be $160 and the plan would collect $360 (assuming its bid for the 1.0 enrollee was still $400). Thus paradoxically, as the HCFA's cutoff price goes down, plan A's total reimbursement goes up for enrollees in all demographic cells with weights less than 1.0.

This example should clarify another important point: when the beneficiary contribution is fixed, the HCFA's choice of the 1.0 beneficiary becomes vitally important. If a relatively low-cost cell is chosen, the out-of-pocket premium for all beneficiaries is likely to be lower than if a high-cost cell is chosen. For example, suppose an aged, institutionalized beneficiary were chosen as the 1.0 beneficiary. Then the plans' bids probably would be distributed at wider intervals. The winning bidder might be $900, with plan A bidding $1,200. Thus all enrollees in plan A would have to pay $300, regardless of their risk class.

REIMBURSEMENT PREDICTABILITY REQUIRES VARIABLE HCFA CONTRIBU-
TIONS. The only way to make the plans' reimbursement predictable for all cells—and to have its total reimbursement go up or down in strict proportion to the demographic factor—is to vary either HCFA or beneficiary contributions. If the beneficiary contribution is fixed, the HCFA would have to pay the residual, after the plan's bid is multiplied by the demographic factor. The implications of this second approach to calculating the HCFA contribution are set forth next.

For a 1.5 enrollee, a $400 bid, and a $300 cutoff, the HCFA would pay $500, as determined by the formula: HCFA contribution = (demographic factor × plan's bid) – beneficiary premium. Under this system, total reimbursement for every enrollee would be predictable. Plan A would be paid its bid times the demographic factor for every enrollee. After subtracting the beneficiary contri-bution of $100, the HCFA's payment is determined as the residual. This formula leads to the HCFA's paying more to higher-priced plans than to lower-priced plans for demographic cells with weights more than 1.0. Con-versely, for cells with weights less than 1.0, the agency would pay more to lower-priced plans.

The problems illustrated here (plans facing uncertain reimbursement or the HCFA's making larger contributions to high-priced plans for high-cost demo-graphic cells) arise because the out-of-pocket premium differences between any pair of plans (though *not* across *all* plans) would be the same for all beneficiaries regardless of their demographic cell. An additional problem is that this formula violates the objective of risk adjustment, namely, that each beneficiary should face prices that reflect efficiency differences among health plans *for that beneficiary*. In fact, this additional problem is almost intractable. Equal out-of-pocket premium differences are efficient only if the efficiency differences among plans are equal across all demographic cells. If this is not the case, then having beneficiaries face equal out-of-pocket premium differences across health plans will produce inefficient choices.

An efficient risk adjuster is easy to describe: each plan's total revenue for an enrollee in a demographic cell would be determined by multiplying the cell weight times the plan's bid for a 1.0 beneficiary; the HCFA would pay the cell weight times the cutoff price; and the beneficiary would pay the difference. In our example, plan A receives $600 for the 1.5 enrollee and the HCFA pays $450, leaving the beneficiary to pay $150. However, this efficient system might violate commonly held concepts of equity because it requires that sicker beneficiaries pay higher out-of-pocket premiums.

The principal results from our analysis of risk adjustment can easily be summarized. Under the first formula, the HCFA's contributions are fixed multiples of the cutoff price and beneficiary premiums are a fixed amount for all cells. In that event, plans will face an uncertainty as to their reimbursement because they will not know the relation of their bid to the cutoff price. They will have to guess the cutoff and hedge their bids to ensure that they cover their costs. The implications of these influences need to be worked out in greater detail. But the incentive for plans to hedge their bids is likely to mean higher bids and greater difficulty for the HCFA in explaining to plans how they are to formulate their bids.

Under the second approach, the HCFA pays the residual after the beneficiary premium is subtracted from the product of the demographic factor times the plan's bid. Total reimbursement becomes predictable for all plans, and it changes in exact proportion to the demographic factor. But HCFA contributions are variable in that different plans receive different amounts from the agency. In addition, HCFA contributions for enrollees in cells with demographic weights greater than 1.0 are greater for the higher-priced plans; for enrollees in cells under 1.0, its contributions are less for the higher-priced plans.

An efficient risk adjuster requires different out-of-pocket premium contributions depending on the beneficiary's demographic cell. This system might be perceived as unfair. In this case the goal of efficiency in health plan reimbursement might have to be sacrificed to achieve equity for Medicare beneficiaries.

Administering a Competitive Pricing System for Medicare

The idea of administering a competitive pricing system may seem paradoxical. Isn't competition an alternative to administered pricing? As we explained in our book, *Competitive Pricing for Medicare*, competition is an alternative to administered pricing, but there are different ways to structure a competitive market. For example, one might leave making choices and negotiating prices entirely up to individual consumers. Automobile purchases usually take that form. Consumers are free to purchase any automobile that manufacturers choose to supply. Consumers canvass the market, take bids from dealers of the models in which they are interested, and choose the brand that offers the best combination of price and quality (which can include features of the automobile itself, financing arrangements, and other aspects of customer service). Some consumers prefer to delegate some of these shopping activities to other organizations, for example, choosing to purchase their cars through credit unions that negotiate fixed profit margins with dealers. Consumers "hire" the credit union to overcome a source of market failure in the new-automobile market, namely limited information (and perhaps their lack of skill in the negotiating process itself). Even after delegating some shopping activities to the credit union, however, consumers still discipline the market by choosing one make of automobile over another.

Similarly, many employees find it desirable to hire their employer to overcome market failure in the health insurance market. The employer collects information on health plans and negotiates prices on behalf of employees. By requiring annual open enrollment periods with restrictions on plan switching at other times during the year, employers can arrange for health plans to accept any employee at a fixed premium without health screening or exclusions for preexisting conditions. Employees want employers to perform these services because the employer can provide them at a cost lower than the individual employees can.

Medicare beneficiaries may also wish to delegate some shopping activities to a third party. Alain Enthoven has referred to the organizations that assume this role as "sponsors." He believes that a sponsor is not only desirable, but necessary: "without carefully drawn rules and active management by sponsors, health plans could pursue profits or survival using competitive strategies that would destroy efficiency and equity. Individual consumers would be powerless to counteract them."[67]

Enthoven lists the following activities of sponsors:

—Sponsors obtain prices from insurers and manage the enrollment process. To attenuate the incentives for health plans to enroll low-risk individuals, the sponsor obtains competitive bids for individuals in each of a number of risk-rating cells.

—Sponsors provide information to individuals to facilitate comparisons of health plans. This information is most easily collected and distributed when there is a single enrollment date for everyone in the group. Health plans are prevented from seeking favorable selection through a prohibition on direct contact with individuals.

—Sponsors standardize the benefit packages so that health plans cannot use specialized or unusual benefits to attract low-risk consumers. Standardization also facilitates comparisons among plans. The standardized package includes guaranteed renewability.

—Sponsors monitor health plan performance by gathering evidence on inappropriate risk-selection behavior and on the plan's success at maintaining the health of its enrollees. The latter activity requires statistical data that cannot be known with accuracy by individual consumers.

—Sponsors foster competition by supporting the marketing efforts of new HMOs. They can insist that HMOs adopt the staff model (or at least contract with only a subset of the providers in the market area).

—Sponsors manage subsidies to promote efficiency by making a premium contribution that leaves individuals facing the full marginal cost of more expensive plans. Sponsors also promote fairness by making larger contributions for high-risk individuals.

In our analysis of competitive pricing, we agreed with much of Enthoven's analysis, and we said that the concept of an active sponsor is "relatively uncontroversial." But in fact there is substantial distrust of sponsors in some quarters. For example, proponents of medical savings accounts view sponsors with suspicion and believe that the accounts are (in part) a way to circumvent limitations on consumer choice that might be imposed by a sponsor. The primary limitation may be the sponsor's failure to offer a plan with unlimited access to medical providers. The fate of the 1993 Health Security Act also shows that there is significant public distrust of sponsors. The proposed National Health Board and regional health alliances were successfully portrayed by opponents as bureaucracies that would impose more government control on the health care system.

These observations suggest that proponents of sponsorship need to address several concerns over the level of sponsorship and the proper roles of government and private sponsors. A primary concern is to ensure that the sponsor will be responsive to the preferences of Medicare beneficiaries. In the following two sections, we discuss the questions of who should administer the competitive pricing system and how the HCFA should view its role as administrator of traditional fee-for-service Medicare.

WHO SHOULD ADMINISTER THE COMPETITIVE PRICING SYSTEM? There are two basic models for promoting sponsor accountability to consumers. The first is political accountability. The sponsoring organization could consist of representatives elected by consumers or it could be accountable to a body of elected representatives. If this model is acceptable, the government is the natural sponsor for Medicare.

The second model of accountability relies on the market to ensure that sponsors are responsive to consumer preferences. In the market model, several competing sponsors could offer different combinations of activities, and consumers could choose among sponsors on a regular basis.[68] Sponsors who failed to meet consumers' demands would be driven from the market. If this model is acceptable, employers could compete with the government to be Medicare sponsors. New market entrants such as organizations of senior citizens and other private entities might also compete effectively in the sponsorship market. The American Association of Retired Persons (AARP) has moved closer to that role with its recent endorsement of selected health plans.

Within the federal government, the HCFA is the likely sponsor. The agency already performs many of the sponsoring activities recommended by Enthoven: it collects data on health plans' service areas, prices, and supplementary benefits; administers a qualification process for health plans that wish to participate in Medicare; and has several quality assurance programs already in place. However, the HCFA does not provide beneficiaries with comparative information on health plans (in part, because there is no coordinated open enrollment in Medicare).

Many large employers also perform some sponsoring activities for their retired employees. For example, the state of Minnesota offers several health plans for its retirees and holds an open enrollment period during which it provides information comparing the plans. The state makes no contribution to health plan premiums for retirees; it simply functions as a sponsor.

Could large employers and the HCFA compete as sponsors? One difficulty is that some employers subsidize health plan premiums for their retirees, and if the subsidy were conditional on staying in the employer's group, real competition between the employer and the HCFA could not be expected to develop. It is possible, however, that if the HCFA offered the same advantages that retirees of large firms enjoy (that is, open enrollment periods, improved information, and attractive prices), an HCFA-sponsored group could offer real competition for employers.

If employers or other organizations compete with the HCFA, how much freedom should they have to set the terms of health insurance offerings to the elderly? Should sponsors be able to negotiate premium discounts with health plans? Should sponsors have the option of not offering some plans approved by the HCFA?

As we discussed earlier, we do not think it is advisable to allow other sponsors to negotiate separate premiums with health plans as long as the government's contribution to premiums is based on bids that health plans quote to the government. Otherwise, health plans might quote high prices to the government, extract a high government premium contribution, and then discount their prices to other sponsors. However, equal premiums do not necessarily imply that the total cost of purchasing health insurance through each sponsor would be the same. For example, suppose that all sponsors had to itemize the cost of administration and charge beneficiaries for those services. In that case sponsors would be able to compete on the basis of efficient administration of the competitive pricing system.

If sponsors competed on the basis of administrative costs, they might not offer all health plans approved by the HCFA. Unpopular plans that increased the sponsor's administrative costs might be dropped. Similarly, some sponsors might offer health plans that the agency did not approve if those plans were popular with consumers. Then it would be important to determine how the government's contribution to premiums would be set for unapproved plans, but the lowest price of an approved plan would be one alternative.

In addition to administrative costs and the menu of offered plans, sponsors might compete on the quality of information provided to their members. One example of such information would be lists of providers in each health plan who are accepting new Medicare patients. Some sponsors might also produce better data than others on consumer satisfaction with health plan services or quality of care.

ADMINISTERING TRADITIONAL FEE-FOR-SERVICE MEDICARE. In addition to its potential role as sponsor of the competitive pricing system, the HCFA needs to resolve its role as administrator of the traditional Medicare fee-for-service sector. The agency could run the fee-for-service plan as an employer manages its own self-insured fee-for-service plan. Currently, the HCFA calculates the "price" of the basic fee-for-service benefit package in each county in the nation as part of the AAPCC payment formula. That process could be used to set the premium for the fee-for-service option under a competitive pricing system. Administration of the fee-for-service plan is not an intrinsic part of being a sponsor, however. The HCFA could contract with a third-party administrator to run fee-for-service Medicare.

If medigap insurers are converted into fully capitated health plans, whoever administers fee-for-service Medicare would need to develop optional supplementary benefit packages and manage them in a way that resolves the medigap spillover problem (that is, by charging a higher price for basic benefits to beneficiaries who buy a supplement).

Finally, Medicare would have to develop the ability to bill beneficiaries choosing the fee-for-service sector for the cost of their coverage. Currently, the program collects only the part B premium, which is the same for all beneficiaries. Under a competitive pricing system, the fee-for-service premium would differ by market area and for beneficiaries choosing and not choosing fee-for-service supplementary coverage.

Any of the sponsoring tasks performed by the government, or administration of the fee-for-service sector, could take place at the federal, regional, and state level. In March 1991 Medicare reorganized responsibilities for its coordinated care programs and established the Office of Prepaid Health Care Operations and Oversight. In January 1992 the HCFA released a statement recognizing that regional offices "are in a better position to be knowledgeable about local market conditions and to be more timely aware of potential problems."[69]

As a part of this reorganization, Medicare regional offices are taking responsibility for contract application review and ongoing monitoring. Included under contract application review will be

—health services delivery (availability, accessibility, and continuity of care),

—organization and administration,

—adequacy of internal quality assurance programs,

—enrollment, disenrollment, and membership processes,

—marketing materials and practices,

—claims processing timeliness and accuracy, and

—appeals and grievances.

When the regional office identifies a problem with an HMO in its region, the office will work with Medicare to develop a corrective action plan and, if necessary, the specification of penalties for noncompliance. Moving these functions to the regional level should improve Medicare's ability to manage and monitor its health plan market areas. Certainly, in monitoring the performance of the health plans market and its effects on consumers, specific knowledge of local markets is important.

Conclusions

Our analysis began with an attempt to clarify the problems facing the Medicare program. We concluded that Medicare is unfair, primarily across generations rather than within the generation of currently eligible beneficiaries. We also concluded that Medicare is inefficient.

We identified two types of inefficiency in the current program. First, the government's price of Medicare benefits is distorted because it pays what the benefits would cost in the fee-for-service sector. Because the fee-for-service sector is less efficient than most HMOs, the government will purchase too few Medicare benefits. The second inefficiency results from distorted prices faced by beneficiaries when they choose the fee-for-service sector or a Medicare HMO. Allowing Medicare HMOs to give cash rebates would solve the second inefficiency problem, but not the first.

The problems of fairness and efficiency are related. The intergenerational fairness problem arises because current noneligible taxpayers cannot expect to receive the same subsidy they are providing to current beneficiaries. The fairness problem can be resolved only by redesigning the program to make it sustainable for the next generation of beneficiaries. Cutting benefits or raising taxes (if either was politically feasible) would extend Medicare's life but would not improve the efficiency of the program.

A better way to extend Medicare's life is to improve its efficiency by ridding the program of distorted prices and addressing the information problems that currently plague it. To achieve those ends, we proposed a competitive pricing system consisting of annual open enrollment periods (with good information on competing health plans distributed to consumers before open enrollment) and limits on plan switching between open enrollment periods. Another element of our proposal is a government premium contribution that is set no higher than the lowest bid for the basic benefit package in each market area.

The remainder of our discussion addressed two broad design issues and a number of technical points that arise in creating a competitive pricing system for Medicare. The first design issue is monitoring the benefits offered by health plans. In our competitive pricing proposal the government defines a basic benefit package on which health plans submit bids, but the plans also may sell supplementary coverage. We identified a problem with this proposal: health plans may include the cost of some supplementary benefits in their bid for basic coverage in order to increase the government's contribution to premiums. Our analysis of that problem revealed an important difference between Medicare and employment-based health insurance.

Workers have an incentive to keep the cost of employment-based health insurance low because higher insurance costs result in lower wages. There is no counterpart to wages for Medicare beneficiaries, however, so beneficiaries have no natural incentive to limit the government's cost of Medicare benefits. Beneficiaries would like the government to pay for both basic Medicare benefits and supplementary benefits, and health plans may try to accommodate that wish. Under some situations, health plans may build the cost of "efficient" supplementary benefits into their bid for basic benefits. (Efficient supplementary benefits are worth to beneficiaries at least what they cost to produce). We explored several methods of ensuring that health plans' bids are limited to the cost of the basic benefit package, but none of the methods appears foolproof.

The second design issue—employer participation in a Medicare competitive pricing system—turned out to be more complicated that we first thought. If HMOs are allowed to submit one price to the government (thereby determining the government's contribution to premiums) and another price to employers, the first price may become meaningless in markets where a large percentage of beneficiaries obtain supplementary Medicare coverage from their former employers. We suggested that the government may have to require that health plans charge all buyers the price that is submitted to the government.

Beyond application of basic quality criteria, we found little reason to restrict the number of participating plans in a market area. Arguments in favor of restricting health plan choice between open enrollment periods (so called lock-in provisions) are compelling, however. In the absence of a lock-in, consumers will view health plans solely as health care providers, with resulting harm to the market for insurance. We propose a one-year lock-in initially because it is the norm in employment-based insurance.

The most important consideration in choosing the government's premium contribution method is that the government make a defined contribution (one that does not vary with the plan chosen). The government can announce that the contribution will be based on the bids received. The lowest-bid method is simple and accomplishes the maximum correction of distorted prices.

We examined the issue of risk-adjusted payments to health plans. The analysis of risk adjustment is different in competitive pricing systems, where plans set their prices, than in administered pricing systems (for example, the current AAPCC), where the government determines prices. Risk adjustments are virtually nonexistent in employment-based competitive pricing systems, whereas one-year lock-in periods, not coincidentally, are virtually universal.

A feasible method of building risk factors into the competitive pricing system is to have plans bid on a standardized beneficiary, with multipliers for other risk categories that are known by health plans before they submit their bids. Although feasible, risk adjustment is not likely to satisfy the objectives of fairness and efficiency for Medicare. The efficiency objective of risk adjustment (having beneficiaries face out-of-pocket premiums that reflect only differences in health plan efficiency) is incompatible with the fairness objective of having beneficiaries in all risk groups face the same out-of-pocket premiums for any pair of health plans, unless the efficiency differences across plans are equal for beneficiaries in all risk categories.

Finally, we looked at the administration of a competitive pricing system. Although the government is the natural candidate to sponsor a Medicare competitive pricing system, we see no reason why private organizations could not serve as sponsors as well. Detailed knowledge of local market conditions is essential to administer a competitive pricing system efficiently in any health insurance market.

In summary, a careful and thoughtful transfer of the "large employer" model of competitive pricing for health insurance to Medicare can succeed. Three features of this model—annual open enrollment periods, good information about plans, and beneficiaries facing the marginal cost of more expensive health plans—will improve the efficiency of the Medicare program. This will extend the program's life, thus providing an opportunity to address the problem of intergenerational fairness.

Notes

1. Paul Starr, *The Social Transformation of American Medicine* (Basic Books, 1982), p. 369.

2. Section 1801, Title 18 (Health Insurance for the Aged) of Public Law 89-97 (Social Security Amendments of 1965) specifically guarantees free choice by patients: "Any individual entitled to insurance benefits under this title may obtain health services from any institution, agency, or person qualified to participate under this title if such institution, agency, or person undertakes to provide him such services."

3. Before the program started, Social Security Administration actuaries estimated that the annual cost of the program would reach $8.3 billion (in 1983 prices) by 1983. This estimate was massively wrong: federal spending on Medicare benefits in 1983 was $57.4 billion. *1985 Economic Report of the President* (Government Printing Office, 1985), chap. 4.

4. For a detailed analysis of these themes, see Bryan E. Dowd, Roger Feldman, and Jon Christianson, *Competitive Pricing for Medicare* (Washington: AEI Press, 1996).

5. Of course, not all employees had access to an HMO. Thus, guaranteed access to HMOs for Medicare beneficiaries would have given them a broader range of choices than that enjoyed by many workers younger than 65.

6. *Health Maintenance Organizations—Reauthorization,* Hearings before the Subcommittee on Health and the Environment of the House Committee on Energy and Commerce, 97 Cong. 2 sess., March 18–19, 1981. As explained by Dowd, Feldman, and Christianson, in *Competitive Pricing for Medicare*, a clearly expected sequence of events would take place: HMOs would provide the standard package of Medicare benefits at lower cost to the federal government than fee-for-service Medicare would, and the resulting savings could be used to expand the benefit package. There is no indication that the purpose of HMO involvement in Medicare was to expand benefits if doing so increased the cost to the federal government.

7. See Dowd, Feldman, and Christianson, *Competitive Pricing for Medicare*; and Joseph P. Newhouse, "Policy Watch: Medicare," *Journal of Economic Perspectives*, vol. 10 (Summer 1996), pp. 159–67.

8. Only 9 percent of Medicare beneficiaries were enrolled in risk-contract HMOs in 1995, with almost half of them concentrated in California and Florida. In contrast, 19 percent of all Americans were enrolled in HMOs. Under a broader definition of managed care plans that includes preferred provider organizations and point-of-service plans as well as HMOs, 69 percent of insured workers in firms with more than 200 employees were in managed care in 1995. *1996 Annual Report to Congress* (Washington: Physician Payment Review Commission, 1996).

9. Randall S. Brown and Jerrold W. Hill, "The Effects of Medicare Risk HMOs on Medicare Costs and Service Utilization," in Harold S. Luft, ed., *HMOs and the Elderly* (Ann Arbor, Mich.: Health Administration Press, 1994).

10. *Report of the Working Group on Health Policy and Economics* (Washington, 1985). The group's proposals seem to have grown out of unease over the Medicare prospective payment system (PPS), rather than directly from the desire to improve HMO payment. "In short, the hospital PPS system does not deal with total Medicare spending for all services for all beneficiaries nor does it provide incentives for overall system efficiency" (p. 17). Nevertheless these proposals would have represented significant changes in the Medicare HMO program had they been implemented.

11. In 1995 the HCFA announced that it would conduct a demonstration of competitive bidding *for HMOs only*, with no change in access and cost for beneficiaries choosing to remain in fee-for-service Medicare. Baltimore was selected as the first site for the demonstration. Even this limited form of competitive pricing was delayed because of objections from HMO trade groups and Maryland's congressional delegation. "Medicare HMO Pilot Programs Face Practical, Political Hurdles," *American Medical News*, vol. 39 (July 29, 1996).

12. "Reforming Medicare: Comparing the House and Senate Legislation," Heritage Foundation, *Issue Bulletin*, no. 220 (November 9, 1995).

13. Dowd, Feldman, and Christianson, *Competitive Pricing for Medicare*, p. 3.

14. The discrepancy between Medicare and personal income tax rates can be substantial. Consider two people earning $20,000 and $150,000 a year, respectively. Both pay Medicare payroll taxes at 2.9 percent of earnings, but their respective income tax rates (based on actual tax payments in 1992) would be approximately 7.6 percent and 18.3 percent. If the two taxes were equally progressive and the low-income person paid 2.9 percent of earnings to Medicare, the high-income person would pay 7.0 percent. *Statistical Abstract of the United States: 1995* (Bureau of the Census, 1995), table 534.

15. Offsetting this bias toward the wealthy, poorer beneficiaries may be more likely to qualify for Medicare benefits because of disability.

16. Congressional Budget Office, *Who Pays and When: An Assessment of Generational Accounting* (1995).

17. Guy King, "Health Care Reform and the Medicare Program," *Health Affairs*, vol. 13 (Winter 1994), pp. 39–43.

18. We will not analyze the alternative of letting Medicare run a permanent deficit. This would force the government to raise other taxes or cut back non-Medicare federal outlays.

19. *The 1995 Annual Report of the Board of Trustees of the Hospital Insurance Trust Fund* and *The 1995 Annual Report of the Board of Trustees of the Supplemental Medical Insurance Trust Fund* (Washington: Government Printing Office, 1995). These projections use the trustees' intermediate assumptions.

20. Most recently, David Cutler and Sarah Reber analyzed health plan choices among Harvard University employees, who are offered a PPO (with the most extensive choice of providers) and five HMOs. Employee salaries were found to be positively related to PPO demand. David M. Cutler and Sarah Reber, "Paying for Health Insurance: The Tradeoff between Competition and Adverse Selection," *Quarterly Journal of Economics* (forthcoming).

21. Robert H. Miller and Harold S. Luft, "Managed Care Plan Performance since 1980: A Literature Analysis," *Journal of the American Medical Association*, vol. 271 (May 18, 1994), pp. 1512–19.

22. Health Care Financing Administration, *Monthly Report: Prepaid Health Plans* (February 1996).

23. "PacifiCare HMO to Buy FHP in $2.1-Billion Deal," *Los Angeles Times*, August 6, 1996, p. A14.

24. For example, President Clinton's 1993 health care proposal included $80 billion (over five years) of expanded long-term care benefits for Medicare. To save $15 billion, the White House pushed back implementation of these benefits to 2002, not 2000 as planned. "Costs Delay Long Term Care Benefit," *Medicine and Health*, vol. 47 (November 1, 1993), p. 1.

25. In an unusually blunt assessment, economist Stuart Altman said of the HMO overpayment problem, "It's become a giant bribe." "Medicare Beneficiaries Flock to HMOs," *St. Paul Pioneer Press*, June 4, 1996, p. 1A.

26. Roger Feldman and Bryan Dowd, "The Effectiveness of Managed Competition in Reducing the Costs of Health Insurance," in R. B. Helms, ed., *Health Policy Reform: Competition and Controls* (Washington: American Enterprise Institute, 1993).

27. The cost of health insurance for workers is subsidized by the tax system. For simplicity, we ignore the effects of this distortion in the present discussion, although we recognize its importance in influencing the choice of health insurance versus wages.

28. This example is based on a presentation by Mark Pauly, "Voucherizing Medicare: How Much Good Will It Do?" paper prepared for the conference, Medicare Reform: What Can the Private Sector Teach Us?, American Enterprise Institute, Washington, 1995.

29. The HMO actually receives $4,000 × 0.95 or $3,800 from the government. We ignore the 5 percent discount. This keeps the example simple but does not affect the point. Pauly assumes that the 5 percent "discount" obtained by the HCFA represents administrative costs that Medicare incurs for all beneficiaries, so that the example deals only with the cost of health services.

30. The optional benefits that cost the HMO more than they are worth to beneficiaries are offered only in counties where HMOs charge no premium for supplementary benefits. As of February 1996, 63 percent of all risk plans did not charge for supplementary benefits.

31. An HMO that included $600 of supplementary benefits in its bid for basic benefits would lose those customers who wanted to purchase only the basic package, and it would not gain any advantage over the low-priced HMO for those customers who wanted the complete package.

32. Roger Feldman and others, "An Empirical Test of Competition in the Medicare HMO Market," in R. J. Arnould, R. F. Rich, and W. D. White, eds., *Competitive Approaches to Health Policy Reform* (Washington: Urban Institute Press, 1993).

33. Employers as a group may purchase a large share of Medicare HMO policies in a market without posing the threat of monopsony buying power, provided that no single employer has a significant share of the market and the employers do not collude with one another.

34. This form of "community rating" is inefficient, but that may be the price employers must pay for having taxpayers pay the bulk of their retirees' health insurance expenses.

35. Roger Feldman and others, "The Demand for Employment-Based Health Insurance Plans," *Journal of Human Resources*, vol. 24 (Winter 1989), pp. 115–42.

36. Jon Christianson and others, *Managed Care and Competitive Health Care Markets: The Twin Cities Experience,* OTA-BP-H-130 (Washington: GPO, July 1994).

37. Jack A. Meyer and others, *Employer Coalition Initiatives in Health Care Purchasing* (Washington: Economic and Social Research Institute, February 1996).

38. Congressional Budget Office, *Reducing the Deficit: Spending and Revenue Options* (1996), p. 304.

39. Ibid.

40. In 1995 there were 567 separate HMOs offered nationwide, with 19 in the Washington, D.C., area alone. For more information on FEHBP, see Walton Francis, "Federal Employees' Health Benefits Program: Promise and Pitfalls," paper prepared for the conference, Medicare Reform: What Can the Private Sector Teach Us? Washington, July 1995.

41. James R. Price and James W. Mays, "Biased Selection in the Federal Employees Health Benefits Program," *Inquiry*, vol. 22 (Spring 1985), pp. 67–77.

42. James R. Price and James W. Mays, "Selection and the Competitive Standing of Health Plans in a Multiple-Choice, Multiple-Insurer Market," in R. M. Scheffler and L. F. Rossiter, eds., *Advances in Health Economics and Health Services Research*, vol. 6 (Greenwich, Conn.: JAI Press, 1985).

43. "Can the Federal Employees' Health Program Survive the Wiles of Health Reform?" *Medicine & Health Perspectives*, vol. 48 (February 21, 1994), pp. 1–4.

44. Ibid.

45. W. Peter Welch, "Restructuring the Federal Employees Health Benefits Program: The Private Sector Option," *Inquiry*, vol. 26 (Fall 1989), pp. 321–34.

46. Walton Francis, "The Political Economy of the Federal Employees Health Benefits Program," in R. B. Helms, ed., *Health Policy Reform: Competition and Controls* (Washington: American Enterprise Institute, 1993).

47. Bryan E. Dowd and others, *Health Insurance Purchasing Practices of City and County Governments: Analysis of Managed Competition* (Institute for Health Services Research, University of Minnesota, 1995).

48. Personal communication from Peter Hickman, director of the Division of Medicare Part B Analysis, Office of Legislation and Policy, Health Care Financing Administration, 1990.

49. Matthew J. Eichner, Mark B. McClellan, and David A. Wise, "Insurance or Self-Insurance?: Variation, Persistence, and Individual Health Accounts," Working Paper 5640 (Cambridge, Mass.: National Bureau of Economic Research, June 1996).

50. This requirement is less onerous than it sounds and simply satisfies a state law requiring participation in an insurance program to participate in open enrollment. The employee takes $10,000 from his or her pension fund and purchases the annuity, which

yields a guaranteed income. The state department for employee benefits reports that most retirees exercise the option.

51. The state does not contribute to the cost of retiree health insurance. Because retirees do not get a premium subsidy if they stay within the system, the nonparticipating plans represent a realistic alternative to the state's plans for healthy employees.

52. Dowd, Feldman, and Christianson, *Competitive Pricing for Medicare.*

53. F. H. Easterbrook, "Predatory Strategies and Counter Strategies," *University of Chicago Law Review*, vol. 48 (1981), pp. 263–337.

54. Feldman and others, "Demand for Employment-Based Health Insurance Plans."

55. The second-lowest bid has a slight advantage over the Dutch auction: the government actually gets to see the winner's cost in a second-lowest-bid system, whereas the winner in a Dutch auction does not have to reveal its cost. This extra bit of information might come in handy during subsequent rounds of bidding.

56. Plans below the 50th percentile might be allowed to give cash rebates or add supplementary benefits.

57. To illustrate the disincentive for submitting low bids under the 105 percent rule, consider the example of two hypothetical health plans with monthly costs of $320 for plan 1 and $350 for plan 2, a $30 difference. If both plans bid their costs, the effect of the state subsidy is to cut that difference by more than half, to $14. Because the extra 5 percent payment dampens the effect of offering a low-priced product, more than one Wisconsin health plan described the lowest-priced health plan as "leaving money on the table." In general, plans believed that the optimal pricing strategy is to guess the lowest bid that will be submitted by any plan and to set their premium at 105 percent of that bid. That would leave the employee with no out-of-pocket premium for their plan but would increase their plan's revenue by 5 percent.

58. Joseph P. Newhouse, "Patients at Risk: Health Reform and Risk Adjustment," *Health Affairs*, vol. 13 (Spring 1994), pp. 132–46.

59. One of the authors has served on committees to purchase insurance for 60,000 University of Minnesota students and employees. Fee-for-service insurers bidding for these groups have implemented care management programs that focus on members identified as having diseases or conditions that pose significant health risks (for example, all high-risk obstetrical patients may be assigned a case manager). HEDIS and preventive care guidelines, provider profiling, utilization review, and complex-case management (for conditions such as HIV/AIDS) are also practiced by fee-for-service insurers. Insurers are implementing these techniques because they realize that 2 to 3 percent of their members may generate as much as 70 percent of health care expenditures and because buyers in a competitive market demand them.

60. Roger Feldman, "Is Risk Adjustment Essential For Medicare Reform?" paper prepared for the conference Medicare Reform: What Can the Private Sector Teach Us? sponsored by the American Enterprise Institute, July 1995.

61. Bryan Dowd and others, "Health Plan Choice in the Twin Cities Medicare Market," *Medical Care*, vol. 32 (October 1994), pp. 1019–39.

62. Stuart A. Butler and Robert E. Moffit, "The FEHBP As a Model for a New Medicare Program," *Health Affairs*, vol. 14 (Winter 1995), pp. 47–61.

63. Dowd, Feldman, and Christianson, *Competitive Pricing for Medicare.*

64. AAPCC ratios are based on fee-for-service costs and therefore do not necessarily reflect the costs of treating the same patients in HMOs. However, the analysis in this

section also applies to other systems of cost weights developed specifically for HMOs. The "1.0 beneficiary" could be selected from any demographic cell (for example, the cell with the largest number of beneficiaries). Alternatively, it could represent the "average" Medicare beneficiary. Bidding on the 1.0 beneficiary then would be identical to bidding on the whole Medicare population.

65. Strict application of this principle would mean that beneficiaries in every eligibility category (aged, disabled, and ESRD) pay the same premium. To simplify matters, we will confine our attention to equal payments within each category. The strict case could be viewed as an extension of our example with more demographic cells.

66. The cutoff price could be determined by any of the systems described in the section "Setting the Government's Contribution to Premiums" (for example, cutoff price equals the lowest bid).

67. Alain C. Enthoven, *Theory and Practice of Managed Competition in Health Care Finance* (North Holland, 1988), p. 2. See also "Managed Competition: An Agenda for Action," *Health Affairs*, vol. 7 (Summer 1988), pp. 25–47.

68. Protection against risk redefinition generally is made possible by an agreement by consumers to remain in the pool for a certain period of time. Employees achieve that agreement implicitly since it is unlikely that person would leave a job that offers insurance just to change insurance products. Movement among sponsors, therefore, might need to be relatively infrequent, but there is some anecdotal evidence that two-year commitments to pools are sufficient to offer risk-redefinition protection.

69. Health Care Financing Administration, Office of Prepaid Health Care Operations and Oversight, January 16, 1992.

Restructuring Medicare: The Role of Public and Private Purchasing Alliances
James C. Robinson and Patricia E. Powers

MEDICARE HAS LED the field of indemnity health insurance in extending benefit coverage, minimizing administrative costs, and rationalizing hospital and physician payment methods. Its progress in doing so has been far outstripped, however, by organizational and financing innovations in the private sector, where health maintenance organizations (HMOs) and other managed care plans have largely displaced indemnity coverage. Medicare has taken modest steps toward widening the range of choices available to its beneficiaries through the HMO risk-contracting program, which enrolls 13 percent of seniors nationwide and much more substantial percentages in states such as California, Oregon, and Arizona. However, the program has been burdened by an inefficient pricing system, inadequate compensation for risk selection, limits on the types of plans available, meager initiatives to improve

This paper was commissioned by the National Academy of Social Insurance.

quality, and inadequate consumer protection. More generally, Medicare's risk-contracting program has a regulatory orientation emphasizing uniformity and stability rather than a market orientation emphasizing diversity and innovation.

A consensus is growing among policy analysts that the Medicare program needs to be restructured in favor of managed competition in which the Health Care Financing Administration (HCFA) is a referee rather than a claims processor and micromanager.[1] The risk-contracting program is a first step in that direction. Medicare can be improved further by disconnecting the payment methodology from fee-for-service expenditures, improving risk adjustment, offering a wider range of plan types, and structuring the enrollment process to make beneficiaries' informed and cost-conscious choices easier. These changes can bring Medicare into line with the best current practices in the private sector, but will not ensure that the program continues to respond to new developments in the health care marketplace. In this era of managed care, the marketplace changes rapidly in ways that are difficult to anticipate. Medicare needs to adopt an administrative structure that permits it to evolve with the marketplace and to keep up with new payment methods and plan types while ensuring beneficiary access and quality of care.

The risk-contracting program has successfully incorporated HMOs, a major innovation from the private insurance and delivery system, into Medicare. The logical next step is to consider ways of incorporating the experience and innovations of the public and private purchasing alliances into the program. This paper examines the experience of purchasing alliances as sponsors of managed care programs, including public and private employers and large and small firms. In particular, we focus on experiences in California, which exhibits a diversified system with multiple sponsors and with the largest number of Medicare HMO enrollees of any state. The business coalition in Minneapolis and the Federal Employees Health Benefits Program (FEHBP) also provide a rich source of experience. We compare the potential advantages and disadvantages of allowing purchasing alliances to function as sponsors for Medicare beneficiaries, especially the retired members of the work forces they already sponsor. Three possibilities are considered. The Health Care Financing Administration could continue as the sole sponsor for Medicare beneficiaries, albeit with some functions delegated to the regional level. Alternatively, large firms and purchasing alliances could seek certification to sponsor their Medicare-eligible retirees, with the HCFA remaining the sponsor for beneficiaries who lack employment-based benefit programs. Finally, Medicare beneficiaries could choose among multiple certified sponsors, which could include retiree associations and labor unions as well as employers.

Limitations of Medicare's Risk-Contracting Program

Medicare's risk-contracting program has permitted a rapidly increasing number of beneficiaries to leave the costly fee-for-service program in favor of HMOs that offer more extensive benefits at lower cost in exchange for limitations on choice of network.[2] Despite its undeniable accomplishments, the program has been plagued by structural problems that threaten to undermine the gains from managed competition. The problems include the program's payment method, the range of plan types, the paucity of attempts to improve quality, and the nature of the enrollment process.

The HCFA's administered pricing system provides perverse incentives to HMOs that frustrate the original intent of the program. The payment for each HMO enrollee is set at 95 percent of what the average Medicare beneficiary in the same county would spend in the fee-for-service system. This links HMO revenues to fee-for-service expenditures, perpetuating the tradition of shadow pricing of indemnity premiums by HMOs in the commercial sector. Costs in the fee-for-service system are driven by excess capacity in hospital beds and specialist physicians, retrospective reimbursement that rewards unnecessary treatment, and the medical arms race of spiraling technology and use. There are dramatic geographic variations in Medicare expenditures per enrollee because of regional differences in system capacity and physician practice styles.[3] These unjustifiable differences create major differences in Medicare HMO payment rates, encouraging health plans to avoid markets with efficient delivery systems and low costs. Public and private purchasers in the commercial health insurance market have fought shadow pricing by using competitive bidding. Despite their differences, many large private employers, public purchasing alliances, and small-firm cooperatives establish a contribution level that is independent of (and typically lower than) the premiums charged by the fee-for-service plans. Employees can choose among plans, but must pay all or part of the incremental premiums charged by the higher-cost options.

In many areas of the nation, the HCFA's premium contributions exceed the cost to the HMO of providing the standard Medicare benefit package. The health plans are not permitted to refund the excess payment to beneficiaries. Rather, the plans must devote the surplus to enriching the benefit package through lower premiums and cost sharing, reduced limitations on hospital days, and the coverage of additional services such as outpatient drugs, vision care, and dental care. This restriction on premium rebates limits price competition among health plans and stimulates nonprice competition through ever richer benefits. Nonprice competition harnesses market forces to increase expenditures rather than to moderate them.[4] On a more philosophical level, the restriction on premium rebates to enrollees in low-cost plans embodies a paternalistic judgment that consumers must spend their disposable income on more medical care benefits rather than on other goods and services. In the context of commercial managed care, sponsors often set their contribution no higher than the average premium of several plans, thereby stimulating price as well as non-price competition among them.

Payments to HMOs are adjusted for the age, gender, disability, Medicaid eligibility, and institutional status of each Medicare enrollee. These demographic factors account for only a very small part of the variance in health status and use of medical services among beneficiaries. Health plans that through good fortune or targeted marketing enroll a mix of enrollees who are healthier than average earn undeserved profits; plans that enroll especially sick people suffer undeserved losses. This risk-selection problem is aggravated over time as plans with sicker enrollees drop their Medicare contracts, forcing the enrollees back into the fee-for-service plan. It is estimated that Medicare beneficiaries enrolled in HMOs are 10 percent healthier that those remaining in the indemnity plan, measured in terms of expenditures per person on medical care.[5] The problem of adverse selection in the indemnity plan further undermines the efficiency of the risk-contracting program because the higher average fee-for-service costs are used as the benchmark for establishing HMO payment rates in the subsequent year. In the private sector some purchasing alliances have developed risk-adjustment methods that go beyond demographic factors to capture the effects of high-cost illnesses. Others contract with only a limited number of plans to concentrate both the high- and low-cost employees in the same risk pools. This is currently a focus of widespread experimentation.

The risk-contracting program has limited the types of health plans that can compete for Medicare beneficiaries. Until very recently, only plain vanilla HMOs qualified. In some markets point-of-service (POS) options have been accepted. Preferred provider organizations (PPOs), managed indemnity plans, and other hybrid forms have been locked out. These limitations on type of plan are particularly a problem in areas of the nation where the commercial insurance industry has been slow to evolve and where local managed care options consist mostly of PPOs. It has also prevented the development of provider-sponsored networks that use local delivery systems without going through an HMO intermediary. In the commercial sector, sponsors typically offer a range of plans. In some communities such as Minneapolis, large sponsors are contracting directly with physician groups and hospital systems.

Medicare provides only weak incentives for HMOs to improve the clinical quality of the services they provide. It is difficult to monitor performance at the regional and, especially, national levels. Egregious acts of omission or commission can result in fines or contract termination, but the severity of contract termination ensures that this punishment will rarely be applied. More generally, the HCFA's quality protections have historically highlighted the small number of worst offenders while ignoring the large number of mediocrities. Medicare's peer review organizations have focused on assisting providers to improve quality, rather than on assisting beneficiaries to understand and act on quality differences. The HCFA does not tie health plan or provider payment rates to quality or other dimensions of performance. Most sponsors in the private sector are refocusing from the worst offenders to continuous quality improvement (CQI), which emphasizes the potential for quality improvement among all providers and all health plans. Some sponsors have initiated their own quality studies while others evaluate those that the health plans and their affiliated providers initiate. Many sponsors use performance information as one criterion for selecting health plans and disseminate quality data to consumers to assist in their choice of plan.

The enrollment process used by the risk-contracting program offers both too much protection and too little to Medicare beneficiaries who consider switching health plans. On the one hand, beneficiaries may switch plans every month. This offers the protection of easy exit but undermines the plans' incentive to invest in preventive services and allows beneficiaries to take unfair advantage of the benefit packages (for instance, switching plans after exhausting the annual limit on outpatient drug coverage). On the other hand, beneficiaries do not have the protection of a sponsoring organization that can monitor undesirable health plan activity at the local level. They receive very little information from the HCFA comparing the plans' quality, networks, benefits, and prices. In the private sector, individual companies and purchasing alliances typically structure beneficiaries' choices through annual open enrollments. Employees must stay with their plan for an entire year, but their choices are abetted by extensive materials comparing plan options. Innovative sponsors are demanding that plans provide performance guarantees for consumer service, grievance processes, quality of care, and network access.

Medicare's risk-contracting program is a major step forward from its exclusive reliance on the unmanaged fee-for-service plan. Many of its features compare favorably with those developed by public employers, private corporations, and small-firm alliances. But the cumulative lesson from the diverse problems is that Medicare's risk program suffers from excess uniformity of plans and insufficient innovation. It is cut off from many of the payment methods, plan types, quality initiatives, and enrollment methods being pioneered by other sponsors. As a health plan, Medicare has much to offer but also much to learn from managed care plans in the private sector. As a sponsor seeking to manage competition among health plans, the HCFA similarly has both much to offer and much to learn from purchasing alliances elsewhere in the economy.

Single or Multiple Sponsors?

The Medicare risk-contracting program to date has functioned as a single sponsor for beneficiaries who choose to enroll in HMOs. There is a single set of criteria for plan participation, single contracting strategy, single payment method, single enrollment system, and single oversight framework. Most policy analysts envision the retention of this uniform structure, albeit with an expansion in the number and type of health plans that are eligible for participation and with other reforms to improve performance. Some anticipate retention of the single-sponsor framework, but advocate the replacement of the HCFA by the FEHBP, which is less wedded to an indemnity insurance culture. President Clinton's proposed Health Security Act envisioned expanding the single sponsor to represent Medicare beneficiaries and all other citizens in each geographic region.

Reliance on a single administrative entity to manage competition has several important advantages. Experiences in the commercial HMO market suggest, however, that a single sponsor is not necessary to stimulate competition and innovation. California has many major sponsors, including the HCFA and FEHBP but also the California Public Employees Retirement System (CalPERS), the Pacific Business Group on Health (PBGH), and the Health Insurance Plan of California (HIPC). In addition, many large firms serve directly as sponsors for their employees and retirees. The presence of multiple sponsors contributes to plan performance in ways that offset many of the advantages of the single-sponsor framework. Sponsors may represent different constituencies, as is the case with major purchasing and negotiating alliances in California, or they may compete for the same enrollees. When considering structural reform of the Medicare system it is important to compare the relative strengths and weaknesses of the single-sponsor and multiple-sponsor approaches. If the multiple-sponsor structure is adopted, the advantages and disadvantages of competition among sponsors must be evaluated.

Advantages of the Single-Sponsor Framework

An administrative framework composed of a single sponsoring agency offers the advantages of uniformity and the potential for economies of scale.

the HCFA can develop and enforce a single benefit package, single payment method, single set of quality measurements, single set of financial and utilization reporting requirements, and single mechanism for consumer grievances. This uniformity facilitates comparisons of plans and simplifies the responsibilities of those that otherwise might face different demands from different sponsors. The size of the Medicare program implies that the single sponsor would enjoy large economies of scale in developing ways of managing competition. The most pressing need is for more quality measures that can be gathered in a timely fashion, constitute valid indicators of the course and outcome of care, and permit comparisons of plans. Better methods for evaluating the health status of beneficiaries are also needed; these data can be used to risk-adjust the payments to particular health plans and to risk-adjust Medicare contributions to particular regions if risk mix varies geographically.

The single sponsor also offers important, albeit more controversial, advantages for financing the Medicare program. Reliance on a single sponsor keeps all Medicare beneficiaries in a single risk pool, which facilitates the cross-subsidy of the sick by the healthy. Health plans have to bid a single rate (adjusted for risk mix) for the entire pool in the county, rather than bid different rates for different sponsors' enrollee populations. This reduces the pressure on the HCFA to develop a finely tuned risk-adjustment method that links premium contributions to health status for each beneficiary. As in the large group market, health plans can set their revenue targets based on the group as a whole rather than ensure that revenues match expected costs for each enrollee. A single sponsor possesses huge potential bargaining leverage with health plans, given that Medicare accounts for one-third of U.S. health care spending. It will be increasingly difficult for large health plans to market their services solely in the commercial market. As Medicare contracts become essential to health plans, the plans' ability to extract high rates by threatening contract termination diminishes. Bargaining leverage has not been prominent in Medicare risk contracting because the HCFA has used an administered pricing method rather than a competitive pricing method. If it disconnects its HMO payments from fee-for-service expenditures, however, the agency would rely more on bargaining leverage to achieve savings.

The final and perhaps most obvious advantage of the single sponsor is that the HCFA's risk-contracting program already exists in most metropolitan areas. The only program with a comparable scale and scope is the FEHBP. Other potential sponsors currently are concentrated in geographic areas with extensive managed care penetration. For this reason, any movement toward multiple sponsors would need to begin with regional demonstration projects.

Advantages of the Multiple-Sponsor Framework

Enumerating the potential advantages of a single sponsor immediately exposes the system's greatest weakness. For twenty years the Medicare program has had the technical expertise and market power to function as the preeminent sponsor of managed competition, yet has been hobbled by political resistance and conservative programming. Many of the innovations in methods of contracting, payment, quality measurement, and risk adjustment have come from much smaller sponsors in the commercial sector. Thus there is a fundamental trade-off between uniformity and size on the one hand and diversity and innovation on the other. A multiplicity of sponsors has augmented rather than diminished the vitality of managed competition in the commercial sector; comparable advantages may be achievable from encouraging multiple sponsors in the Medicare sector. Four potential benefits of such a framework deserve consideration.

First and most important, the presence of multiple sponsors permits diversity and encourages innovation in managing competition. Sponsors differ in the number and type of plans with which they choose to contract. Some contract with most, if not all, local HMOs to expand consumer choice. Others limit contracts to only a few plans, thereby encouraging mutual investments in the partnership and creating performance incentives for the plans. Some sponsors contract only with HMOs, some with both HMOs and PPOs, some with a full range of plan types. Some use only insured plans, while others are self-insured or combine insured with self-insured plans. Sponsors also differ in their payment mechanisms and in the ways they encourage price competition. Some accept whatever premiums the plans request but require individual enrollees to pay the difference above the sponsor's baseline contribution. Others prefer to use bargaining leverage to negotiate favorable rates with plans and place less emphasis on consumer switching to reward plans that offer low premiums. Sponsoring organizations have pioneered various methods for structuring enrollee choice, providing comparative data on health plans, monitoring for quality, and surveying consumer satisfaction. Some rely on consumer choice to motivate administrative efficiency among plans while others bargain explicitly for performance guarantees and impose financial penalties for noncompliance. Some sponsors impose a single-benefit design while others offer several options or leave wide latitude for health plans to establish their own benefit designs. Sponsors exhibit a wide variety of approaches to measuring risk differences among plans and compensating those that suffer from adverse selection.

Second, and more controversially, a framework with multiple sponsors avoids monopsonistic concentration on the buyer's side of the managed care marketplace.[6] This deconcentration appears controversial in health policy circles because so much has been made in recent years of the advantages of purchasing power in promoting market performance. This monopsonistic perspective, according to which purchasing alliances can never grow too large, echoes the single-payer proposals that evolved in the context of indemnity insurance. Insights into the problems potentially afflicting a true government monopsony in managed care can be derived from examining the military procurement industry, in which there is a dominant government buyer. The industry is characterized by the lobbying of government officials by the firms whose viability rests on a single decision, up to the point where some observers talk of agency "capture," in which the agency comes to depend on only a few suppliers. Were this framework to be extended to health care, where plans and providers are well organized politically in every state and locality, it would inevitably produce myriad legislative and judicial interventions that uphold due process and other protections for private entities against arbitrary government decisions. These rules and regulations would limit the flexibility of public procurement entities in deciding which entities should receive contracts and under what terms.

Third, the multiple-sponsor framework is consistent with the nation's commitment to diversity and choice. Diversity permits a better matching between heterogeneous health care systems and heterogeneous citizen preferences. The ability of Medicare beneficiaries to elect sponsorship through their erstwhile employer or another entity would stimulate competition in better ways of managing competition, counteracting the tendency toward bureaucratization that inevitably afflicts organizations with captive memberships. On a more philosophical level, government refusal to permit citizens to use the services of independent sponsoring organizations limits initiative in a manner that requires justification. Differing views on the relative importance of autonomy and choice on the one hand and of community and uniformity on the other underlie much of the apparently technical debate on Medicare policy.

Finally, and as a practical matter, many sponsoring organizations are well established and have strong records of performance in their regions. Some have developed innovative programs for early retirees or Medicare-eligible retirees or both. The HCFA would need to establish criteria according to which these organizations could become certified to sponsor Medicare beneficiaries and would need to establish a uniform contribution formula and other structural supports. The HCFA program would continue to function as the sole sponsor in those geographic regions where no alternatives are available and would remain an option for Medicare beneficiaries even in areas with multiple sponsors.

Choice among Sponsors?

There are two variants of the multiple-sponsor framework. The first builds directly on the current retiree benefit programs of large firms, allowing them to evolve from a supplemental program for the Medicare fee-for-service plan to a sponsor for HMOs and other managed care plans, and will here be termed the employment-based sponsor system. The second permits a wider range of organizations to seek certification as Medicare sponsors and allows individual beneficiaries to choose among sponsors; it will here be termed the competing-sponsor approach.

Many large firms currently offer supplemental health insurance benefits for their Medicare-eligible retirees, using the same administrative framework developed for the health benefits programs for active employees and early retirees. As retirees move to HMO plans, these employer-based systems continue to offer various supplemental benefits. The scope and cost of the HMO supplemental benefits often are modest compared with those offered to retirees choosing Medicare fee for service because the HMOs already have lower cost sharing and offer richer benefits than does the indemnity Medicare plan, and there is less need for supplements. Some of these firms, or alliances of firms, could serve as sponsors for their Medicare-eligible retirees that choose an HMO plan. The firms thereby assume responsibility for the full range of premium negotiations, quality monitoring, open enrollment, and other sponsor functions. These would not be new tasks because the firms and alliances already perform such functions for their active employees and early retirees. Indeed, they are better set up than the Health Care Financing Administration to perform many of these functions. In this employment-based sponsor framework, individual Medicare beneficiaries could choose to be sponsored by the firm that provides retiree benefits or to be sponsored by the HCFA, in somewhat the same manner in which they currently choose to participate in the firm's retirement health program or go purely with Medicare. However, the employment-based sponsors would not cover Medicare beneficiaries other than their own retirees; individual beneficiaries would not have a choice among multiple sponsors (aside from the basic choice of employment-based sponsor or the HCFA).

In the competing-sponsor approach, a wider range of organizations could be certified as sponsors for Medicare beneficiaries. These could include senior citizen groups such as the American Association of Retired Persons (AARP), labor unions, professional associations, and churches. Multiple sponsors could be certified in each locality, and beneficiaries could choose among them. The HCFA would continue to operate as a backstop sponsor for beneficiaries who decline to elect an independent sponsor. This framework approximates the small-firm insurance market in California, where individual businesses can purchase coverage directly from a health plan, go through an insurance broker, join the public purchasing alliance (HIPC), or join a private purchasing alliance (operated by industry associations and brokerages). This option would be susceptible to greater problems of risk selection across sponsors than would the option of employment-based sponsor and would require commensurably greater supporting regulation (open enrollment) and risk adjustment of Medicare premium contributions. Its advantage over the employment-based system lies in the greater potential for innovation and performance competition among sponsors, and the greater number of choices available to beneficiaries. It would offer choices to Medicare beneficiaries who do not have retiree benefit programs.

Examples of Sponsor Organizations

Many organizations perform one or more of the functions of a sponsor. Large corporations and government entities purchase coverage for their employees and sometimes join with other entities to increase leverage and gain economies of scale. Purchasing cooperatives for small firms and individuals can be run by public agencies, industry associations, labor unions, insurance brokers, or professional associations. Some sponsors perform a wide range of functions, including eligibility verification, plan enrollment, improvement of care, benefit standardization, claims payment, information dissemination, and premium negotiation, while others perform only one or two. Very few currently include Medicare beneficiaries. We focus our discussion on four large alliances that operate successfully in markets with very high HMO penetration. Two of these alliances represent Medicare-eligible retirees as well as active employees and early retirees. We then consider the Federal Employees Health Benefit Program, the largest nationwide sponsor of managed and unmanaged care.

California Public Employees Retirement System

Established in 1962, CalPERS manages health insurance benefits for the state of California and for cities, counties, school districts, and other public agencies that elect to participate. It covers 1 million active employees, dependents, and retirees from almost 1,000 public agencies that vary in size from 600,000 employees (the state of California) to 2 (Antelope Valley Mosquito Abatement Program). CalPERS contracts with fourteen HMOs and four association plans (for example, the firefighters union) and manages two self-insured PPO plans. Covered enrollees can choose among plans at the annual open enrollment without regard to which public agency is their sponsor; more than 80 percent have selected HMOs. CalPERS is a quasi-public entity governed by a thirteen-member board appointed by the governor, the state legislature, nonstate public agencies, public employee labor unions, and others.

CalPERS was the first purchasing alliance to develop a standard benefit package, which all contracting plans must offer. The package was standardized to improve consumers' abilities to compare plans and to limit risk selection created by subtle differences in benefits. The state and other public sponsors set their premium contribution at a level lower than PPO premiums but similar to many of the HMO premiums. Enrollees pay the difference themselves if they choose a high-cost PPO but typically have no out-of-pocket contribution if they choose an HMO. CalPERS does not rely primarily on price-conscious consumer demand to discipline HMOs. Rather, it negotiates premiums each year and is willing to freeze enrollment in particular plans or drop plans altogether if it believes that unreasonable rates are being charged.

The transition of CalPERS from a passive payer of insurance premiums to an active sponsor with a defined benefit package, limited employer contributions, and aggressive premium bargaining, a change that has occurred only in the past five years, has achieved significant cost savings for program beneficiaries.[7] After a decade of double-digit premium inflation, CalPERS achieved actual reductions in HMO premiums of 0.4 percent in 1994, 0.7 percent in 1995, 5.3 percent in 1996, and has negotiated a decrease of 2.5 percent for 1997.[8] CalPERS uses consumer satisfaction surveys covering preventive services, satisfaction with care, and satisfaction with administrative aspects to facilitate enrollee comparisons among plans. Recently, it has developed health plan performance scores based on beneficiaries that are high users of services (those who, for example, have been hospitalized during the previous year) in addition to scores based on all beneficiaries.

Pacific Business Group on Health

The Pacific Business Group on Health is a coalition of thirty-three large public and private purchasers that together have 3 million covered employees, dependents, and retirees. A subgroup of eighteen PBGH firms in California negotiates with HMOs over premiums, quality improvements, and other performance features. In 1996 this Negotiating Alliance represented 380,000 active employees, dependents, and early retirees. The alliance also negotiates for 40,000 Medicare-eligible retirees, 30 percent of whom are enrolled in Medicare HMO plans. Participation in the Negotiating Alliance is limited to those firms that are willing to use the PBGH standard benefit package, which resembles the CalPERS package. Prices for modifiers to the package, such as for varying copayment levels and for mental health or prescription drug carve-outs, also are negotiated by the alliance on behalf of firms with individual needs. Companies agree to use the rates negotiated by the alliance without seeking firm-specific rates based on firm-level differences in risk mix; demo-graphic risk differences among firms are small. The University of California and some other entities with different benefit packages (typically the result of union negotiations) choose not to participate in the Negotiating Alliance, but participate in the coalition's quality-improvement and data-sharing activities. CalPERS and the state's small-firm purchasing alliance are members of the PBGH but conduct their HMO negotiations separately.

Firms participating in the PBGH Negotiating Alliance include Pacific Telesis, Bank of America, Stanford University, Bechtel, Mervyns, Wells Fargo Bank, Varian, and Chevron. The PBGH entities also maintain self-insured plans outside the Negotiating Alliance; approximately two-thirds of all beneficiaries have chosen HMO coverage, with a range among employers of 50 percent to 97 percent. All member employers are committed to basing their premium contributions on the rates charged by the lower-cost plans, but they are phasing in this defined contribution over several years. The PBGH realized average HMO premium decreases of 9.4 percent in 1995 and 4.3 percent in 1996 and negotiated level premiums (no increase or decrease) for 1997.[9] Many PBGH members have employees in other states who are offered regional HMOs and the employer's national self-insured plans. The Negotiating Alliance is beginning to expand to other states where member firms have sizable numbers of employees.

The PBGH is a negotiating alliance rather than a purchasing alliance such as the FEHBP or CalPERS. It negotiates premium rates and performance requirements with all HMOs. Each member entity, however, contracts with only a few plans, using PBGH-negotiated premiums. This preserves their autonomy but at the cost of narrowing choices for individual employees. Gradually the Negotiating Alliance is coming to resemble a purchasing alliance as employers contract with larger numbers of HMOs and as the HMOs themselves consolidate. Participation in the alliance has permitted member employers to achieve bargaining leverage, lower administrative costs, reduced concern for adverse selection, and other advantages of scale that previously were available only if they severely restricted the number of plans with which they contracted. Employers are also expanding their offerings to encourage market entry and growth of additional HMOs.

The PBGH has steadily increased the range of issues over which it bargains with health plans. In addition to premiums, it has negotiated performance levels for customer service, quality, enrollee satisfaction, and data reporting that HMOs must achieve or risk losing 2 percent of the premiums.[10] Until recently, the PBGH focused on employees, dependents, and early retirees, but now it is actively increasing its attention to Medicare-eligible retirees. It is negotiating with Medicare HMOs over network scope and composition, administrative issues, and supplemental benefits. Employers are very interested in having the plan design for Medicare-eligible retirees mirror the design for active employees and early retirees as a means of ensuring continuity of care and cost-conscious choice. Negotiated performance criteria for Medicare HMOs include flu shots, health risk assessments, and maintenance of good communications and relations with medical groups and hospital systems.

Health Insurance Plan of California

The Health Insurance Plan of California is a purchasing alliance for small firms with 3 to 50 employees that is managed by the state of California. It currently includes 6,185 employers with 115,000 employees and dependents and is growing at the rate of 5,000 enrollees a month. The HIPC contracts with twenty HMOs and nine other managed care plan types (PPOs, POSs), all of which are fully insured. More than 95 percent of enrollees have chosen HMOs. The HIPC offers two HMO and two PPO plan designs. As a state entity it seeks to include a very large number of plans. It does bargain over premiums, but prefers to discipline plans by exposing them to price-conscious consumer choices instead of terminating their contracts. The HIPC is a purchasing alliance rather than merely a negotiating alliance and assumes marketing, eligibility, and enrollment functions. A distinguishing feature of the alliance within the small-group insurance market, where most businesses offer only one health plan choice to employees, is that employees can choose from the full set of health plans regardless of employer. Employers are required to contribute a minimum of 50 percent of the premium for their employees. Many pay the full premium, which reduces the element of cost-consciousness in enrollees' choices.

The HIPC has had a significant effect on the small-firm insurance market in California. HMO premiums declined by 3.6 percent in 1995, 2.8 percent in

1996, and 0.2 percent in 1997.[11] It has pioneered a risk-adjustment method that transfers premium dollars from health plans enrolling especially healthy populations to plans enrolling sicker populations. Employers pay premiums based on age, gender, and region but not on diagnoses. The alliance then monitors high-cost hospitalizations and retrospectively transfers funds from plans with few such admissions to plans with many. In practice this has implied shifting premium dollars (less than 1 percent) from several HMOs to several PPOs, with the majority of HMOs attracting enrollees with average risk profiles.[12]

The HIPC continues to enroll only a small minority of its target constituency, in part because of resistance from health insurance brokers and agents, who are reimbursed less generously under the alliance than in the outside market. The principal reason for the modest rate of growth in enrollment, however, is that premiums outside the HIPC have declined due to spillover of competitive incentives. Two HMOs with large enrollments in the small-group market, Blue Cross and Foundation Health, have declined to contract with the HIPC but work closely with brokers and offer rates similar to those available through the alliance. The HIPC does no underwriting and charges a community rate adjusted for age, family size, and region to all enrollees. Health plans selling outside the HIPC structure are prohibited by California law from denying coverage or charging especially high rates to high-risk employers. There is considerable controversy over whether plans and brokers are engaged in subtle forms of risk selection outside the HIPC. Currently the organization does not represent Medicare-eligible retirees from its member entities.

Buyers Health Care Action Group

The Buyers Health Care Action Group is an alliance of twenty-two large private firms with 250,000 employees and dependents in the Minneapolis area. An additional 150,000 state employees are affiliated. All twenty-two firms participate in a self-insured POS plan operated by the alliance that contracts directly with medical groups and physician-hospital organizations (called care systems) in the Twin Cities. A few member firms also contract with HMOs outside the BHCAG structure. Unlike their California counterparts, there is little use of capitation payment methods. Approximately 100,000 of the total 250,000 employees and dependents currently participate in the BHCAG plan, but this number is rising rapidly as member firms terminate contracts with outside HMOs.

The BHCAG has pioneered a strategy of contracting with care systems rather than primarily with health plans. It uses the services of the HealthPartners HMO to provide claims processing and other administrative backup services to the care systems and to member firms. Each care system establishes its own target payment rate per enrollee, which is then used to establish a fee schedule for that system based on utilization patterns and the care system's target rate. Because the BHCAG plan is self-insured, it is prohibited from capitating care systems but must reimburse on a fee-for-service basis. The use of budget targets to set fee schedules mimics the incentives of capitation (creating a budget within which the care system must operate), while allowing the alliance to remain exempt from state insurance regulation. The payment system combines the virtues of prepayment incentives (virtual capitation) with the data advantages of retrospective fee-for-service payment. Each member firm sets its contribution below the level of the lowest care system premium, thereby forcing employees to make price-conscious choices using their own money. At present, the care systems are grouped into three categories for determining premium contributions by employees. The BHCAG does not negotiate premiums (claims targets) with the care systems; systems with high rates are expected to lose market share because of consumer choices.

The BHCAG assesses risk differences among provider organizations based on fee-for-service claims data processed through the Ambulatory Care Group's (ACG) software.[13] The fee schedules for each provider organization are adjusted up or down from their budget-based target depending on whether their risk mix is above or below the average for all organizations. This transfers monies among providers but not among employers (each employer pays all the claims for its own employees). A major advantage of this system is that it adjusts payments for medical groups and hospitals, not payments for health plans. Differences among health plans in risk mix may be fairly small, while differences among provider organizations may be large. For example, there is a 35 percent difference in ACG risk among the fifteen care systems with BHCAG contracts in Minneapolis.[14]

The BHCAG system has had major effects on the Minneapolis health care market. Medical groups and hospital systems have coalesced into fifteen care systems, each providing or contracting for the full range of medical services. This offers the benefits of system coordination while avoiding the extremes of oligopolistic concentration; in the non-BHCAG insurance market, three HMOs account for 80 percent of insurance enrollment. The BHCAG system can be thought of as a mechanism for dispensing with health plans as intermediaries in favor of direct provider contracting. The costs of components of the system, such as service delivery and administration, are made transparent. The BHCAG system reduced member firm costs by an average of 9 percent for 1997, its first year of direct contracting with providers. In collaboration with the care systems and with the HealthPartners HMO, the BHCAG has developed extensive information on each care system—its medical groups, primary care providers, specialty referral panels, and hospitals—that is made accessible to consumers choosing among systems. The BHCAG cooperates with major provider organizations, such as the Mayo Clinic and Park Nicollet, on clinical pathways and protocols that will improve health care. It works closely with the Minnesota Health Data Institute, a public-private partnership created by the Minnesota legislature, to obtain community data for comparison of clinical and service quality at the care center level.

The Federal Employees Health Benefits Program

The Federal Employees Health Benefits Program has a distinguished record of managing competition among health plans while maintaining a national scope of operations.[15] It oversees the health insurance benefits for 9 million federal employees, dependents, and retirees, contracting with more than 400 HMOs, PPOs, and indemnity plans. Approximately 40 percent of active employees and 20 percent of retirees have chosen HMOs. All health plans contracting with the FEHBP must cover a core set of benefits, but they are allowed discretion in adding others, which increases the range of choices for beneficiaries but makes comparisons among plans difficult. The Office of Personnel Management (OPM), which manages the FEHBP, does not bargain with health plans over premiums. Instead, plans are required to assure OPM that their FEHBP rates do not exceed the rates offered to any other purchasers in the market. Plans also submit rates with the understanding that the FEHBP sets its contribution at 60 percent of the average premiums of six large plans, which implies that beneficiaries must contribute toward premiums for all plans and pay the full difference when choosing a high-cost plan.[16] Low-cost plans receive the lowest FEHBP premium contribution because the government cannot contribute more than 75 percent of any premium. The most expensive plans receive the highest dollar contributions, although these cover only half the premium. The result is a wide range in employee contributions, with most choosing plans with mid-range premiums. Although this contribution strategy limits price-conscious consumer choice, it mitigates the effects of adverse selection that have afflicted indemnity plans in the FEHBP.

Beneficiaries choose among health plans in an annual open enrollment season. Detailed information on the benefits, premiums, and other features of each plan is prepared in different forms by the OPM, the National Association of Retired Public Employees, and independent publications such as *Consumer Checkbook's Guide*. The FEHBP has encountered adverse selection among some health plans because of its community rating payment method, according to which plans receive the same premium for each enrollee regardless of age or health status. A risk-adjustment method is needed to protect health plans with large numbers of older enrollees. Aside from this technical problem, the FEHBP has proved its ability to sponsor choice and competition in all fifty states and among all forms of health plans. During the 1980s it enjoyed lower premiums than those found in the outside market despite improving benefits and covering an increasing number of retirees. Premium inflation has declined sharply in recent years, with an average increase of only 3 percent in 1994 and an average decrease of 3 percent in 1995.[17] In California the program experienced HMO premium increases of 6.2 percent in 1993 and 2.9 percent in 1994, then decreases of 5.8 percent in 1995 and 4.5 percent in 1996.[18]

Criteria for Sponsors in a Multiple-Sponsor Model

The Medicare risk-contracting program could benefit greatly from closer links with public and private sponsors. In the employment-based version of the multiple-sponsor model, large firms and purchasing alliances that sponsor HMO coverage for their active employees would be allowed to extend their sponsorship to cover their Medicare-eligible retirees. Many large firms already offer retiree benefits that supplement Medicare's benefit package under the fee-for-service plan, but play no commensurate role in supporting retirees that choose HMO plans. (The HMO benefit packages already cover at no extra cost many of the cost-sharing, prescription drug, and ancillary benefits that the employer-paid supplementary packages cover for Medicare fee-for-service enrollees.) In the competing-sponsor version, consumer cooperatives, retiree groups, and other independent organizations, as well as employers, could be authorized to sponsor the coverage of Medicare beneficiaries with whom they had no previous employment relationship. In either case the HCFA would need to establish criteria against which to evaluate applications by public and private organizations to become sponsors for Medicare beneficiaries.

Employment-Based Sponsors

In principle, large employers that sponsor active employees' and early retirees' choices among competing health plans could extend their programs to cover Medicare-eligible retirees. Many offer health insurance to retirees older than age 65. In the past this almost exclusively took the form of supplemental benefits such as outpatient prescription drugs that fill in the holes in the Medicare package. Even where the majority of active employees have chosen HMO coverage, most retirees have stayed with fee-for-service Medicare and the employer's supplemental benefits. There has been no financial incentive for these retirees to choose the HMOs because the employers already offer the extended benefits through which the HMOs compete for enrollment in the individual Medicare market. HMOs are not permitted to compete for enrollees by offering rebates of premiums. An additional factor influencing retiree choice has been the limited geographic scope of most HMO networks and restricted benefits for out-of-area use. This is unattractive to retirees who spend the winter months in a warm state and the summer months in their state of origin.

Many large employers are moving toward a defined contribution payment strategy for retiree benefits. In the new format the full cost of retiree coverage is paid by the employer if the retiree chooses an employer-sponsored HMO plan, but only a fraction of the cost is paid if he chooses an indemnity (medigap) supplement. (The actual dollar contribution by the employer is the same in either case; the medigap premium is much higher than the HMO premium for similar benefits.) A defined contribution encourages retiree migration to the more efficient plans. Migration is also facilitated by the growing enrollment in and familiarity with HMOs among the active employees, who often choose to stay with their HMOs after becoming eligible for Medicare. Some employers are limiting employer-paid health benefits to retirees who select HMO coverage. In more extreme circumstances, some large employers are dropping retiree health insurance coverage altogether as a means of containing spiraling premium costs.

Criteria for certifying individual employers as sponsors for Medicare beneficiaries will differ from criteria for purchasing alliances or other noncorporate sponsors. Most obviously, it would be impossible to demand that corporate sponsors be nonprofit organizations or that they be governed by a consumer board. Private sector sponsors are structured as taxable nonprofit membership corporations or for-profit organizations owned by participating employers and management. It is unlikely that a purchasing organization in the commercial market would qualify for tax-exempt status because of the private benefits that accrue to participating businesses.

Competing Sponsors

The Institute for Health Policy Solutions, a Washington, D.C., association that monitors and assists small-employer purchasing pools, has developed criteria for sponsoring organizations. They should be publicly operated or governed by a board of employers and consumers with no financial conflicts of interest. They should offer standardized benefits and a choice among competing health plans (several plan products within one carrier would not qualify). Interested sponsors for Medicare beneficiaries might include:

—a public or quasi-public agency (CalPERS, FEHBP, HIPC);

—a private sector business group (BHCAG, PBGH, The Alliance in Madison);

—a private sector industry or union purchasing pool (the meat packers Taft-Hartley trust);

—a senior citizen or consumer organization (the American Association of Retired Persons, the California Group Insurance Trust of United Way); and

—a private brokerage or benefits organization (California Choice, developed by brokers; National HMO Group, developed by the William M. Mercer consulting firm).

An important consideration is whether a qualified sponsor would be required to offer its plans to all Medicare beneficiaries or only those who meet its own criteria. For example, a sponsor that represents entities with at least 1,000 employees, or one that serves only nonprofit organizations, may be very interested in becoming a qualified sponsor for its own members retirees but less interested in opening up its pool to all Medicare beneficiaries.

Corporate Status and Ownership

In health care debates nonprofit organizations once seemed to wear halos. Nonprofits often are perceived as providing a social good and placing the organization's constituents first. In contrast, for-profit organizations often are perceived as placing shareholders' interests above those of customers. However, many nonprofit health care organizations have come under criticism for their failure to provide evidence of social contributions that justify their tax exemption and by behavior patterns that mirror those of their for-profit counterparts. In recent years many nonprofit health care organizations, such as Blue Cross/Blue Shield associations and community hospitals, have become for-profit entities. To remain competitive in a fast-moving health care marketplace, access to capital is essential and is most readily obtained through such conversions.

Nonprofit or for-profit status may be less important than ownership. Public ownership by state or local government is a possibility, although public entities are subject to lobbying and capture by plans and organized provider groups. Texas and Florida have created unique models by chartering alliances that are managed by private not-for-profit organizations. Given the recent debate surrounding physician self-referrals, it is unlikely that owners with any financial conflict of interest would qualify. For example, a sponsor owned by providers or others directly involved in the delivery of health care would present a conflict of interest. One solution would be to set forth ownership principles and then evaluate individually those candidates that pass a preliminary screening. Alternatively, the HCFA could specify the kinds of representatives (for example, consumers or employers) to serve on a sponsor board. This was the approach taken by President Clinton's Health Security Act.

Sponsors would assume many activities currently performed by the HCFA, and thus the federal government would have an interest in overseeing their viability and integrity. Financial oversight may include reserve, capital, and deposit requirements. Examples may be found in states that have formed purchasing pools in recent years, as well as in federal and state regulations governing health plans. At a minimum, the HCFA should require an annual audit and public report of each sponsor's financial condition and retain the right to conduct an audit or inspection at any time.

Scale and Geographic Scope

The geographic scope of an organization may be a criterion for whether it should be designated as a sponsor for Medicare beneficiaries. Nationwide, state, regional, and city-specific organizations and alliances could apply to sponsor Medicare beneficiaries in their market areas. Allowing sponsors to define their own geographic boundaries would increase flexibility and build on their experience with the commercial market. It would also avoid creation by the HCFA of what might be arbitrary geographic boundaries. The major drawback is that some areas could be highly competitive, while others could lack any sponsor.

An alternative would be for the HCFA to create geographic areas paralleling its current regions or to examine each market on a local basis. For example, although the California HIPC itself is statewide, health plans compete within six geographic areas. Theoretically, each of these six could be covered by one or more sponsors. Several brokerage alliances are attempting to compete with the HIPC in narrow geographic areas.

Should the HCFA control the number of sponsors in a given area, perhaps by specifying a minimum or maximum number of enrollees? A pure market approach would resolve this issue through the sponsors' own evolution. To remain viable by offering sufficient volume to payers and to cover the sponsor's own costs, a minimum number of pooled beneficiaries would emerge. The HCFA may wish to establish a minimum threshold for other reasons. Fewer sponsors could create economies of scale, limit the opportunity for biased selection by sponsors, ensure that undesirable areas would be covered, and keep the HCFA's oversight responsibilities manageable. These considerations must be balanced with the goals of stimulating and maintaining competition. Size does not pose a problem for government sponsors with respect to antitrust laws; however, a public monopoly would raise questions of efficiency. The PBGH requested a formal review and letter of approval from the Department of Justice, demonstrating that its membership comprised less than a quarter of any health plan's or geographic area's commercial market. In general, the department tends to view organized purchasing favorably.

Sponsor Administrative Fees

On average, purchasing pools use 1 to 3 percent of their enrollees' premiums to cover administrative costs. Sponsors with a very large pool of enrollees could keep this fee very low. The Health Security Act capped administrative fees at 2.5 percent. It would be difficult, however, to develop a reliable working definition of what is included in administration. For example, although one large public sector sponsor asserts that it adds a mere 0.5 percent onto its premium, the full costs of the state's staffing are not considered in this figure. This dilemma is similar to that faced by sponsors that have attempted to evaluate the administrative fees of health plans. There is sufficient wiggle room in the definition that the spread in HMO administrative fees and profit presently ranges from 30 to 3 cents on the dollar (a medical loss ratio of 70 to 97 percent). This spread is likely attributable to differences in product, market, and geographic mix rather than substantive differences in the value-added activities of the HMOs.[19]

Selecting and Managing Health Plans

Medicare sponsors could assume two responsibilities in selecting and managing health plans: managing all plans and provider systems that meet specified criteria set by the HCFA or contracting selectively with a more limited number of plans. The first option assumes that consumers rather than sponsors are best suited to motivate competition, efficiency, and quality among health plans. A wide array of health plan choices permits a closer match between the heterogeneous preferences of Medicare beneficiaries and the characteristics of the health plans. Contracting with numerous plans limits the potential for incumbent plans to offer low premiums in the early years of the relationship and then boost premiums in later years when the membership is locked in. In this approach the sponsor is relatively passive, focusing on the collection and dissemination of information on plan structure, price, and quality. It is important, however, for the sponsor to enforce a defined contribution toward the premium because consumer choice on the basis of price is what drives cost consciousness and efficiency among health plans.

Most firms and purchasing alliances contract with a subset of available health plans in each region. Limiting the number of contracting plans reduces administrative costs, makes measurement and adjustment for risk selection easier, and creates an initial stage of competition in which health plans vie for contracts on the basis of premiums and performance.[20] This approach is particularly attractive when sponsors are unwilling to impose a defined contribution because it relies more on sponsor bargaining power than on cost-conscious consumer choice to motivate health plan performance. An extreme example of selective contracting is the Department of Defense's award of a five-year CHAMPUS contract to one plan in each region. Plans bid to provide supplementary services to the department's own health care system within one or more of its twelve regions. DOD represents 8 million enlistees, dependents, and retirees nationally. Sole-source contracts require beneficiaries to switch physicians when the sponsor switches health plan contracts unless the physicians and medical groups contract with the new health plan.

If selective contracting were applied to Medicare, sponsors could compete for beneficiaries based in part on their strategies for selecting and managing plans and providers. Not all health plans in a given market would be offered by all sponsors. Differences in plan choices among sponsors would create a perceived clash with the philosophy of equal treatment for all beneficiaries in the federal entitlement program. The reality of Medicare, in contrast to its rhetoric, is that beneficiaries face very different health care options depending on whether they have an employer's retiree program to fill in the gaps of the benefit package, whether they are eligible for Medicaid as well as Medicare, or whether they are personally responsible for paying an individual medigap insurance premium or directly paying for noncovered benefits. A significant difficulty with selective contracting is that it magnifies the information requirements for individual Medicare beneficiaries, who now would need to understand the differences among sponsors and the health plans they offered.

The private sector offers several examples of diverse strategies for creating plan competition. The Mercer National HMO group, which negotiates in twenty-seven cities nationwide for half a million people, typically selects four HMOs in each market. Participating businesses are required to offer all these plans to their employees. If a participating company had an HMO in place that was not selected by the group, it must freeze its enrollment in that plan. The AARP takes a similar tack, offering a select few medigap carriers to its members nationwide. The association is deploying this strategy for selecting

Medicare HMOs as well. Several coalitions with large employers, including the PBGH and the St. Louis Gateway Purchasing Association, allow any licensed HMO to participate in negotiations. Each participating employer then chooses plans to offer its employees.

Some employer-driven purchasing arrangements were formed because of a lack of health care competition in their marketplace. In Memphis and Houston, where there have been few managed care plans and little provider competition, employers decided to contract directly with hospitals and physician groups. In the Twin Cities, the earlier BHCAG exclusive contract with one plan produced a consolidation of the market as HMOs merged to bid for the sole-source contract. To undo this oligopoly as well as to create informed consumer choice of physicians, the BHCAG created a self-insured plan owned by the employer alliance rather than by a health plan. Business coalitions in rural states such as Iowa that do not have managed care and in states threatened by HMO oligopoly, such as California, are closely monitoring this approach.

Ground Rules for Competition

Ground rules need to cover criteria for contracting health plans, premium negotiations and enrollment, adjustment of payments to reflect differences in risk, and customer service and quality of care.

Criteria for Contracting Health Plans

Most sponsors that contract with HMOs use competitive bidding. Some use state licensure as a criterion for bidding. For Medicare beneficiaries federal qualification may be appropriate. The HCFA could take the best state licensure requirements and expand them to all states. This would ensure that consumer protections are upheld through financial, administrative, and quality assurance requirements without duplicating or creating new regulations.

In addition to establishing criteria for HMO participation in sponsored-choice programs, the HCFA could set ground rules to ensure that every beneficiary retained access to a fee-for-service plan. This would maintain the current extent of choice while subjecting the fee-for-service plan to a competitive market where costs and quality can be compared to those available through HMOs. The agency could require that all sponsors offer the standard Medicare fee-for-service plan as one option along with the HMO, PPO, and POS plans. Most purchasing pools in the public and private sectors today offer a range of plan types. In markets with high managed care penetration, PPOs have replaced indemnity carriers as the option that combines higher premiums with broader provider networks compared with HMO coverage. There is, however, no compelling reason to offer more than one indemnity plan or other broad access plan. National insurance carriers experienced in offering indemnity coverage typically contract with large employers to serve as third-party administrators for the self-insured broad access plans. By working with one national carrier, the firms' administrative burdens are reduced and the standardization of benefits and contributions across state lines is simplified.

For Medicare beneficiaries, sponsors could be allowed to select a private insurer or other third-party administrator for the indemnity plan or contract with the HCFA and its fiscal intermediaries. Alternatively, the HCFA could oversee the Medicare fee-for-service plan outside of the sponsored-choice framework, while determining contributions toward the fee-for-service and HMO plans in an unbiased manner. Maintenance of an indemnity option may be especially important for public and private sponsors with Medicare-eligible retirees who reside part of the year outside their home state. Reciprocity agreements among HMOs and other managed care plans is another potential solution to this snow bird phenomenon.

Premium Negotiations and Enrollment

Nearly every sponsor conducts an annual evaluation of the bidding health plans and then determines rates. Because of the long time horizon that sponsors need to develop open enrollment materials, health plans typically bid eighteen months before enrollment opens. Some sponsors conduct more frequent in-depth reviews of health plan financial records or audit the quality of care biannually. Many large employers offer Medicare risk plans to their retirees outside the calendar year cycle. This allows them to concentrate on communications to retirees apart from the busy season with active employees and early retirees. Medicare sponsors could consider conducting their negotiations off-cycle as well to avoid the health plans' busiest times of year.

Although employers prefer an annual lock-in enrollment cycle to ease administration, many health plans are not opposed to allowing Medicare beneficiaries to enroll and disenroll on a monthly basis. In the commercial health insurance market, people can disenroll when they expect not to use medical services and then reenroll when they anticipate use, but Medicare beneficiaries remain continuously insured. This mitigates the adverse selection problems potentially posed by monthly enrollment and disenrollment. Annual open enrollment and lock-in facilitates informed consumer choice because the sponsors can gather and publish comparative information on premiums, networks, quality, and patient satisfaction. This should be weighed against the advantages of beneficiaries' being able to respond quickly to dissatisfaction by switching plans. The ability to switch monthly is likely to be viewed by the elderly as a significant safeguard against the possibility of a mistake in health plan choice. The annual lock-in may discourage seniors from experimenting with managed care.

Many of the states that created small-group purchasing pools simultaneously enacted insurance underwriting practices for this market. Insurance carriers who participate in these pools, as well as competitors who do not, must guarantee issue and renewal for small businesses and limit clauses for not covering preexisting conditions. Most insurers still medically underwrite individuals; it would be important for the HCFA to disallow this for Medicare beneficiaries to avoid competition based on risk selection.

Most sponsors ask health plans to price a core benefit for HMO and non-HMO products. Some request prices for options to the core design, such as higher or lower copayments, carve-outs for mental health, or such extra services as alternative healing. The prices of these additional benefits are also negotiated by the sponsor. The greater the clarity in the definition of the product, the less room for creating competition based on biased selection and the easier it is for consumers to compare options.

Adjusting Payments to Reflect Differences in Risk

Much has been written about selection bias with respect to Medicare beneficiaries. This has also been an important issue for the small-group market, in which health plans avoided businesses perceived as high risk. Most of the sponsors that pool small firms use traditional rating practices to address differences in risk. These sponsors tend to operate in markets that have created uniform rules with respect to issuing and renewing insurance and medical underwriting. Adjusting enrollee premiums by age and family size, and in some instances allowing health plans to bid competitively in defined geographic areas, ensures that most of the differences in plans risk are taken into account. Large sponsors such as the FEHBP, CalPERS, and PBGH have successfully managed competition among health plans with little or no adjustment of payments for risk. One advantage of a multiple-sponsor framework, however, is that it permits experimentation in risk-measurement and risk-adjustment methods. The HIPC and BHCAG have developed the most innovative risk-adjustment methods for active employees; these could potentially be adapted for Medicare-eligible retirees.

Customer Service and Quality of Care

A key feature of a sponsored-choice structure is that consumers must be able to compare health plans on the basis of both price and nonprice criteria. Many sponsors currently demand extensive information from health plans concerning customer service, satisfaction, utilization rates for preventive services, network breadth, and techniques for managing use. This information helps sponsors select plans for contracting, improve consumer understanding of their options, and develop incentives for rewarding plans'performance improvement. The HCFA has begun to form partnerships with private sector organizations to develop new information on the quality of care in HMOs. In collaboration with the National Committee on Quality Assurance, the agency is developing Medicare-specific measurements for the HEDIS database. It is requiring health plans to administer the Consumer Assessment of Health Plans Survey, developed by the Agency for Health Care Policy and Research.

Conclusion

The Medicare risk-contracting program relies on three oversight mechanisms to protect beneficiaries and ensure quality of care. The HCFA uses regulatory powers to control benefit design, network breadth, grievance procedures, and related structural facets of HMO performance. Beneficiaries may use the tort liability system under traditional malpractice law and new legal doctrines to gain compensation in cases of negligent performance.[21] Most important, perhaps, beneficiaries may switch plans every month if dissatisfied. Each of these mechanisms for oversight and beneficiary protection has strengths, but each has significant limitations. Command and control regulation can impose severe penalties, up to and including contract termination, but is often slow moving, bureaucratic, and subject to political influence. Litigation can exact high damages and attract unfavorable publicity, but is unpredictable and uneven in its treatment of patients with similar problems. Plan switching is a quick and low-cost means of expressing dissatisfaction, but consumers may not understand the technical aspects of care and may quit only in response to minor problems in amenities or service. Moreover, health plans can profit from the disenrollment of particularly sick or demanding patients.

The private sector lacks the regulatory powers of government and relies instead on purchasing power to elicit improvements in price and performance from health plans. Medicare has taught private purchasers of health insurance many valuable lessons and developed many important methods to improve health care in traditional fee-for-service coverage. As it moves further into managed care, new problems present themselves and new responses are needed. Here Medicare has much to learn from public and private purchasing alliances. Through its risk-contracting program, Medicare has evolved from a public insurance company to a system of multiple competing health plans for senior citizens. The logical next step is to consider moving the risk-contracting program from a purchasing monopsony to a system of multiple purchasing sponsors.

Notes

1. Alain C. Enthoven, *Theory and Practice of Managed Competition in Health Care Finance* (North Holland, 1988); Henry J. Aaron and Robert D. Reischauer, "The Medicare Reform Debate: What Is the Next Step?" *Health Affairs*, vol. 14 (Winter 1995), pp. 8–30; Marilyn Moon and Karen Davis, "Preserving and Strengthening Medicare," *Health Affairs*, vol. 14 (Winter 1995), pp. 31–46; Stuart M. Butler and Robert E. Moffit, "The FEHBP as a Model for a New Medicare Program, *Health Affairs*, vol. 14 (Winter 1995), pp. 47–61; and Brian E. Dowd, Roger Feldman , and Jon Christianson, *Competitive Pricing for Medicare* (Washington: AEI Press, 1996).

2. C. Zarabozo, C. Taylor, and J. Hicks, "Medicare Managed Care: Numbers and Trends," *Health Care Financing Review*, vol. 17 (1996), pp. 243–62.

3. Mark R. Chassin and others, "Variations in the Use of Medical and Surgical Services by the Medicare Population," *New England Journal of Medicine,* vol. 314 (1986), pp. 285–90; John E. Wennberg and others, "Hospital Use and Mortality among Medicare Beneficiaries in Boston and New Haven," *New England Journal of Medicine*, vol. 321 (1986), pp. 1168–73; and W. P. Welch and others, "Geographic Variation in Expenditures for Physicians' Services in the United States," *New England Journal of Medicine*, vol. 328 (1993), pp. 621–27.

4. G. J. Stigler, "Price and Nonprice Competition," *Journal of Political Economy*, vol. 76 (1968), pp. 149–54; and J. C. Robinson and H. S. Luft, "Competition and the Cost of Hospital Care, 1972–1982," *Journal of the American Medical Association*, vol. 257 (1987), pp. 3241–45.

5. G. Riley and others, "Health Status of Medicare Enrollees in HMOs and Fee-for-Service in 1994," *Health Care Financing Review,* vol. 17 (1996), pp. 65–76; and Physician Payment Review Commission, *Annual Report to Congress* (Washington, 1996), chap. 15.

6. *Monopsony* means single buyer and contrasts with *monopoly* or single seller. Both monopsony and monopoly undermine the primary function of market contracting, which is to stimulate innovation and performance through competition.

7. General Accounting Office, *Health Insurance: California Public Employees Alliance Has Reduced Recent Premium Growth*, GAO/HRD-94-40 (1993).

8. A. C. Enthoven and S. J. Singer, "Managed Competition and California's Health Economy," *Health Affairs*, vol. 15 (Spring 1996), pp. 39–57.

9. James C. Robinson, "Health Care Purchasing and Market Change in California," *Health Affairs,* vol. 14 (Winter 1995), pp. 117–30.

10. H. H. Schauffler and T. Rodriquez, "Exercising Purchasing Power for Preventive Care," *Health Affairs*, vol. 15 (Spring 1996), pp. 73–85.

11. Enthoven and Singer, "Managed Competition and California's Health Economy"; and R. Figeroa, California HIPC, personal communication, October 30, 1996.

12. S. Shewry and others, "Risk Adjustment: The Missing Piece of Market Competition," *Health Affairs*, vol. 15 (Spring 1996), pp. 171–81.

13. J. B. Fowles and others, "Taking Health Status into Account When Setting Capitation Rates: A Comparison of Risk-Adjustment Methods," *Journal of the American Medical Association*, vol. 276, no. 16 (1996), pp. 1316–21.

14. S. Wetzell and A. Rubinow, Buyers Health Care Action Group, personal communication.

15. A. C. Enthoven, "Management of Competition in the FEHBP," *Health Affairs*, vol. 8 (Fall 1989), pp. 33–50.

16. S. M. Butler and R. E. Moffit, "The FEHBP as a Model for a New Medicare Program," *Health Affairs*, vol. 14 (Winter 1995), pp. 47–61.

17. Ibid.

18. Enthoven and Singer, "Managed Competition and California's Health Economy."

19. James C. Robinson, "Use and Abuse of the Medical Loss Ratio to Measure Health Plan Performance," *Health Affairs*, vol. 16 (July-August 1997), pp. 176–87.

20. James C. Robinson, "Health Care Purchasing and Market Changes in California," *Health Affairs*, vol. 14, no. 4 (1995), pp. 117–30.

21. W. M. Sage, "Health Law 2000: The Legal System and the Changing Health Care Market," *Health Affairs*, vol. 15 (Fall 1996), pp. 9–27.

Carve-outs for Medicare: Possible Benefits and Risks

Melinda Beeuwkes Buntin and David Blumenthal

IN RECENT YEARS, pressure has mounted on the Health Care Financing Administration to incorporate successful private sector health insurance strategies into the Medicare program. *Carve-outs,* which are generally separately administered specialized health care programs, are one of the strategies that experts have urged the HCFA to consider. Gail Wilensky, former administrator of the HCFA and current member of the Medicare Payment Advisory Commission, has advocated allowing risk-based carve-outs among other Medicare reforms that would increase the availability of managed care, remove barriers to managed care growth, and provide incentives for beneficiaries to choose cost-effective health plans.[1] Others have advocated using disease management programs for conditions such as diabetes that cause significant disability and mortality in the Medicare population. Specialists see carve-outs as a way to maintain their professional autonomy and their patient volume. Carve-outs appear promising because unlike some comprehensive risk-based contracts that give health plans incentives to avoid or undertreat the chronically ill, these programs can combine incentives to provide cost-effective care with the delegation of responsibility for care to companies that specialize in treating serious or chronic diseases.

Descriptions of selected carve-outs are placed throughout the text to elucidate important points. These examples were chosen because they are particularly relevant to the discussion of using carve-outs in the Medicare program. The first example, the ESRD Managed Care Demonstration, will be a carve-out run and financed by Medicare. The second, SalickNet, is the only capitated cancer care company now operating. It is also the only capitated carve-out company not associated with mental health care. The third example, the Community Medical Alliance, is a highly regarded health plan for the severely disabled and chronically ill. Its success is an example of how carve-outs can deliver high-quality, patient-centered care. Our last example, Control Diabetes Inc., was profiled because improving diabetes care in the Medicare program is a subject of particular interest to legislators and advocates.

What Is a Carve-out?

There is no standard definition of a carve-out. All definitions, however, assume that carved-out care will be separated administratively or legally from other care a patient receives. This means, at a minimum, that carve-outs rely on separate entities employing different providers to deliver care for carved-out conditions, procedures, benefits, or patient groups. Carve-outs also commonly use payment systems (including methods of sharing financial risk) and benefit designs different from those governing the rest of the care received by patients with carved-out conditions, services, or procedures.

One source of confusion in discussions of carve-outs is the terms *disease management* and *carve-in,* which are sometimes used interchangeably with carve-out. By our definition, disease management refers to a systematic effort to improve the management of a condition by applying appropriate guidelines, protocols, and information systems that are specifically designed for a given disease. As efforts to apply such techniques, disease management programs can be used by any provider with the capacity to employ them, including both carve-out companies and patients' usual or routine source of care. Nothing about disease management programs requires that they be used by administratively or legally separate providers.

The term *carve-in* is best used to connote a program of care for a particular disease, condition, or procedure that is organized within a single health plan to improve the quality or reduce the costs of care for the problem in question. A carve-in can range from the application of disease management programs by patients' primary care providers to the assignment of responsibility for care to a distinct group of providers who, nevertheless, are legally and administratively part of the health plan and accountable to the same management. This paper will not deal explicitly with the advantages or disadvantages of either disease management programs or carve-ins.

Types, Methods, and Approaches

Carve-outs vary in the scope or type of services, patients, or conditions covered, the extent of financial risk assumed by responsible entities, the extent of integration between the carve-out and other providers of care, and organizational characteristics of the carve-out entity. In addition, characteristics of the purchaser of carved-out services, the method of contracting between the purchaser and the carve-out, the contracting requirements imposed on it, and the way beneficiaries are enrolled distinguish carve-outs that may be more or less appealing from a policy perspective.

Scope of Services

The scope of services for which the carve-out assumes responsibility is one of its primary characteristics. The scope is the basis for the distinction between the two main types of carve-outs: specialty-benefit carve-outs and population carve-outs.

A *specialty-benefit carve-out* assumes responsibility for care associated with a specific procedure, disease, or condition. It does not assume responsibility for any other care that may be required by patients with the carved-out condition (table 4-2). Specialty-benefit carve-outs constitute the overwhelming majority of carve-outs. They usually involve formal contractual arrangements between an entity with responsibility for purchasing or providing care to a group of consumers and another independently managed corporate entity. The second entity, often an investor-owned company, may share financial risk for the costs of care in question. Specialty-benefit carve-outs have been used for years for vision and dental care, although the term *carve-out* was coined to describe the pharmacy and mental health and substance abuse specialty-benefit programs that have proliferated recently. Another example of a specialty-benefit carve-out is the Medicare Coronary Artery Bypass Graft Surgery (CABG) Demonstration, which is a carve-out for a specialty procedure.

The second type of carve-out referred to in discussions about the Medicare program is a *population carve-out*. A population carve-out connotes the admin-

Table 4-2. *Carve-outs and Scopes of Service*

Type of carve-out	Scope of services	Example
Specialty benefit	Education	Self-care and monitoring for diabetes
	Procedure	Coronary Artery Bypass Graft Demonstration
	Disease entity	Cancer care carve-out
	Group of related diseases	Behavioral health carve-out
Population	Comprehensive care	ESRD Manged Care Demonstration

istratively or legally separate provision of all the health care needed by patients who share a health-related characteristic. The Medicare End-Stage Renal Disease (ESRD) managed care demonstration is perhaps the best current example of a population carve-out (box 4-1). The unique feature of a population carve-out is that it permits a group with a special health care problem to receive integrated and comprehensive care, including primary and specialty care, from a single group or network of providers. This is, by definition, impossible under a specialty-benefit carve-out, which assumes responsibility only for the care required for a particular disease, condition, or procedure.

Financial Gains or Losses and Carve-out Risk

The extent of risk assumed is another distinguishing factor of carve-out entities or contractors. A carve-out contractor may assume no risk: for example it may receive simple fee-for-service compensation for health care services. It may assume minimal risk by receiving fee-for-service compensation with a withhold or other incentive payment, or it may assume modest risk by accepting partial capitation or capitation with risk corridors (which are a way of sharing profits and losses between a purchaser and a provider of services). A carve-out may also assume extensive risk: full capitation with no risk-gain corridor in the case of a contractor or full risk (insurance provision) in the case of a government program or health plan insuring a carved-out population. The extent of risk will affect the carve-out's incentives regarding risk selection, cost reduction, and quality improvement.

Integration of Care with the Primary Health Care Provider

Carve-outs can also be integrated to a greater or lesser extent with other entities caring for a patient, including, especially, primary health care providers. Obviously, the level of integration is most pertinent to specialty-benefit providers, who provide only a portion of any particular patient's care. For

Box 4-1.   *The End-Stage Renal Disease Managed Care Demonstration:*
A Population Carve-out

The ESRD managed care demonstration was congressionally mandated under the Social HMO legislation. Under the demonstration the HCFA awarded four contracts to health plans to develop and implement comprehensive managed care plans for ESRD patients. The plans chosen were either existing HMOs or subsidiaries of HMOs. One of the awardees, PacifiCare of California, later withdrew from the demonstration.

The demonstration is designed to test whether year-round open enrollment of Medicare's ESRD patients in managed care is feasible, integrated acute and chronic care services and case management for ESRD patients improves health outcomes, capitation rates reflecting patients' treatment needs increase the probability of patients' receiving kidney transplants, and the additional benefits offered by the awardees are cost effective.

The demonstration project is intended to be cost neutral for the Medicare program while offering expanded benefits to enrollees. The three awardees will bear the full risk for all the health care costs of those ESRD patients who choose to enroll. One capitation rate will be paid for patients receiving maintenance dialysis, a higher payment will be made for patients while they are undergoing a transplant, and a lower rate will be paid for those who have been successfully transplanted. The first and third types of payment will be risk adjusted based on a patient's age and whether diabetes was the cause of kidney failure. However, despite this risk adjustment there could be risk selection that increases costs for the Medicare program. Because the program is voluntary, enrollees may differ from nonenrollees in ways unaccounted for by the risk-adjustment system.

Awardees will have responsibility for all of the care of their enrollees. Health Options Inc. in southern Florida and Phoenix Healthcare of Tennessee intend to have nephrologists act as primary care physicians for enrolled ESRD patients. The remaining awardee, Kaiser of Southern California, will integrate the ESRD demonstration into its existing case management structure.

The awardees have one year to develop their capabilities, and the planned implementation date for enrollment to begin is October 1, 1997. They will then provide services for the remaining three years of the demonstration. The Institute for Health Policy at Brandeis University is providing technical assistance during the development period.

Source: "HCFA Information Fact Sheet on the ESRD Managed Care Demonstration," April 7, 1997.

reasons discussed later, the level of integration can affect the coordination of care and thus its overall quality. In principle, more integration is better than less. However, the optimal amount will depend on the scope and type of services provided under the carve-out. Carve-outs' levels of integration may range from no integration to full integration:

—No integration: contractor operates with minimal or no contact with other providers of health care, including primary care providers, for relevant patient population.

—Minimal integration: contractor is required or chooses to provide periodic reports to other providers, including primary care physicians (PCPs) concerning patients under contractor's care.

—Modest integration: contractor is required or chooses to provide detailed, frequent reports to other providers concerning patients under the contractor's care. Such reports include, at a minimum, the diagnoses, medications, pertinent laboratory results, and treatment plans of patients under the joint care of the contractor and other providers.

—Extensive integration: contractor chooses or is required to provide frequent detailed reports, to solicit PCPs' response and approval, and to ensure that the treatment plans of PCP and contractor are integrated and consistent over time.

—Full integration: contractor organizes or provides all care for persons with a given disease or characteristic.

Organizational Characteristics of the Contractor

The primary business, size, diversity of providers, and other organizational characteristics of a carve-out contractor may be relevant to the goals of the Medicare program. The primary business of the contractor could be the provision of a particular service, such as drug delivery or home health or nursing care, or comprehensive health care services, such as a managed care organization. The primary business of the contractor could affect its expertise, preferred methods of treatment, and ability to integrate with other providers. The size of the contractor, its provider network, its service area, and the number of consumers it serves are likely to influence the choice of providers available to beneficiaries, the ability of the contractor to bear risk, and the experience of the contractor in providing care. For example, an ESRD carve-out run by a physician group in conjunction with a local dialysis center would have a limited service area, panel of physicians, and ability to bear risk when compared with a carve-out offered by a statewide HMO, dialysis center chain, or group of hospitals.

Contracting Methods and Requirements

The purchaser of carved-out services, whether a health plan, employer, or public program, can affect the functioning of the carve-out through the methods used to select a contractor, the requirements placed on it, and its skill and investment in supervising and monitoring the care of the consumers on whose behalf the carve-out is purchased.

Purchasers have choices about the numbers of separate populations or conditions for which to seek carve-outs. For each condition or population the purchaser can decide to contract with multiple carve-out vendors or a single vendor. If multiple vendors are selected, purchasers encourage competition among them for enrollees. If a single carve-out is sought, there is competition among vendors for contracts.[2] These different contracting methods have very different implications for the ability of carve-outs to reduce risk selection among vendors, achieve integration and coordination of care, and contain costs or improve quality.

Purchasers also face choices in their ways of managing carve-outs once contracts are assigned. The purchaser can monitor the contractors heavily, include incentive payments in the contract for meeting goals, or rely more heavily on market competition to ensure that quality is maintained and costs contained. Health plans acting as purchasers may be better able to monitor the care that beneficiaries receive and ensure that it is properly coordinated with primary care and other specialty services than other purchasers who may have to rely more on correctly aligning the incentives of carve-outs.

For example, state Medicaid agencies have taken different approaches to contracting with mental health carve-out companies. Massachusetts has chosen to contract with a single vendor of mental health services. This vendor is paid, monitored, and evaluated by the state. In contrast, Connecticut has placed responsibility for mental health services on contracted HMOs, many of which subcontract to mental health carve-out companies. Each of these HMOs is responsible for monitoring and integrating with its contractor.

Beneficiary Choice

Purchasers of carve-outs can also choose the method of beneficiary enrollment. If there are multiple carve-out vendors of the same services, beneficiaries can be allowed to choose among them. Beneficiaries can also be given the option to choose not to enroll in a carve-out. If enrollment is mandatory, beneficiaries can be exempted if they choose to enroll in an HMO. Alternatively, all beneficiaries can be required to enroll in a single carve-out plan.

Options Available to the Medicare Program

Given the ways carve-outs and the methods of managing them can vary, the Medicare program would face a range of options in designing carve-out initiatives for its beneficiaries. To illustrate these options, figures 4-1 to 4-7 show

Figure 4-1.   *Current System*

Beneficiaries choose traditional Medicare or an HMO; HMOs contract with carve-out vendors at their discretion.

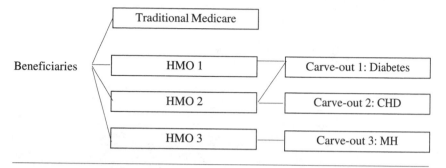

Figure 4-2.   *Beneficiaries Electing Traditional Medicare Are Directed to Carve-out Vendors for Certain Types of Care*

HCFA chooses a single carve-out vendor for certain types of care; all beneficiaries must receive care from that vendor; HMOs contract with carve-out vendors at their discretion.

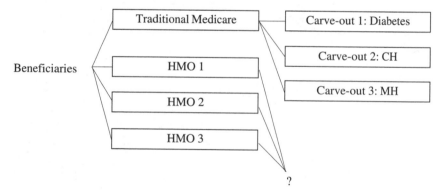

some of the alternatives that Medicare could pursue by varying just two characteristics of its approach: the methods of contracting it chooses and its requirements (or lack of requirements) for beneficiary choice. We focus on these aspects of any carve-out strategy because methods of contracting are readily controlled by the Medicare program, and requirements for beneficiary choice are likely to be politically sensitive. However, each of the options can vary along other dimensions, including extent of risk sharing by the contractor, integration required of contractors (especially for specialty-benefit carve-outs), and the scope of services for which the contractor is responsible. The carved-out diseases—diabetes, congestive heart failure (CH), and mental health (MH)—are chosen for illustrative purposes only.[3]

Figure 4-3. *Beneficiaries Electing an HMO Are Directed to Carve-out Vendors for Certain Types of Care*

HCFA chooses a single carve-out vendor for certain types of care; all HMO enrollees must receive care from that vendor; traditional Medicare beneficiaries are unaffected.

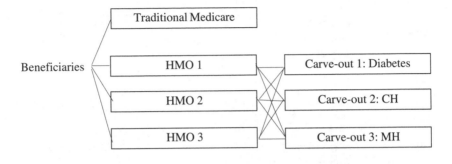

Figure 4-4. *All Beneficiaries Are Directed to Carve-out Vendors for Certain Types of Care*

HCFA chooses a single carve-out vendor for certain types of care; all beneficiaries receive certain types of care from a carve-out vendor regardless of whether they are enrolled in an HMO.

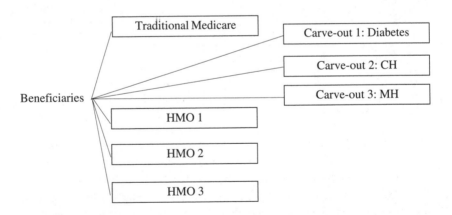

Potential Strengths of Carve-outs

The potential advantages of carve-outs are that they may offer a way to improve the quality of services delivered to Medicare beneficiaries, contain costs, and expand beneficiaries' choices. The potential drawbacks of carve-outs are discussed in the next section

Figure 4-5.   *Beneficiary Choice of Carved-out or Integrated Care*

HCFA chooses a single carve-out vendor for certain types of care; beneficiaries choose traditional Medicare, traditional Medicare plus carve-outs, or an HMO that may or may not use carve-outs.

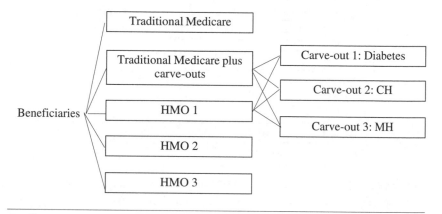

Figure 4-6.   *Population Carve-out*

HCFA chooses a single carve-out vendor for certain types of care for beneficiaries with certain diseases; beneficiaries with that disease receive all care through the carve-out vendor.

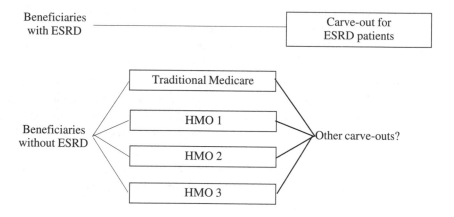

Implications for Quality of Care

Carve-outs may increase the quality of care received by Medicare beneficiaries. To begin with, they may increase the percentage of beneficiaries receiving needed specialty services within a risk-contracting environment. The tendency of managed care organizations to require patients to use primary care

Figure 4-7. *Variation on All Figures, Beneficiary Choice of Carve-out Vendor*

HCFA makes available more than one carve-out vendor for a type of care; beneficiaries choose from among two or more carve-out vendors for certain types of care.

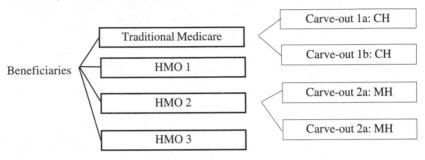

physicians for a large portion of their health care services, or at a minimum to get approval from a PCP before seeing a specialist (so-called primary care gatekeeping), has focused increased attention on the comparative quality of services provided by primary care and specialist physicians.[4] Substantial research now suggests the shortcomings of primary care physicians and the superior competence of specialty physicians in caring for particular chronic and acute conditions, including diabetes, cardiac disease, depression, diagnosis of malignant melanoma, ulcer disease caused by helicobacter pylori infection, and asthma.[5] Other studies have documented the tendency of primary care gatekeeping to reduce the use of specialists and to substitute primary care services.[6] Because of the increased expense associated with specialty care, less use of specialists is appealing.[7] If carve-outs facilitate access to specialty services for patients who will genuinely benefit from them, yet at the same time maintain pressures to contain costs, they could avert any quality problems created by gatekeeping arrangements. The carve-out models in figures 4-3 and 4-4 may be most attractive in this regard.

By facilitating access to specialty care, carve-outs could overcome a problem that has troubled some observers of managed care organizations: evidence that the organizations may have been less effective than traditional fee-for-service arrangements in treating chronic illnesses prevalent among Medicare beneficiaries. Studies by John Ware and colleagues demonstrate inferior outcomes of care for poor elderly and chronically ill patients treated in managed care as compared with fee-for-service settings.[8] Other studies suggest that unlike healthy patients, chronically ill patients are less satisfied in managed care arrangements than in fee-for-service settings.[9] To the extent that inferior outcomes or reduced satisfaction flows from barriers chronically ill patients face to receiving specialty care under traditional managed care arrangements, carve-outs could allow the benefits of risk contracting for healthy patients to be realized while circumventing the risks posed by managed care for chronically ill beneficiaries.

A second way carve-outs could improve quality of care would be to concentrate patients with certain complex problems under the care of a limited number of physicians or health care organizations. This channeling could permit purchasers or health plans to direct patients to providers with proven records of providing high-quality services. Carve-outs could also ensure that providers encounter sufficient numbers of patients to take advantage of the relationship between greater volume and improved outcome of care: in effect, the providers become so-called centers of excellence.[10] In several disease areas, including the care of HIV patients and the provision of specialized cardiac services, the number of cases treated by physicians and health care organizations has correlated strongly with better outcomes of care.[11] This volume-quality relationship may not exist for all conditions, however. Contracting and enrollment models that direct patients to a limited number of plans, such as those in figures 4-4 and 4-6, could improve quality of care for conditions in which such a volume-quality reinforcement exists.

The concentration of patients with particular illnesses in carve-out arrangements may have still another quality-improving effect. Organizations with responsibility for a particular illness may be more likely to develop strategies for disease management that have for some conditions, including asthma and diabetes, improved outcomes.[12] This potential effect might be observed in any of the carve-out models in the figures shown earlier.

A recent proposal for a Medicare demonstration put forward by the Center to Improve the Care of the Dying at George Washington University would also seem to show the potential for carve-outs to improve the quality of care, but in a different way.[13] People in the last phase of life are not well served by the traditional fee-for-service system. They may see too many specialists, receive too many medical interventions, and not receive basic advance care planning, palliative primary care, and social services. A carve-out for this population could improve care planning and primary care for the dying by channeling higher volumes of patients to organizations that have developed expertise in serving their needs and by trading specialty medical care for specialized supportive care.

Carve-outs as Cost-Containment Devices

Carve-outs may have advantages in containing the costs of care without compromising quality. First, by specializing in the management of a particular complex, costly disease or condition, vendors may become better at devising methods for containing the costs associated with it.[14] The argument here is closely analogous to the argument for the quality-enhancing effects of carve-outs: practice makes perfect. The likelihood that vendors will invest in such strategies, of course, will increase with the incentives provided to reduce costs. The incentives are easily developed through paying carve-outs on a risk-sharing basis (box 4-2).

Second, by virtue of the volume of care they provide for a particular condition, carve-outs may enjoy economies of scale for complex, high-cost procedures. Third, and perhaps most intriguing, they may improve the functioning of health care markets under circumstances in which providers share financial risks for the care of patients. The primary appeal of carve-outs in this regard is that they may reduce incentives and opportunities for risk selection on the part of competing health care providers.[15]

The potential deficiencies in market functioning that carve-outs may remedy are illustrated by the experience with risk contracting under the Medicare program. Medicare attempts to reduce its expenditures by paying health plans a fixed amount that is less than would have been paid in its traditional fee-for-service program. The fixed payment is intended to give health plans incentives to deliver cost-effective care, since they retain the difference between the fixed payment (plus any premiums charged to beneficiaries) and their actual costs. In addition, managed care organizations must compete for beneficiaries with the traditional Medicare program and other managed care providers in their region. Ideally, this competition should force them to become as efficient as possible.

However, managed care organizations can also increase their income in another, less socially efficient way by enrolling patients whose expected costs of care are less than the amounts Medicare pays. This practice is formally referred to as risk selection. Numerous studies have shown that Medicare HMOs do indeed enroll Medicare recipients who are healthier than average.[16] In fact, the Medicare risk program seems to cost the Medicare program about 5 percent more than the fee-for-service system because of the risk-selection phenomenon.

Carve-outs can mitigate the effects of risk selection and thereby capture the benefits of competitive markets. If high-cost enrollees or types of care are carved out, the health plan will have less incentive to engage in risk selection. A specialty-benefit carve-out would relieve the plan of the costs associated with a given disease or condition, thus reducing the difference in expected costs between chronically ill and healthy patients. A population carve-out would eliminate the sicker enrollees from the pool of potential enrollees altogether, leaving plans to compete for patients with less variable expected costs of care.

Box 4-2. *Carve-outs as Cost Containment Devices:*
          Salick Cancer Care

SalickNet Inc. is the only cancer care vendor that has signed a capitated contract with an HMO. In 1994 it contracted with the Physician Corporation of America, a financially troubled HMO with 140,000 members in the Miami area. The contract covers all cancer care, including radiology, chemotherapy, home therapy, hospice stays, and psychosocial counseling. Bone marrow transplants, however, are paid for separately, and children are not covered under the contract. SalickNet is paid between $6 and $7 per member per month for these services, although this amount could change as the company gains experience and opportunties arise for it to renew or renegotiate its contract.

SalickNet was able to sign a capitated contract because cancer care fits most of the criteria for a good carve-out. Cancer is expensive to treat and occurs with an appropriate frequency in the commercially insured population. As a disease it has a reasonably clear beginning and end. Primary care physicians willingly turn patients over to cancer specialists, although SalickNet's medical oncologists do deliver some primary care and its physicians have been given the authority to refer patients to providers in the HMO's network for noncancer care. Cancer care is complex and varies by condition, so there is the potential to improve care through guidelines and channeling high volumes of patients to a limited number of physicians.

Salick Health Care, the parent company of SalickNet, owns and manages 10 cancer centers, contracts with 200 oncologists, and also operates dialysis centers. Salick Health Care has developed a comprehensive information system that integrates all patient records, provides guidelines to physicians, and tracks treatment plans. It has also developed comprehensive treatment protocols by compiling existing guidelines, meta-analyses, and the results of Delphi method physician focus groups.

Initial data collected by SalickNet on patient satisfaction and process measures look very good when compared to national and Florida benchmark data. However, reliable data on survival and other outcome measures will not be available until late in 1997.

Although the initial data are promising, SalickNet has not yet managed to sign any other capitated contracts. It is, however, engaged in discussions with Cigna Health Plan of Arizona, Oxford Health Plan, and Humana.

Source: SalickNet Inc.

Enrolling patient populations with more similar health-related risks, managed care organizations might then compete more on the basis of quality and efficiency and less on the basis of which plan could attract or enroll a healthier group of beneficiaries.[17] This could improve the quality of care for all managed care enrollees if, for example, plans put fewer restrictions on access to specialty care or tried to demonstrate improved health outcomes to attract new members.

Reducing risk selection could also allow the Medicare risk program to realize the savings it was designed to achieve. Because the real costs of care for enrollees in managed care would be less variable (after carved-out costs and populations are excluded), the average prices paid by Medicare would be more likely to approximate the true costs incurred. Medicare would be less likely than under its current at-risk arrangements to pay more for managed care enrollees than these patients would have cost under the fee-for-service system.

In adjusting its payments to managed care organizations, Medicare would also benefit from carve-outs in another way. By separating the Medicare population into groups with similar risks, a carve-out strategy is likely to improve the technical capabilities of risk adjusters or severity indexes used by Medicare to adjust prospective payments to account for the expected costs of enrollees' health-related conditions. Because of the great variability in costs among Medicare enrollees, current risk adjusters have poor technical capabilities, predicting at most 10 to 20 percent of the variability in expected costs of care. Reducing the inherent variability in populations for which risk adjusters are developed is likely to improve the performance of these indexes. This would not only reduce plans' incentives to risk-select, but would also improve Medicare's ability to monitor and regulate residual efforts by plans to avoid high-cost patients.

Finally, a carve-out might promote competitive markets in high-cost illnesses (box 4-3). Paid a fair price to treat expensive illnesses and populations, enterprising providers might find financial opportunity in treating unhealthy patients. This would encourage them to compete for Medicare beneficiaries who under current at-risk arrangements are shunned by competing managed care providers.[18] Such competition should reduce the cost and increase the quality of care provided to carve-out populations.

Potential Weaknesses of Carve-outs under Medicare

The potential drawbacks of carve-outs include fragmentation of care and problems with contracting and cost containment.

Quality of Care

The foremost concern about quality of care in a program that uses carve-outs is that they may interfere with the quality of primary care received by patients. Ideally, primary care should have four attributes.[19] As the patient's usual source of initial contact with the health care system, it should be accessible. It should also be coordinated, comprehensive, and longitudinal. Coordina-

Box 4-3. *Community Medical Alliance: An HMO Exclusively Serving Disabled and Chronically Ill Patients*

The Community Medical Alliance (CMA) in Boston was the first HMO developed exclusively for severely disabled and chronically ill patients, including AIDS patients. CMA began in the Urban Medical Group, which specialized in caring for frail elders and the severely disabled. The Urban Medical Group pioneered the use of nurse practitioners as primary care providers for homebound or institutionalized patients and made care available twenty-four hours a day, seven days a week. Giving nurse practitioners the responsibility and time for case management, allowing them to make home visits, and offering continuous availability improved patient care and reduced hospitalizations and emergency room visits.

In 1992 CMA entered into a capitated agreement with the Massachusetts Medicaid Agency to care for severely disabled and end-stage AIDS patients. Dr. Robert Master, the medical director of CMA, felt strongly that capitation would give the organization the freedom to develop special systems of care. This included continuing its home care and case management programs and providing flexible durable medical equipment benefits.

The praise for CMA has been widespread. A review by the National Committee for Quality Assurance found that enrollee satisfaction was "impressively high" and that members of an enrollee focus group could not think of any way to improve CMA's services. Although an appropriate comparison group is difficult to find, a review concluded that CMA's patients seem to use more primary and home care and less inpatient and specialist care than comparable patients. CMA has been held up as a model program by the Department of Veterans Affairs, and Dr. Master was recently given an award by the Health Care Financing Administration for his work in the care of AIDS patients. In another indication of support, CMA was given approval to expand its service area to cover all severely disabled patients in Massachusetts (it currently serves only 300 patients in the Boston area). To finance this expansion, CMA merged with the Neighborhood Health Plan, another HMO in Massachusetts.

According to Dr. Master, CMA "would feel strongly that the plan-within-a-plan framework has strong applicability" to the Medicare program but that a specialty-benefit carve-out would "not fit the clinical reality" of severely disabled or chronically ill patients. He hopes that partnership with the Neighborhood Health Plan will demonstrate that the plan-within-a-plan concept is "the next generation of capitated plans."

Sources: Telephone interview with Robert Master; and Master and others, "The Community Medical Alliance: An Integrated System of Care in Greater Boston for People with Severe Disability and AIDS," *Managed Care Quarterly,* vol. 4, no. 2 (1996), pp. 26–37.

tion allows for the integration of information and diagnostic and therapeutic plans among all caregivers involved. Comprehensiveness means that a broad range of needed services is available at one site. Longitudinality is the development of a continuous relationship between a patient and a single provider over time. Primary care with these attributes, particularly accessibility and longitudinality, has beneficial effects on patients' health status and satisfaction with care, and it reduces health care expenditures.[20] Similarly, lack of coordination and longitudinality seems to increase the risk of problems with quality. For example, the greater the number of physicians prescribing medications for elderly patients, the greater the possibility that they will be given inappropriate combinations of drugs and will be admitted to a hospital because of noncompliance with drug regimens.[21]

Carve-outs could undermine primary care by reducing both the coordination and the longitudinality of these services. The requirement that patients with particular conditions receive their care from providers or organizations that are administratively separate from primary care physicians and not accountable to them creates barriers to coordinating the management of care. Problems of coordination may be overcome in theory through better communication across organizational boundaries, but this will certainly require added administrative effort and expenditure. By introducing additional providers who care for problems that primary care physicians might otherwise manage, carve-outs also reduce the longitudinality of services.

In addition, some studies suggest that outcomes of care for a number of chronic illnesses, including diabetes, chronic obstructive pulmonary disease, and hypertension, do not differ significantly when primary care physicians as opposed to specialists are in charge.[22] If such care were carved out, there would be costly duplication of services because primary care physicians would not be able to manage the care in the context of regular visits for checkups or medical complaints. All types of carve-outs except the population carve-out model shown in figure 4-6 could have a deleterious effect on the coordination, comprehensiveness, and longitudinality of primary care.

Problems with Contracting and Cost Containment

The ability of carve-outs to save money for the Medicare program is far from certain. The achievement of savings could be frustrated by the administrative, political, and technical problems likely to arise in the implementation of any carve-out program.

Carve-outs may reduce risk selection by Medicare managed care providers, but it is also possible that they will merely transfer the problem from the general Medicare market to the new carve-out market. Although carving out high-risk patients may create groups with similar expected costs of care, variability will persist.[23] Thus some opportunity for risk selection will remain and will be particularly a problem within carve-out markets, where the consequences of enrolling higher-than-average risks could be especially painful to vendors. Vendors sharing financial risk will have the incentive to enroll patients with lower-than-expected costs for their group.

To prevent this problem, Richard Frank, Thomas McGuire, and Joseph Newhouse advocate "competition for contracts not enrollees."[24] Under this structure Medicare would require that all beneficiaries with carved-out conditions in any given market receive care from a single vendor. The benefits of competition would be realized through competitive bidding in which the purchaser (Medicare or its designee) would choose the plan with the best proposal, based on price and quality. This form of contracting and enrollment is shown in figures 4-3 and 4-5.

The problems with such a strategy are that it requires limiting choice on the part of Medicare enrollees and it may impede the development of truly competitive markets for carve-out services. Medicare patients have never been receptive to limits on their choice of a provider, and it is not clear they would accept such limits for treatment of the chronic conditions with which so many of them live. Competing for contracts rather than enrollees has the further problem that once a particular contractor has won the business in a particular area, there will be significant costs associated with awarding the contract to an alternative vendor in the future. The prospect of losing a contract will reduce vendors' incentives to invest in care, including preventive services, with distant payoffs. Picking a new vendor will also require severing physician-patient relationships and will impair coordination and longitudinality of care. As result, Medicare will encounter disincentives to put the carve-out business out to bid and could become captured by a particular vendor in a particular market.

The potential for carve-outs to improve the technical ability of risk-adjustment systems may also face problems. The two most promising risk-adjustment systems being considered by the HCFA for the at-risk HMO program are based on administrative data because such data are relatively inexpensive to collect. However, it is not yet certain that risk-adjustment methods for carve-outs based on these data will prove significantly superior to current methods.[25] Much of the potential for improving risk adjusters may lie in the use of clinical data that are unique to the conditions in question. Unfortunately, collecting such data would likely be very expensive.

Carve-outs face other administrative problems, many of which could be called "boundary issues" because they result from the difficulty of drawing lines and assigning responsibility efficiently and fairly between different organizations caring for the same patients.

To implement any carve-out, including the single-vendor variety, Medicare would have to be able to define exactly which conditions, services, and treatments would be covered. Vagueness will create opportunities for taking advantage of the system. For example, diabetics often have concomitant problems with other organ systems, including nerves, eyes, kidneys, and heart. A diabetes carve-out would have every incentive to interpret its responsibility for these other ailments as narrowly as possible so as to avoid their huge costs. At the same time, failure to control blood sugar can aggravate these conditions, especially over the long term. Diabetes carve-outs are likely to insist that PCPs or other carve-outs care for these conditions, while physicians will want carve-outs to accept some of the responsibility. Adjudicating such disputes could keep a new bureaucracy of Medicare officials busy for decades. Patients could find themselves bounced between finger-pointing providers.

The use of population carve-outs, in which vendors take responsibility for all care of patients with particular illnesses (such as end-stage renal disease) is a potential solution to the boundary problem. However, population carve-outs have their own boundary issues. Under some capitated arrangements, they create incentives for providers to move patients too readily into carve-outs, thereby costing Medicare money and unnecessarily increasing fragmentation of care.

Consider a patient who straddles the boundary between being in good health and having a chronic condition such as early heart disease, early diabetes, or mild rheumatoid arthritis. Under a system in which a carve-out vendor was paid a capitation or management fee for each patient, both the mainstream provider and the carve-out have incentives to define the patient as sicker than he or she may really be, if it allows the condition to be carved out. The PCP escapes the costs of care associated with this condition, and the carve-out picks up a patient whose expenditures are likely to be low compared to the payment the vendor receives. Paying the carve-out on a fee-for-service or per-eligible-beneficiary basis would minimize the contractor's incentives to manipulate the system in this way, but would sacrifice cost-constraining incentives or place greater financial risk on the contractor. The proposed Medicare end-of-life demonstration described earlier would fall into this category because of the difficulty of defining when a patient is in the last stage of life. This example demonstrates how critically interwoven carve-out enrollment and payment systems are and how carefully they must be designed.

Administrative solutions may be devised for many boundary issues and other implementation problems that could jeopardize the feasibility or cost-reducing potential of carve-outs. But if the solutions become complex, they will also become costly and could defeat the purpose for which carve-outs are created. Administrative costs of existing managed behavioral health carve-outs are estimated at 10 to 15 percent of benefit costs.[26] Imagine the administrative costs likely to be incurred by a patient who is subject to three or four carve-outs simultaneously. Imagine also the administrative costs of achieving the necessary integration of information among multiple vendors.

In addition, administering and monitoring vendors would be new responsibilities for the HCFA and its fiscal intermediaries. New regulations would be required for the agency to implement carve-outs outside a demonstration project. Choosing a single vendor for a service or mandating enrollment in a carve-out would be a new, difficult, and potentially controversial task for the agency to perform. The HCFA's fiscal intermediaries would have to track enrollment and disenrollment and analyze claims to ensure that Medicare did not pay for services under the jurisdiction of carve-out vendors. All these tasks are possible, but they are very different from the tasks Medicare administrators perform now.

Other Problems

Other problems with carve-outs include segregating vulnerable populations and sharing confidential patient information between health organizations. Placing only the sickest and most vulnerable Medicare beneficiaries in a relatively untested type of health plan could be dangerous because the beneficiaries may be least able to detect, report, or fight problems with quality of care. The requirement that health care organizations share information to coordinate care between carve-outs and mainstream vendors also multiplies the number of people and organizations with access to confidential patient information. This is likely to be an increasingly sensitive issue at a time when privacy is already a concern for many patients.

Experiences with Carve-outs

After examining the theoretical strengths and weaknesses of carve-outs, it would be useful to examine how they have performed. Unfortunately, little is known about their performance, especially about those that are relevant to the Medicare program.

What Services Are Carved Out?

Dental and vision care have been carved out of general health plans for decades, and pharmacy and mental health carve-outs have become commonplace in recent years. Other carve-outs are being developed as part of the disease management movement, although few have begun delivering services.

Developers of these specialty-benefit plans expect that private employers and managed care organizations will be their primary customers. The diseases targeted, therefore, are those that affect the employed population, have costs that are rising faster than general health care costs, interfere with job performance, and are likely to respond well to increased management. Centers of excellence for heart surgery and organ transplants have sprung up virtually nationwide (although depending on the structure of these programs they may or may not qualify as carve-outs by our definition).

Some experience is also accumulating with carve-outs for publicly insured populations. Medicaid agencies, seeking to enroll high-cost disabled beneficiaries in managed care, have encouraged the growth of specialized health plans to serve patients with exceptional needs. The Medicare program has itself embarked on a population-specific managed care plan for ESRD patients and is expanding its program of centers of excellence for coronary artery bypass graft surgery to cover more cardiac procedures and joint replacement (see box 4-1).

Who Uses Carve-outs?

Large and sophisticated purchasers are the dominant clients of carved-out health care services. These include private employers such as Dow Chemical and Delta Airlines and state employee health plans, some of which use managed behavioral health carve-outs and centers of excellence. An exception is the giant California Public Employees Retirement System (CalPERS), which believes that carve-outs offer it nothing that it cannot get by working with contracted HMOs and will cause confusion and loss of coordination of care for its beneficiaries.[27] Medicaid agencies and the Civilian Health and Medical Program of the Uniformed Services (CHAMPUS) have contracted with managed behavioral health companies.

Accounts in the literature on business and employee benefits would lead one to think that carve-outs and disease management programs are widespread. But although many of these programs are under development, few other than managed behavioral health and managed pharmacy programs have actually been sold to employers or managed care companies.

The prevalence of managed behavioral health care plans is well documented. Towers Perrin estimated that in April 1995 about 80 percent of Fortune 500 companies carved out employee assistance services, mental health care, or both.[28] Richard Frank, Jacob Glazer, and Thomas McGuire have reported that fourteen state employee health plans and twelve state Medicaid agencies are using MBHC.[29] Monica Oss calculated that 53 million patients were enrolled in MBHC programs and that 20 million to 25 million of them were in risk-based carve-outs.[30] Another source reports that 44 percent of employers with more than 20,000 employees offer a separate preferred provider organization for mental health care. However, many companies that offer carved-out mental health care offer it as an option, not a requirement, for their employees.[31]

Pharmacy benefits programs and centers of excellence are also widespread. There are 107 pharmacy benefit managers operating in the United States, a dozen of which serve more than 10 million clients each.[32] Thirty state employee health plans use vendors for pharmacy benefits and discounted pharmacy networks, and seven carve out pharmacy benefits on a cost-plus or capitated basis. Twenty-one states use centers of excellence for high-cost procedures such as transplants.[33] Sixty-six percent of very large employers offer prescription drug plans.[34] Although pharmacy programs and centers of excellence are not what proponents of carve-outs for Medicare envision, they are among the few types currently serving large numbers of beneficiaries.

A recent survey by William Mercer, Inc., showed that 77 percent of employers planned to install a disease management program.[35] Whether these plans will materialize and whether they will involve true carve-outs as we have defined them remains to be seen.

How Successful Are Carve-outs?

Many employers report that they consider their carve-outs successful, but there are few rigorous evaluations. Here again, information is limited almost entirely to behavioral health and pharmacy carve-outs.

Employers claim that behavioral health carve-outs have saved them large amounts of money. The National Railway Labor Conference says it has saved $38 million a year. U.S. West boasts of saving 25 percent of what it used to spend on behavioral health without reducing covered benefits. The Orange County, Florida, school board cut mental health spending in half, and the Dow Chemical manufacturing division reduced mental health spending from $5.2 million to $1.4 million in five years.[36] A CHAMPUS behavioral health carve-out demonstration program had costs that were nearly one-third below what was expected, and the carve-out program was subsequently expanded nationwide.

Some pharmacy benefit managers and their clients report that the rate of growth in their pharmacy costs has slowed. There is, however, little public information about the cost savings or outcomes achieved by these companies.[37]

Despite these claims, employee benefits analysts have decidedly mixed views of these carve-outs. Kirk Strosahl and Michael Quirk of the Group

Health Cooperative of Puget Sound argue that "carving out mental health as a separate benefit leads to the provision of care only for the minority of people willing to seek specialty mental health service."[38] Consultant Richard Heller worries that carve-outs will fail to meet employee mental health needs and lead eventually to higher employer costs.[39] In addition, most benefits analysts warn that too many carve-outs are certain to cause problems and that communication and coordination are the keys to successful programs because mental and physical health problems are often coincident. There are also some signs that employers may be disappointed in the performance of carve-outs, which may be increasing indirect costs and not providing the savings the employers had anticipated.

In summarizing the evidence on the success of behavioral health carve-outs, Richard Frank, Thomas McGuire, and Joseph Newhouse noted that published case studies of mental health carve-outs are a nonrepresentative sample, may be biased by regression to the mean, and rely largely on before and after comparisons. Overall, however, they say it is "reasonable to conclude that cost savings result from risk contracting and managed behavioral health care, but the magnitude of those savings is highly uncertain, as are the determinants of those savings."[40] It should also be noted that most studies have been of employers and other purchasers who have given exclusive contracts to vendors, which can have cost and risk-selection advantages over awarding multiple contracts.[41]

Some information is available concerning the performance of procedure-specific carve-outs. Delta Airlines contracts with six centers to provide cardiac valve or bypass surgery, angioplasty, cardiac catheterization, pacemaker insertion, and heart transplants.[42] The centers are paid 35 percent less than their standard rates, and Delta employees are given strong incentives to use them (they must pay a $2,000 deductible if they wish to be treated outside the network). So far, Delta claims the program has saved it $20 million. The Medicare CABG demonstration project was very similar and is also considered successful. In fact, it is currently being expanded, and new centers of excellence will provide hip and knee replacement and additional cardiac services. These centers, like the CABG centers, will receive a negotiated bundled payment.

Other employer carve-outs and disease management programs are still in development. One journalist found that "interviews with about 100 organizations involved in disease management revealed that few of these programs have been sold or developed to the point of having outcomes measures in place."[43] An example of one disease management company that has been providing services for a year and hopes to sign at-risk contracts in the future is provided in box 4-4.

Box 4-4. *Control Diabetes Inc. Hopes to Sign At-Risk Contracts*

Control Diabetes Inc., an independent subsidiary of Eli Lilly, is one of a limited number of disease management companies that is actually delivering services, but its attempts to sign capitated contracts with managed care organizations have been unsuccessful.

Control Diabetes has offered intensive outpatient education to diabetic HMO enrollees for more than a year. The HMOs that contract with the company refer patients to it for an individual assessment, ten hours of training in a classroom, including training on how to monitor and control their own insulin levels, and instruction from dietitians. Patients are then followed up after one month and six months to ensure compliance. Control Diabetes also offers a complete line of supplies for diabetics, a range of special programs for those with gestational diabetes and those with varying levels of proficiency with self-management, meal planning, and use of an insulin pump. The company also provides a phone number for participants to call when they have questions.

Like SalickNet, Control Diabetes has promising initial data on costs and outcomes. In its first year of operation, it saw 3,000 patients as part of its thirty contracts with HMOs covering 40 million people. Average hemoglobin levels, hospitalizations, emergency room visits, and days of lost work all dropped. The company's before and after comparison of hospitalizations and emergency room visits among patients who received training showed reductions of 45 and 58 percent, respectively. Annual per patient costs of diabetes management dropped by 9 percent after the cost of the training ($580), increased outpatient visits, and increased amounts of drugs and supplies were factored in.

The satisfaction rate among Control Diabetes patients was 95 percent, and three of its HMO clients have presented the Control Diabetes program to the HCFA as one of the innovative strategies that they are using for their Medicare risk enrollees (30 to 40 percent of Control Diabetes patients are Medicare risk enrollees).

Still, Control Diabetes is not finding HMOs willing to sign at-risk contracts for diabetes care and training. David Lance, the company's vice president for sales and marketing, thinks this is because HMOs want to keep any savings from reduced utilization for themselves. But it may be that because diabetes is associated with so many comorbidities and can be managed by primary care physicians, it simply does not fit the criteria for a good carve-out program. Lance intends, however, to keep looking for HMOs interested in at-risk contracting and may even take his programs directly to employers.

Telephone interview with David Lance; and Control Diabetes Inc..

Evaluation of Carve-outs

The attractiveness of carve-outs for the Medicare program and its beneficiaries must be evaluated based on their costs, the quality of care they would deliver, and their long- and short-term effects on competition in the rest of the

Medicare program. The main difficulty with evaluating carve-outs in these ways is that so little is known about them. And much of the experience to date may not be applicable to the Medicare program.

The most common specialty-benefits carve-outs are, unfortunately, those that are the least relevant to Medicare in its current form. Vision and dental programs cannot be used by Medicare because routine vision and dental care are not covered. Outpatient drugs are also not covered, making pharmacy benefits managers a less useful model than they might otherwise be. Some of these benefits are now included, of course, under the package of services offered by at-risk Medicare contractors. Thus the private sector and Medicaid experiences with these benefits, such as they are, may prove more relevant to Medicare in the future.

Mental health services are covered by Medicare, but the mental health needs of Medicare beneficiaries differ from those of the rest of the population. For example, dementia is a problem that does not fit neatly into a mental health carve-out. Many of the mental complaints of the elderly are the effects of medication or illnesses such as poststroke depression that are far less prevalent in younger people, making projections difficult. In addition, many elderly patients may be unwilling to seek specialty care for their mental illnesses.[44] Mental health is not now a high-cost program for Medicare and so may not be the most attractive candidate for initial experimentation.

Models do exist of carve-outs of diseases prevalent in the Medicare population such as cancer and diabetes (boxes 4-2 and 4-4), and the ESRD demonstration shows promise (box 4-1). However, decisions about contracting for these carve-outs would have to be governed more by the issues we have raised than by actual information on the carve-outs' performance.

How then, should the Medicare program evaluate potential carve-outs? It is easier to define poor candidates than good ones. All else equal, carve-outs should avoid conditions that are low cost, simple to care for in a primary care setting, common, associated with comorbid conditions, insensitive in terms of cost and quality to the volume of patients that providers see with the conditions, and have a gradual onset that is difficult to pinpoint.

The reasoning behind these recommendations is straightforward. Low-cost conditions are unlikely to be factored into risk-selection efforts by managed care organizations, so carving them out does not confer benefits associated with reduced risk selection. Carving out conditions whose care is simple or well within the proven abilities of primary care providers will not produce the quality benefits that carve-outs may confer by facilitating access to specialists' services under managed care. Very common conditions, if carved out, would require that very large numbers of Medicare beneficiaries participate, increasing the administrative costs and the potential for fragmenting care within the Medicare population. Illnesses that are very likely to be associated with interacting comorbid conditions will be highly susceptible to the boundary issues described earlier and thus also to be associated with costly requirements for monitoring and regulation and with patient dissatisfaction. A potential benefit of carve-outs is that they may channel large numbers of patients to select providers, which takes advantage of volume-related effects on quality and cost. If there are no volume-related effects, carve-outs will be less attractive. Finally, carve-outs of conditions with gradual, subtle onset will be susceptible to vendor attempts to shift responsibility to other providers.

Once a good candidate for carve-out has been defined, the method of contracting and beneficiary enrollment must be chosen. The strengths and weaknesses of each of the contracting and enrollment strategies pictured in figures 4-1 to 4-7 are summarized in table 4-3. Models 4-4 and 4-6 may have the greatest advantages.

Model 4-4 requires that all Medicare beneficiaries in each market, including those enrolled in at-risk plans, receive care for the carved-out condition through a single contractor. This is the model for contracting and enrollment referred to as competing for contracts as opposed to competing for enrollees. The model has the advantage of potentially reducing risk selection by Medicare managed care providers while also forestalling the risk selection likely to develop among competing contractors. Also, the number of beneficiaries using the carve-out could be predicted fairly accurately, and the volume of beneficiaries could allow the contractor to bear a significant degree of risk and to achieve price discounts.

Model 4-6, the population carve-out, also has advantages over the other models. It would achieve all of the advantages of model 4-4 and would avoid the disadvantages caused by lack of integration between primary and specialty care. Opportunities for displacing costs between mainstream and carve-out providers would be minimized if the number of carve-outs were limited.

Nevertheless, both models have limitations, some of which have already been discussed. Both, for example, would be problematic if more than one disease were carved out. ESRD seems an attractive candidate for a carve-out, at least to the extent that it has few of the properties that a bad prospect would have. (The one exception is that its onset is subtle and often prolonged, but that problem can be managed because there are well-defined, easily monitored, objective indicators of the progress of renal failure, such as serum creatinine. Thus, defining laboratory criteria for eligibility for a carve-out is technically feasible.) However, an ESRD carve-out might run into problems if the Medicare program were to create additional carve-outs for such likely prospects as

Table 4-3. *Evaluation of Carve-out Models*

Criterion	*Model 4-1: current system*	*Model 4-2: traditional Medicare enrollees directed to single-vendor carve-outs*	*Model 4-3: Medicare HMO enrollees directed to single-vendor carve-outs*	*Model 4-4: all Medicare enrollees directed to single-vendor carve-outs*	*Model 4-5: enrollee choice of Medicare or HMO with or without carve-outs*	*Model 4-6: population carve-out*	*Model 4-7: beneficiary choice of multiple carve-out vendors*
Efficiency							
Risk selection							
Reduces incentive, opportunity for risk selection between traditional Medicare and carve-outs or HMOs	Baseline	?	—	+	—	+	?
Reduces incentive, opportunity for risk selection between carve-outs and HMOs	Baseline	n.a.	+	+	?	+	-
Difficulty in pricing carve-out due to boundary issues	Baseline	-	-	-	-	-	—
Potential for cost reduction	Baseline	+	?	+	-	+	?
Quality							
Primary care quality	Baseline	-	-	-	-	+	—
Disease-specific technical care	Baseline	+	+	+	+	+	+
Institutional capability for integration	Baseline	-	+	n.a.	+	+	?
Beneficiary choice							
Enrollment choice for those with carved-out condition or disease	Baseline	-	+	-	+	-	?

Note: - some detrimental effect; — large detrimental effect; + some positive effect; ++ large positive effect; ? effect could be positive or negative; n.a. not applicable.

heart disease, diabetes, high blood pressure, peripheral vascular disease, mental and behavioral health, and hyperlipidemia. All these conditions (including depression) are common complications of end-stage renal disease, and they interact to make ESRD the costly and challenging condition it is. Treatments and payments for them would have to be continually allocated among contractors.

Judgments and Conclusions

The general principle that Medicare should take advantage of successful private sector innovations such as carve-outs is certainly a sound one. There is, however, an equally sound principle that Medicare's decisions concerning the adoption of new health care strategies should be based on evidence that these strategies will promote the distinctive objectives of the program.

If Medicare does proceed with carve-out experiments, as it has with ESRD, the current plan to begin with a population carve-out as opposed to a specialty-benefit carve-out seems well advised, given our analysis of the risks and benefits of alternative options. The major problem with the ESRD demonstration program is that enrollment will be voluntary. Thus it may attract an atypical group of patients, which will limit the generalizability of its findings. Furthermore, it is unclear whether voluntary population carve-outs can succeed in addressing the risk-selection problems that carve-outs are partly intended to ameliorate.

There would almost certainly, however, be very real political difficulties with the mandatory enrollment of beneficiaries in a carve-out, especially if they are not given a choice of vendors. Unfortunately, those models judged most likely to succeed in improving risk selection and achieving savings by channeling high volumes of patients to at-risk providers (models 4-5 and 4-7) feature mandatory enrollment in a single plan.

The problems with the use of carve-outs would not just be political. The promise of the strategy is limited by the administrative difficulties and threats to quality of care associated with multiple carve-outs for potentially overlapping illnesses. The Health Care Financing Administration would have to develop capitation payments and quality standards for new types of plans when its current payment methodologies and standards are being questioned. Overall, given the problems they could create and the paucity of evidence concerning the record of carve-outs, their widespread adoption would seem premature.

Nevertheless, given the current interest in the use of carve-outs in Medicare, some experiments seem likely. And indeed, careful experimentation with them for particular illnesses that are important and prevalent in the Medicare population and that meet other criteria for a potentially successful program would seem reasonable. We have outlined the criteria for a successful Medicare carve-out. Those are that

—the carved out condition is relatively high-cost;

—the condition is best cared for in a specialized setting;

—the condition is not associated with interacting comorbid conditions;

—the condition is best treated, in terms of cost and quality, by a provider who sees a high volume of patients with it; and

—the condition does not have a gradual onset that is difficult to pinpoint.

Any carve-out that does not meet all these criteria would run the risk of creating more problems than it would solve.

What kind of carve-outs might fulfill these requirements? Although it was beyond our scope to apply these criteria rigorously to specific diseases or conditions, several would seem to be good candidates. One attractive program might be solid organ transplantation (likely to be relatively common among disabled Medicare beneficiaries) for which the monitoring of immunosuppression requires the intimate involvement of transplant physicians in primary care. Another possibility would be the care of certain cancers that have chronic courses or very rapid and predictable ones. Finally, if a way to reasonably define the onset of the last phase of life were developed, a population carve-out for those at the end of life would likely meet the other criteria for a good carve-out.

It is important to note that good carve-outs for Medicare may not be the same as those for which the private sector has chosen to begin carve-out initiatives. In particular, because of the differing causes of behavioral health problems in the Medicare and general population, it may not be desirable for Medicare to start with the adoption of mental and behavioral health carve-outs.

The cautious experimental approach to adopting carve-outs that we have outlined is likely to maximize the chance that their benefits can be captured and their risks, both political and to the patient, minimized. However, a cautious approach will also make it unlikely that carve-outs will realize significant short-term savings or improvements in the current problems of adverse selection in the at-risk Medicare market.

Notes

1. Gail Wilensky, "Bite-Sized Chunks of Health Care Reform: Where Medicare Fits In," in Henry J. Aaron, ed., *The Problem That Won't Go Away: Reforming U.S. Health Care Financing* (Brookings, 1996).

2. Richard Frank, Thomas McGuire, and Joseph Newhouse, "Risk Contracts in Managed Mental Health," *Health Affairs,* vol. 14 (Winter 1995), pp. 50–64.

3. The format of these figures is due to Richard Frank, Jacob Glazer, and Thomas McGuire, Harvard Medical School, September 1996.

4. Marsha R. Gold and others, "A national survey of the arrangements managed-care plans make with physicians," *New England Journal of Medicine,* vol. 333 (1995), pp. 1678–83; and Jerome P. Kassirer, "Access to specialty care," *New England Journal of Medicine,* vol. 331 (1994), pp. 1151–53.

5. For diabetes see Kevin A. Peterson, "Diabetes care by primary care physicians in Minnesota and Wisconsin," *Journal of Family Practice,* vol. 38 (1994), pp. 361–67; E. R. Ettinger and others, "Referral patterns of primary care physicians for eye care," *Journal of the American Optometric Association,* (1993), 468–70; and Joseph C. Konen and others, "Symptoms and complications of adult diabetic patients in a family practice," *Archives of Family Medicine,* vol. 5 (1996), pp. 135–45. For cardiac disease see Theodore L. Schreiber and others, "Cardiologist versus internist management of patients with unstable angina: treatment patterns and outcomes, *Journal of the American College of Cardiology,* vol. 26 (1995), pp. 577–82; Peter D. Friedmann and others, "Differences in generalists' and cardiologists' perceptions of cardiovascular risk and the outcomes of preventive therapy in cardiovascular disease, *Annals of Internal Medicine,* vol. 124 (1996), pp. 414–21; Steven J. Borowsky and others, "Effect of physician specialty on use of necessary coronary angiography," *Journal of the American College of Cardiology,* vol. 26 (1995), pp. 1484–91; and John Z. Ayanian and others, "Knowledge and practices of generalist and specialist physicians regarding drug therapy for acute myocardial infarction," *New England Journal of Medicine,* vol. 331 (1994), pp. 1136–42. For depression see Kenneth B. Wells and others, "Detection of depressive disorder for patients receiving prepaid or fee-for-service care. Results from the Medical Outcomes Study," *Journal of the American Medical Association,* vol. 262 (1989), pp. 3298–3302. For malignant melanoma see Gerbert B. and others, "Primary care physicians as gatekeepers in managed care. Primary care physicians' and dermatologists' skills at secondary prevention of skin cancer," *Archives of Dermatology,* vol. 132 (1996), pp. 1030–38; and A. Mark Fendrick, Richard A. Hirth, and Michael E. Chernew, "Differences between generalist and specialist physicians regarding Helicobacter pylori and peptic ulcer disease," *American Journal of Gastroenterology,* vol. 91 (1996), pp. 1544–48. For asthma see Robert S. Zeiger and others, "Facilitated referral to asthma specialist reduces relapses in asthma emergency room visits," *Journal of Allergy and Clinical Immunology,* vol. 87 (1991), pp. 1160–88.

6. Stephen H. Moore, Diane P. Martin, and William C. Richardson, "Does the primary-care gatekeeper control the costs of health care? Lessons from the SAFECO experience," *New England Journal of Medicine,* vol. 309 (1983), pp. 1400–04.

7. Sheldon E. Greenfield Jr. and others, "Variations in resource utilization among medical specialties and systems of care. Results from the medical outcomes study," *Journal of the American Medical Association,* vol. 267 (1992), pp. 1624–30; and Daniel C. Cherkin and others, "The use of medical resources by residency-trained family physicians and general internists. Is there a difference? *Medical Care,* vol. 25 (1987), pp. 455–69.

8. John E. Ware Jr. and others, "Differences in 4-year health outcomes for elderly and poor, chronically ill patients treated in HMO and fee-for-service systems. Results

from the Medical Outcomes Study," *Journal of the American Medical Association,* vol. 276 (1996), pp. 1039–47.

9. Karen Donelan and others, "All payer, single payer, managed care, no payer: Patients' perspectives in three nations," *Health Affairs,* vol. 15 (1996), pp. 254–65.

10. Harold S. Luft, Sandra S. Hunt, and Susan C. Maerki, "The volume-outcome relationship: practice-makes-perfect or selective-referral patterns?" *Health Services Research,* vol. 22 (1987), pp. 157–82.

11. For HIV patients see Mari M. Kitahata and others, "Physicians' experience with the acquired immunodeficiency syndrome as a factor in patients' survival," *New England Journal of Medicine,* vol. 334 (1996), pp. 701–06. For specialized cardiac services see Stephen E. Kimmel, Jesse A. Berlin, and Warren K. Laskey, "The relationship between coronary angioplasty procedure volume and major complications [see comments], *Journal of the American Medical Association,* vol. 274 (1995), pp. 1137–42.

12. For asthma see Zeiger and others, "Facilitated referral to asthma specialist reduces relapses"; Dirk K. Greineder, Kathleen C. Loane, and Paula Parks, "Reduction in resource utilization by an asthma outreach program," *Archives of Pediatric Adolescent Medicine,* vol. 149 (1995), pp. 415–20; and Paul H. Mayo, Julieta Richman, and William H. Harris, "Results of a program to reduce admissions for adult asthma," *Annals of Internal Medicine,* vol. 112 (1990), pp. 864–71. For diabetes see Barry H. Ginsberg, "Preliminary results of a disease management program for diabetes," *JCOM,* vol. 3 (1996), pp. 45–51.

13. Anne Wilkinson and Joanne Lynn, "Quality End-of-Life Care: The case for a Medicaring Demonstration," George Washington University, May 2, 1997; and personal communication with Dr. Joanne Lynn, May 1, 1997.

14. This assumes that there is variation in the treatment of patients with the same condition.

15. Frank, McGuire, and Newhouse, "Risk Contracts in Managed Mental Health."

16. Randall S. Brown and others, "Do Health Maintenance Organizations Work for Medicare?" *Health Care Financing Review,* vol. 15 (Fall 1993), pp. 7–21; and Physician Payment Review Commission, *1996 Annual Report to Congress* (Washington, 1996). There is no evidence, however, about the extent to which this reflects self-selection versus deliberate plan selection.

17. Frank, McGuire, and Newhouse, "Risk Contracts in Managed Mental Health."

18. Comprehensive health plans would also be willing to compete for high-risk patients if they received well risk-adjusted payments.

19. Barbara Starfield, *Primary Care: Concept, Evaluation, and Policy* (Oxford University Press, 1992).

20. David Blumenthal, Elizabeth Mort, and Jennifer Edwards, "The efficacy of primary care for vulnerable population groups," *Health Services Research,* vol. 30 (1995), pp. 253–73.

21. Robyn M. Tamblyn and others, "Do too many cooks spoil the broth? Multiple physician involvement in medical management of elderly patients and potentially inappropriate drug combinations," *Canadian Medical Association Journal,* vol 154 (1996), pp. 1177–84; and Nananda Col, James E. Fanale, and Penelope Kronholm, "The role of medication noncompliance and adverse drug reactions in hospitalizations of the elderly," *Archives of Internal Medicine,* vol. 150 (1990), pp. 841–45.

22. Sheldon Greenfield and others, "Outcomes of patients with hypertension and non-insulin dependent diabetes mellitus treated by different systems and specialties. Results from the medical outcomes study," *Journal of the American Medical Association,* vol. 274 (1995), pp. 1436–44.

23. For example, there is enormous variability within mental health diagnoses.

24. Frank, Glazer, and McGuire, Harvard Medical School, September 1996.

25. Joseph Newhouse, Melinda Beeuwkes Buntin, and John Chapman, "Risk Adjustment and Medicare," *Health Affairs,* vol. 16 (September-October 1997), pp. 26–43.

26. Frank, Glazer, and McGuire, Harvard Medical School, September 1996.

27. Personal communication with Margaret Stanley of CalPERS.

28. Shari Caudron, "Carving Out Healthcare Savings," *Personnel Journal* (April 1995, pp. 38–48.

29. Frank, Glazer, and McGuire, Harvard Medical School, September 1996.

30. Monica Oss, *Managed Behavioral Health Market Share in the United States* (Gettysburg, Pa.: Open Minds, June 1994).

31. Caudron, "Carving Out Healthcare Savings."

32. David Kreling and others, "Assessment of the Impact of Pharmacy Benefit Managers," HCFA Master Contract HCFA-95-023/PK, September 30, 1996. There is double counting of individuals covered by more than one PBM.

33. Clark J. Yaggy and Daniel Jackson, "Report on the Segal Company's 1995 Survey of State Employee Health Benefit Plans," 1995.

34. Caudron, "Carving Out Healthcare Savings."

35. "Formularies, my dear Watson," *Risk Management,* vol. 43 (June 1996).

36. Caudron, "Carving Out Healthcare Savings."

37. Kreling and others, "Assessment of the Impact of Pharmacy Benefit Managers."

38. Kirk Strosahl and Michael Quirk, "The Trouble with Carve Outs," *Business and Health,* vol. 12 (July 1994), p. 52.

39. Vicki Gerson, "Chomping at the health care system," *Business and Health* (August 1996), pp. 29–33.

40. Frank, McGuire, and Newhouse, "Risk Contracts in Managed Health Care."

41. Frank, Glazer, and McGuire, Harvard Medical School, September 1996.

42. Geoffrey Leavenworth, "Four Cost-Cutting Strategies," *Business and Health,* (August 1994), pp. 26–33.

43. Greg Muirhead, "Disease state management falling short," *Drug Topics,* vol. 140 (July 8, 1996), pp. 80–82.

44. Personal communication with David Whitehead of MCC Behavioral Health.

5

Fee-for-Service Medicare
in a Managed Care World

R EJECTING THE IDEA that fee-for-service and managed-care services are mutually exclusive, the authors in this chapter explore their compatibility, whether in the application of managed care techniques to the traditional fee-for-service Medicare program to achieve greater cost effectiveness or in the coexistence of fee-for-service and capitated payments within one Medicare managed care model.

The Medicare Fee-for-Service System:
Applying Managed Care Techniques
Peter D. Fox

THERE IS NO COMMONLY accepted definition of managed care. A broad definition could be: any measure applied by a health plan or purchaser (employers, union-management trust funds, or government programs such as Medicare and Medicaid) that affects the cost, utilization, or quality of health services. This definition would, for example, encompass measures that constrain payment levels for individual items of service but that do not influence utilization. The more common definition, however, entails a relationship between the payer and a defined network of providers, such as

I am deeply grateful to the National Academy of Social Insurance, and particularly the Study Panel on Managing Fee-For-Service Medicare, for its support and guidance. Because I have interviewed dozens of people during the course of preparing this paper, the list of individuals to whom I owe a debt of gratitude is too long to include here. The study panel's efforts are part of the Restructuring Medicare for the Long Term initiative, which is supported by The Robert Wood Johnson Foundation, the Pew Charitable Trusts, the Henry J. Kaiser Family Foundation, and The Commonwealth Fund.

through a health maintenance organization (HMO) or preferred provider organization (PPO).

This paper addresses the ways the Medicare fee-for-service program might employ managed care techniques, particularly those adopted by the private sector, to address utilization and quality of services. It does not restrict consideration to network-based options. However, it does not address measures whose primary focus is price per unit of service.[1] Also excluded from the scope of the paper are the more fundamental reforms being debated such as transforming Medicare into a voucher, or defined contribution, program. Finally, the objective of managed care is viewed as maximizing the value of the health care dollar, not just constraining costs, and thus includes quality and access as goals.

Two factors motivate this discussion. First, despite the rapid growth in Medicare beneficiaries enrolled in HMOs, most enrollees will remain in the fee-for-service system for the forseeable future. As of July 1996, some 38.1 million beneficiaries were enrolled in part A or part B or both.[2] In contrast, at the end of 1996 only 4.2 million were enrolled in HMOs with Medicare risk contracts.[3] To be sure, Medicare risk enrollment is rising rapidly, having increased by 40 percent from the year before. This increase can be expected to accelerate if certain policy changes are adopted that are under serious consideration—in particular, a relaxation of the current requirements that health plans have a minimum of 5,000 commercial enrollees to be awarded a Medicare risk contract and that at least 50 percent of enrollment be other than Medicare or Medicaid beneficiaries.[4] Nonetheless, most Medicare beneficiaries can be expected to remain in the fee-for-service system.

The second factor motivating this discussion is the persistent increases in Medicare expenditures. The federal government has had far greater success in controlling unit costs than it has utilization. For example, for physician services, expenditures have been constrained by reducing payment levels to the extent that expenditures exceed preset targets, known as the Medicare Volume Performance Standards (MVPS). However, there is no evidence that the application of the MVPS significantly affects utilization.

The next section of this paper summarizes managed care techniques that the private sector has adopted. It is followed by a section that addresses the institutional constraints facing Medicare in implementing these techniques. The section after that proposes options for applying managed care techniques to the Medicare program. The concluding section discusses private sector success factors in implementing managed care, followed by a listing of what I regard as some of the more promising strategies.

Managed Care Techniques

This section summarizes some of the techniques that characterize managed care, recognizing that significant differences exist in the extent to which, and how, managed care organizations rely on them. For example, some HMOs rely on financial incentives for providers, whereas others make principally fee-for-service arrangements and depend mostly on administrative oversight such as prior authorization of services to keep costs in line. Thus at one end of the spectrum the HMO retains the full risk for utilization; at the other end it devolves risk to providers. The effectiveness of any given method also depends on how it is implemented and not just the underlying design.

Managed care *techniques* should be distinguished from the *organizations* that undertake them. Important organizational structures include the following, recognizing that the definitions are not hard and fast and the demarcations between them are becoming blurred.

—Health maintenance organizations are organizations that are capitated to provide or arrange for a comprehensive array of services to a defined population of enrollees through a network of providers.

—Preferred provider organizations differ from HMOs in two respects. First, they do not accept risk; rather, risk is retained by the employer, Taft-Hartley trust fund, or insurance carrier. Second, enrollees can self-refer to providers who are not in a PPO's network, but they typically face higher cost sharing when they go to these outside providers.

—Point-of-service (POS) programs represent a hybrid between HMOs and PPOs. Their distinguishing characteristic is that the enrollee has financial incentives to designate a primary care physician (PCP) within the network and obtain referrals from the physician for any services that he or she does not provide.

Purchasers of care may also engage in managed care directly by requiring prior authorization and concurrent review of inpatient stays. Like the Health Care Financing Administration (HCFA), private employers are limited in their ability to engage in managed care because they are commonly reluctant to exercise control over the delivery system. For example, they are generally unwilling to capitate primary care or individual specialty services, both of which are common cost-containment techniques of HMOs.

Financial Incentives

HMOs may place providers at risk to varying degrees for the quantity and intensity of services they deliver or prescribe. The underlying philosophy is to align the incentives of the providers with those of the health plan to achieve common objectives. Many HMOs combine incentives for reducing utilization with payments that reflect measures of quality, access, and patient satisfaction. Examples of financial incentives include

—capitating PCPs for primary care services,

—capitating specialty groups,

—capitating specific services such as behavioral health and laboratory services (sometimes referred to as carve-outs),

—creating incentives for PCPs to be conservative in their referral practices, usually in conjunction with incentives to be concerned with quality, access, and patient satisfaction, and

—sharing with physicians and hospitals the financial risk associated with hospital care.

Administrative Oversight

The most common form of administrative oversight is precertification and concurrent review of inpatient stays as well as of expensive outpatient services that are often discretionary—for example, magnetic resonance imaging (MRI) examinations, administration of growth hormones, and selected ambulatory surgery procedures. Referrals to specialists may also require prior approval.[5] One of the reasons for administrative oversight is to control costs in situations in which the providers lack the incentive to do so. Thus health plans that have financial incentives are less likely to have significant administrative oversight, and vice versa.

Selection and Deselection of Efficient Providers

The idea of limiting the participation of providers in the health plan to those that are efficient works better in theory than in practice. Hospitals can be evaluated in terms of their costs or, more commonly, their willingness to agree to prices that the health plan is willing to pay, in part because of the availability of such data as Medicare claims files and cost reports. With regard to physicians, a health plan is generally able to assess efficiency only after it has contracted with the physician for sufficient time to have adequate data on practice patterns. Obtaining anecdotal information on practice styles is possible, although many physicians report being more comfortable assessing the quality of their professional colleagues than their efficiency. Furthermore, a physician's practice style before joining may not predict performance under a different set of incentives. Once a physician has assumed responsibility for a sufficiently large number of that plan's patients, deselection is more feasible.

Culture of Efficiency

Some medical groups and staff model HMOs seek to achieve savings by fostering a culture of efficiency rather than by adopting administrative controls or financial incentives. Tight-knit medical groups are best able to foster such a culture, in contrast to organizations that bring together otherwise independent physicians largely for purposes of managed care contracting or assistance in office management such as billings and collections.

Prevention and Demand Management

Increasingly, health plans are undertaking prevention and demand management activities oriented to persons with identified illnesses (secondary and tertiary prevention). As with other terms in the managed care field, there are no generally accepted definitions, and the field is evolving. Prominent among demand management methods are the "nurse line" or "advice nurse" services that entail enrollees' calling an 800 number and talking to a nurse to determine how they can care for themselves and whether to see a physician. This service may be combined with written information, such as a book or newsletters, dealing with self-care and symptoms requiring immediate attention.

Secondary and tertiary prevention can take a variety of forms, especially for a chronically ill elderly population. Interventions that health plans have adopted include the following.

—Screening Medicare enrollees to identify those who have chronic illness in order to facilitate early intervention including geriatric assessment and case management.

—Coordinating access with such community-based social services as nutrition programs, support groups, housing, and financial counseling.

—Providing more extensive primary care than typically exists in the traditional Medicare program. In particular, programs directed at custodial-level nursing home patients have been shown to reduce emergency room and inpatient hospital use.

—Promoting friendly visiting and telephoning, particularly to enrollees who live alone. For example, volunteer programs have been undertaken to make sure that congestive heart failure patients take their medications and monitor their weight.

—Providing targeted education and self-care efforts for patients with hypertension, diabetes, arthritis, and other long-term conditions.

—Instituting programs to promote a safer home environment and other measures to reduce falls.

—Creating support groups for cancer patients, grieving spouses, and caregivers.[6]

Data Analysis

Critical to managed care is having data on physicians' practice patterns that are valid and presented in a user-friendly manner. It is a truism that practice patterns are difficult to change without knowing what they are. The past few years have seen major advances in data systems that profile physicians. The systems are sold commercially by such companies as HPR, GMIS, Equifax, and Value Health.

The past few years have also witnessed the development of practice guidelines or clinical care pathways, which are generally disease or condition specific. Many are inpatient oriented, although the more comprehensive ones encompass the full range of settings in which care is delivered. They have been developed by a variety of organizations, including specialty societies and federal agencies. They reflect the perspective that physicians and other providers can come together and think more systematically than has been true historically about what constitutes appropriate care, including the site and timing of care, to reduce undesirable variations in medical practice, thereby improving quality and, more often than not, reducing costs.

Institutional Constraints

In developing options for applying managed care techniques to the Medicare program, one should be mindful of the institutional constraints that face the federal government. For example, consider a physician who has not committed fraud but who has a highly inefficient practice style, including providing services that many in the medical profession view as unnecessary and even potentially harmful to the patient. A private health plan might exclude such a physician from participation, but Medicare would have difficulty doing so. Institutional constraints include the following.

—The size and dominance of the Medicare program. Medicare accounts for more than one-third of the patient volume of many providers, and for ophthalmologists, oncologists, and many internists more than half. Thus punitive measures such as termination from participation can make it difficult for the provider to earn a living, particularly since Medicaid and some private payers are likely to follow suit. One result is the tendency of government to limit its attention to extreme outliers, thus making it less able to influence the norm of practice.

—Due process requirements. Society is reluctant to allow government agencies the level of discretion afforded private sector payers in making judgments on policy and managerial matters. Medicare is subject to requirements that characterize federal agencies in general, such as those set forth in the Administrative Practices Act, as well as those in the Medicare Act. These requirements can be cumbersome and can delay decisionmaking.

—Procurement and personnel policies. Government agencies face restrictions in procurement and hiring that are not faced by the private sector, thus allowing the private sector to operate in a more "businesslike" fashion.

—Government in the sunshine. Many decisions made by private plans are judgmental and made privately. However, government agencies are typically required to justify their decisions in public forums. The concern about criticism from the press, Congress, and various investigative bodies such as the Inspector General and the General Accounting Office is ever present. One consequence is that inaction is encouraged.

—Slowness in decisionmaking. Government agencies are often slow in making decisions because of their size and the way they are organized. For example, it can take the HCFA several years to issue a program regulation or approve a demonstration application. Although the agency, or some successor, could improve its performance, some of the slowness is inherent in the nature of government and the levels of approval required. Juxtaposed against this are health plans that are nimble in their decisionmaking, changing payment mechanisms frequently and making adjustments to reflect the circumstances of individual providers within the network.

—Congressional limitations on flexibility. Congress is often loath to allow the executive branch latitude in decisionmaking. Alternatively, when legislation is first enacted, considerable latitude may exist that gradually becomes constrained. Statutes, except for those that might be repealed altogether, tend to become longer and more prescriptive with the passage of time.

—Lack of points of accountability. HMOs and many other health plans are responsible for defined populations and thus can be held accountable for the health of the population. In theory, the same could be said for Medicare as a health plan. However, the number of beneficiaries in the fee-for-service system is so large that population-based performance measures, such as those that employers and other purchasers of health care may require of the HMOs with which they contract, have less potential to affect the delivery system.[7]

Options for Applying Managed Care Techniques

Despite some drawbacks, there are options for applying managed care techniques to the Medicare fee-for-service system. Table 5-1 rates each option as high (H), medium (M), or low (L) along three dimensions: the extent to which it would be technically feasible for the Medicare program to implement it; its institutional feasibility, which reflects the presence of institutional constraints on the Medicare program; and its potential effect, whether on cost or quality.[8]

In many cases, the ratings entail judgments of which I may be uncertain myself. Nonetheless, they are presented in the hope that they can help inform the reader's thinking. Many of the options have not been fully researched and are presented as concepts for further exploration. Some may warrant being tested using the HCFA's research and demonstration authority. Indeed, a number are already under consideration by the HCFA or represent extensions of what is under way.

Data and Claims Analysis

Because of the size of Medicare and the volume of claims it processes, it has access to a rich array of data, and the HCFA's data systems have improved significantly over time. The following sections explore the potential uses of the data.

COMPARE QUALITY OF CARE AMONG PROVIDERS. Purchasers, including the HCFA for HMOs with Medicare risk contracts, are increasingly requiring HMOs and other managed care entities to provide data on performance, although the extant measures are limited in scope. The most common ones are those developed by the National Committee for Quality Assurance, which accredits HMOs and other managed care plans. Similarly, outcomes or performance data could be published for individual providers for selected high-prevalence conditions. As with the requirements on Medicare risk contractors, these need to be valid but not perfect. Such data can affect patient care two ways. The first is by making objective comparisons available to the providers in question. The second is through public disclosure, which has the potential for inducing patients to seek out the higher-quality providers, who in turn compete for patient volume. As an illustration of the potential for data to affect medical practice, in 1989 New York State started disseminating hospital- and physician-specific data for coronary artery bypass graft surgery. The result was an impressive 41 percent decline by 1992 in risk-adjusted mortality.[9] Providers

Table 5-1. *Managed Care Options for Fee-for-Service Medicare*

Options	Technical feasibility	Institutional feasibility	Impact
Data and claims analysis			
Compare quality of care among providers	M	M	M
Use claims data to identify underservice	H	H	a
Improved prepayment review and services bundling	H	H	M
Improved provider profiling	H	M	a
Conduct studies of areawide variations in utilization	H	H	L
Create PPO arrangements based on practice profiles	M	L	M
Administrative controls on utilization			
Prior authorization and concurrent review	M	M	M
Encourage or require enrollees to elect a PCP as gatekeeper	M	L	a
Clearer medical necessity definition for SNF and home health services (would apply to HMOs as well)		H	H
Package pricing			
Bundling of facility and physician payments for selected procedures	M	L–M	H
Includes SNF payments within the hospital DRG payment	H	H	H
Payment for home health service on a per-episode basis	M	M	M
Prevention and case management			
Enhanced payments for primary care to long-stay nursing home patients	M	H	M
Education of elderly or disabled regarding self-care	H	H	M
Grants to local agencies to conduct secondary and tertiary prevention	H	H	M
Areawide expenditure targets	M	L	M

Note: H = high; M = moderate; L = low.
[a]Depends on how administered.

changed their performance because of the availability of comparisons. The comparative data did not result in patients' changing providers, which would have been evidenced by shifts in market share.[10]

USE CLAIMS DATA TO IDENTIFY UNDERSERVICE. HMOs with Medicare risk contracts commonly use their data systems to identify persons who need care but are apparently not receiving it. These services are oriented toward prevention and in some cases result in documented cost savings. For example, several studies have been performed in HMOs on the effectiveness of reminders to enrollees to get influenza inoculations.[11] Because this is a service covered by Medicare, the Medicare records could be scanned and communications sent to beneficiaries who may not have been immunized. And because of data lags, the communications might be sent in the few weeks before flu season to those who were not inoculated the previous year.[12] Use of pneumonia vaccine could also be encouraged; the *Wall Street Journal* reported on February 3, 1997, that the federal Centers for Disease Control found that less than 5 percent of elderly people in nursing homes had been vaccinated. Claims data might also identify underservice of diabetics, for whom regular retinal and foot exams are important because without them the need for expensive services is probable.[13]

IMPROVED PROVIDER (PARTICULARLY PHYSICIAN) PROFILING.   Recent advances in commercially offered provider profiling systems have been striking. These systems rely on flexible relational databases and have modules that can adjust utilization data to reflect relative patient mix or severity of conditions. The major market for these vendors is managed care plans, particularly HMOs. Although principally oriented toward identifying physicians with expensive practice styles, the systems can also identify quality problems.

The HCFA faces greater constraints than HMOs in using profiling data. The numbers of providers involved is larger. Most HMOs require that enrollees elect a primary care physician who serves as gatekeeper, thereby improving the opportunities to hold a physician accountable for the totality of services received by a given patient. HMOs also have a better ability to contact individual physicians to discuss performance. Finally, a private health plan is not subject to the due process requirements that characterize government agencies, particularly the HCFA, that are administering a national entitlement program.

Nonetheless, several forms of intervention, which vary in their feasibility and effects, might be considered. First, using the peer review organizations or other structures, the data could educate physicians. Most physicians know little about how they compare with their peers, particularly in practice styles. It is important that data affecting performance be presented in a way that is clinically sensitive and user friendly. An open question is the potential effectiveness of providing information not tied to payment. Such information might have considerably greater impact if it were combined with area budget targets, as described later. The data could also be used to sanction physicians who have particularly expensive practice styles. The physicians thus identified could be required to explain their practice styles to a local peer group, become subject to prior authorization requirements for certain services, and be precluded from

Medicare altogether, a measure that has historically been limited to providers who are guilty of fraud, and then only after a lengthy judicial process.

CONDUCT STUDIES OF AREAWIDE VARIATIONS IN UTILIZATION.   The large, and largely unexplainable, variations in Medicare spending, both in the aggregate and by type of service, are well known.[14] Additional efforts to analyze these variations can be valuable only if the analyses will lead to action. At the least the data could be broadly disseminated in hopes that they would stimulate providers, particularly physicians, in high-cost, high-utilization areas to become more restrained in their practice styles. A more effective application of the data would be to target interventions. For example, prior authorization of selected high-cost services might be performed only in areas where utilization is high. Provider profiling, including the application of sanctions, might also be initiated in these areas. Finally, areawide targets for Medicare expenditures might be established that would relate provider payment levels to the achievement of the targets in high-cost areas. Each of these options is discussed elsewhere in this paper.

DEVELOP PPO ARRANGEMENTS BASED ON PRACTICE PROFILES.   PPOs for the commercial population achieve savings through provider discounts, utilization management, and provider selection, although the latter occurs more in theory than in practice. Enrollees face incentives to use network providers, typically in the form of differential cost sharing (copayments, deductibles, or coinsurance).[15] The HCFA could potentially employ practice profiles to identify efficient physicians and negotiate arrangements with those willing to accept rates below those paid by Medicare or those who volunteer to cooperate with selected utilization management requirements such as prior authorization of services. Beneficiaries would have incentives such as reduced cost sharing to use these providers. In practice, this might be difficult to implement, particularly on a scale large enough to achieve meaningful savings. The HCFA has made efforts to enter into PPO demonstrations with understandably limited success, and I am skeptical of the viability of broad-based PPO arrangements for Medicare, notwithstanding private sector experience. Nonetheless, efforts might be devoted to determining whether workable arrangements could be feasible.

Administrative Controls on Utilization

Given the difficulty that the HCFA would have in introducing financial incentives for physicians, administrative controls on utilization warrant particular consideration.

PRIOR AUTHORIZATION AND CONCURRENT REVIEW.   Prior authorization of selected high-cost services can potentially achieve savings. Most private plans, including indemnity plans, review the necessity for admission and continued stay in hospitals or other care facilities. They also review selected diagnostic procedures such as MRI use and elective surgical procedures. In areas with particularly high utilization, Medicare could require that these services be subject to prior authorization. In addition, concurrent review might be appropriate for home health care and stays in skilled nursing facilities. One key to the success of such reviews is to conduct data analyses that target selected geographic areas and services rather than analyses that are comprehensive and unfocused.

ENCOURAGE OR REQUIRE BENEFICIARIES TO ELECT A PCP AS GATEKEEPER. Most HMOs require that enrollees select a primary care physician who is responsible for delivering or authorizing all services except emergency services or those rendered when people are away from home. Many state Medicaid fee-for-service programs require that beneficiaries select a participating PCP who serves as gatekeeper. The PCP is not placed at risk but may receive a monthly case management fee. This system permits tracking most services delivered to any given patient back to a single PCP and offers two advantages. The first is to achieve savings, as the experience of state Medicaid programs has documented.[16] Second, physicians with a geriatric focus have long sought payment for telephone calls to patients and for dealing with family members and local social services agencies. The case management fee could be regarded as compensation for these activities.

If mandating that Medicare beneficiaries designate PCPs is not politically feasible, financial incentives in the form of reduced cost sharing or lower Medicare premiums might be offered enrollees who agree voluntarily to obtain services through a PCP. One problem with reduced cost sharing is that almost 90 percent of the elderly face minimal cost sharing anyway because they have coverage in addition to Medicare, including medigap policies, retiree benefits, and Medicaid.[17]

Package Pricing

Package pricing can take various forms, the most comprehensive of which is capitation, the method of payment for HMOs with Medicare risk contracts. An important example of package pricing in the standard Medicare program is payment to acute care hospitals on a per admission basis using diagnosis related groups (DRGs). Package pricing incorporates incentives to minimize costs within the package and to maximize the number of packages delivered. Cost minimization raises the specter of underservice. However, whether underservice occurs depends on countervailing pressures, in particular, the potential for losing patient volume, the cost of paying for rework if it is factored into the package, and the effectiveness of administrative oversight. For example, Medicare's prospective payment system holds hospitals responsible for the cost of hospital readmission within sixty days of discharge. Package pricing arrangements raise the issues of how the package should be defined, how it should be priced, and how to ensure quality.

BUNDLING OF FACILITY AND PHYSICIAN PAYMENT FOR SELECTED PROCEDURES.   The HCFA has conducted demonstrations yielding promising results of bundled pricing of facility and physician services for coronary artery bypass grafts and cataract surgery.[18] It is soliciting proposals for package pricing, referred to as centers of excellence, for heart and orthopedic procedures. The demonstration would entail a single payment to the hospital that includes physician services and, unlike the earlier demonstrations, post-hospital services such as skilled nursing facilities, rehabilitation, and home health care. The HCFA is also exploring testing bundled payments to hospitals for all DRGs. It anticipates that the developmental phase will take at least a year.

INCLUDING PAYMENTS FOR SKILLED NURSING FACILITY SERVICES IN HOSPITAL DRG PAYMENTS.   Medicare requires that a beneficiary be hospitalized for at least three days to qualify for SNF services. Thus, by law these are post-hospital services associated with an admission. One consequence of acute care hospitals' being paid mostly on a per admission basis while SNFs continue to be paid based on their costs has been an explosive growth in SNF use. In each of the four years ending in 1987, Medicare-covered SNF days ranged between 221 and 296 per 1,000 aged and disabled beneficiaries; since then utilization has climbed steadily, reaching 1,072 days in 1994.[19]

The major arguments against including SNF payments within the DRG payment are that there is wide variability in SNF use within DRGs and making the payment to the hospital would give the hospital considerable control over a major segment of the nursing home industry. However, SNF services commonly substitute for hospital inpatient services, increasingly so with the growth in recent years of subacute care units, and sometime have staffing levels characteristic of community hospitals. This substitutability, combined with the rapid increases in utilization, argues for the inclusion of SNF services in the DRG payment (and inclusion of rehabilitation hospital services when they follow the discharge from an acute care hospital).

PAYMENT FOR HOME HEALTH SERVICES ON A PER EPISODE BASIS. Like SNF services, the use of Medicare-covered home health services has ballooned. In the four years ending in 1987, Medicare-covered visits annually ranged between 1,113 and 1,324 per 1,000 beneficiaries; in 1994 the rate reached 6,122 visits. This more than quadrupling reflects increases in both the number of persons served (which rose 94 percent between 1987 and 1994) and the number of visits per person (which rose 187 percent).[20]

Home health care has been a baffling benefit to control and a difficult one for fiscal intermediaries to administer consistently. Unlike SNF services, the home health care benefit was never intended to be strictly post-hospital.[21] Another problem is the wide geographic variation in per capita costs, which exceeds that of other Medicare services. Furthermore, the need for care may be continuing: there may not be episodes with readily identifiable beginning and end points, although by law the services must be part-time or intermittent, a flexible yardstick in practice. Finally, neither the ordering physician nor the home health care agency has any reason to economize.

One way to contain costs would be to issue guidelines for prevalent conditions. Carriers would be required to provide detailed justification if the guidelines were exceeded, particularly agencies that exhibit a pattern of exceeding the guidelines. Efforts under way in the HCFA to obtain better data on home health services should facilitate the development of clinically sound guidelines.[22] Another means of cost containment is prior authorization of services every few visits, starting perhaps after the first few. However, an effective prior authorization program would likely entail nurses on a sample basis to review medical records or meet with patients because requests for prior authorization can be worded to pass review. A third method would be to pay on a per episode basis, with a limit of perhaps three or six months of service per episode. Thus, someone who reached the end of the time limit would generate another, or a different level of, payment. This would provide incentives for efficiency during the episode. The HCFA is conducting demonstrations in five states of per episode payments, defined as care for a 120-day period, with services beyond 120 days being treated as outliers and reimbursed at a low rate per visit.

Prevention and Case Management

Prevention and case management are considered linked topics. Prevention for elderly or disabled populations can occur across a continuum of health status or level of functioning and can be categorized as:

—primary prevention, directed at those who are fundamentally well and for whom exercise, inoculations, diet, not smoking, and so forth are important;

—secondary prevention, directed at persons with conditions that are largely asymptomatic, such as hypertension or diabetes, for whom self-care classes, outreach programs, and printed materials can be helpful; and

—tertiary prevention, directed at persons with known chronic conditions entailing functional deficits such as heart or pulmonary disease; it is designed to prevent further deterioration. Case management can be viewed as a form of tertiary prevention in addition to being a vehicle for coordinating services and ensuring delivery in the least costly, appropriate setting.

It is with regard to prevention that the experiences of HMOs with Medicare risk contracts and extensive elderly-oriented programs are particularly instructive, although the Medicare fee-for-service program cannot replicate the full range of interventions that HMOs have adopted. Many HMOs believe that the key to financial success is to retard physical deterioration and maintain function to reduce hospital use. A full exposition of these efforts is beyond the scope of this paper; what is presented merely indicates the interventions that might be considered.[23]

However, two shifts in thinking regarding the way the Medicare program functions would be required. First, Medicare has traditionally operated as a financing rather than a health program, although recently it has made efforts to embed geriatric principles in its payment mechanisms. Second, the program generally operates independently of other federal programs. One option, which is explored below, is for grants to community agencies that fall outside the HCFA's traditional purview but that could integrate with the Medicare program. The rationale for so doing is to avoid the increasing costs associated with expanding benefits through an open-ended fee-for-service payment mechanism.

ENHANCED PAYMENTS FOR PRIMARY CARE FOR LONG-STAY NURSING HOME PATIENTS. For (typically, long-stay) patients for whom Medicare does not cover the daily room and board charges because they do not meet the criteria of medical necessity, Medicare coverage rules require physician visits upon a beneficiary's admission to the facility at least every thirty days for the first ninety days and every sixty days thereafter. Visits of greater frequency are often questioned by the fiscal intermediary. Indeed, it is often easier to transfer a resident to the hospital than undertake the effort required to keep him or her in the nursing home. Transferring this resident is also more lucrative for the physician, the nursing home, and the hospital. Evidence also exists that nursing home residents who are transferred back and forth between the nursing home and the hospital experience decreased quality of life and a potential worsening of other physical and mental conditions.[24]

The provision of additional services, whether by physicians or nurse practitioners, has the potential for reducing admissions.[25] HMOs have experienced large reductions in emergency room and hospital inpatient use as a result of better primary care.[26] Thus, it is suggested that the HCFA review its coverage and payment rules to ensure adequate primary care to long-stay nursing home residents.

EDUCATION AND INFORMATION FOR ELDERLY AND DISABLED SELF-CARE. Structured self-management programs and those intended to change behavior have been demonstrated to improve health outcomes and, presumably, reduce use of the medical care system for conditions including diabetes, heart disease, hypertension, and arthritis.[27] A number of HMOs have adopted self-management programs and found them to be cost effective. The challenge, however, is to implement them in a fee-for-service environment. As with some of the other programs, an open-ended payment mechanism is not recommended. However, national informational programs might be undertaken along with grants, perhaps on a pilot basis initially, to local community agencies such as Area Agencies on Aging (AAA), public health departments, or provider groups. One example of a successful program mounted in a fee-for-service enviroment is Medicaid's program in Maryland for diabetics. Through a combination of structured outpatient education programs, which are viewed as the cornerstone of the effort, case management, and primary care providers' undergoing a five-hour course in diabetes management (for which they receive continuing medical education credits), a 40 to 50 percent reduction in inpatient care and emergency room use has been achieved.[28]

Also, "nurse line" or "advice nurse" pilot projects might be mounted whereby enrollees can telephone an 800 number and obtain information on self-care as well as whether medical care is needed and, if so, how immediately it is necessary. In some cases the conversation results in a referral to case management. Significant savings have been claimed for these programs.

GRANTS TO LOCAL AGENCIES TO CONDUCT SECONDARY AND TERTIARY PREVENTION. The Medicare program has little experience with joint endeavors with local agencies such as local health departments or the federally funded AAAs, many of which have health care programs for the elderly. For example, many AAAs perform case management, but it is not integrated with Medicare, nor is it oriented toward reducing use of medical, particularly inpatient, services. Grants might be made to such agencies (or existing funding reoriented) to mount programs to help elderly people who are disabled or have functional limitations. Prospective grantees would have to present detailed plans to be eligible for funding. A block grant with limited strings attached is *not* intended; rather, the grantees should become contract agents of the HCFA. Because many of the functions would be new, modest developmental funds might be desirable.

Case management is one possible function. Research on the costs of case management for the Medicare population has been less than encouraging. The so-called channeling demonstrations of case management, conducted in the 1980s, failed to reduce costs for a frail elderly population, even with the availability of additional funds to purchase community-based services. Carefully controlled research has not been conducted in an HMO setting, although many plans have case management programs, which they justify based on an evaluation methodology that entails comparing actual costs with an estimate of what costs would have been in the absence of case management.[29] For HMOs two frequently encountered problems, which would be worse if the locus of case management were a community agency, are coordination between the case manager and the PCP and patients' refusing case management as an intrusion into their lives.

Nonetheless, one should ask whether the negative findings reflect the inherent shortcomings of case management or the way it has been implemented. In contrast to the Medicare experience, the Maryland Medicaid program instituted case management in twelve large medical centers and reported savings of 24 percent.[30]

Keys to case management's cost effectiveness include careful targeting of the population and limiting the resources that are invested. Also, many HMOs use case management as the gateway to off-policy benefits. For example, the case manager may be authorized to pay for simple home repairs or additions such as fixing steps or adding grab rails in bathrooms to prevent falls. A limited amount of money might be available for such purposes.

Another function of the local grantee agency could be to conduct disease management programs for a limited number of conditions. For example, education and regular follow-up (to check problems with medication and weight, for example) have been found to substantially reduce hospital readmissions for persons with congestive heart failure.[31] Other functions that the community agency could perform, all of which are performed in some HMOs, include

—home assessments to spot problems such as low lighting, loose rugs, or cords that can generate falls;

—developing support or self-help groups for diabetics, cancer patients, grieving widows, and caretakers of Medicare beneficiaries who are frail or disabled;

—developing or arranging for exercise programs that are geared to an elderly or disabled population; and

—mounting volunteer programs such as friendly visiting and telephoning.

As an illustration of such a program, PacifiCare and the Group Health Cooperative of Puget Sound have teamed up with a senior citizens center in Washington state to offer supervised health promotion and chronic illness self-management interventions to chronically ill seniors. The interventions, which entail randomized, controlled trials, include meetings with nurse practitioners to develop individually tailored health promotion plans, medication reviews, classes, support groups, and volunteer mentors. Preliminary, as yet unpublished, findings reveal significant reductions in hospitalizations, higher levels of physical activity, and reductions in the use of psychoactive medications. The intervention group has also experienced fewer disability days and less deterioration in functioning in activities of daily living, although no difference was observed in functional status as measured by the so-called SF-36.

Areawide Expenditure Targets

This proposal on expenditure targets is perhaps the most far-reaching one I offer. It entails establishing areawide targets to which physician (and possibly other provider) payment would be tied to create incentives to constrain utilization. The physician payment reform legislation enacted in 1989 included provisions for creating national expenditure targets for physician services such as the MVPS. Performance nationally relative to the targets results in physicians' payment levels being adjusted upward or downward. Areawide expenditure targets are intended to correct two shortcomings of the current law. First, there is no vehicle or intent under current law for physicians to come together nationally to influence performance other than, perhaps, through a general education campaign. Thus the MVPS serve as a budget control device, not as a mechanism to constrain utilization. Second, the target is based on expenditures for physicians' services only, a subset of part B expenses, and does not, for example, allow physicians to be rewarded financially for constraining use of part A services.

The proposal would entail, starting perhaps with high-expenditure geographic areas, establishing targets for all Medicare expenses within a given area and rewarding or penalizing physicians for how expenditures compare with the targets within that area. The area would be of a size small enough, perhaps a metropolitan area, that physicians could review the care of their peers. The intent is both to constrain overall spending and to reduce the existing wide geographic variations. The plan would entail a fundamental change in incentives within the fee-for-service system and would work best in conjunction with prior authorization for selected services and the timely availability of severity-adjusted data. Demonstrations might be conducted that initially would entail positive incentives only, thus allowing doctors to share in savings but not penalizing them if the savings are not realized.

Conclusion

This paper seeks to serve as a source of ideas, not to present recommendations, particularly because the options described require refinement before they can be implemented. Although presented as individual options, a successful managed care strategy requires an integrated approach. For example, one cannot determine the data analyses that merit being undertaken without knowing how they are to be used. As another example, a program to precertify use of selected high-cost services is more likely to be effective in conjuction with the proposal for areawide expenditure targets, which entails changes in physician payment incentives.

Another determinant of program success is targeting. The geographic variations in expenditure patterns are well known, and greater efforts at program cost savings are warranted in high- rather than low-expenditure areas. Furthermore, the use rates of specific procedures correlate imperfectly with aggregate expenditures. Thus successful interventions require consideration of local circumstances. Indeed, the wide variations are likely to gain attention as a public policy issue as more beneficiaries enroll in HMOs with Medicare risk contracts. These HMOs are able to offer broader benefits at lower premiums in high- rather than low-expenditure areas, leading to benefit variations that reflect accidents of geography. Although cost-management interventions that differ geographically may be regarded as violating an underlying premise of the Medicare Act that the program is to be uniform nationally, that uniformity is already being challenged by the growth in Medicare risk enrollment and the resulting variations in benefit packages.[32] Recognition of the need for different approaches to cost management, which will largely be invisible to the beneficiary, would appear to be far less problematic.

Yet another determinant of success in managed care is the manner in which a program is implemented. Even the terminology often has different meanings in different situations. For example, most HMOs have case management programs, but they are not alike.[33] Finally, successful managed care plans are characterized by flexiblity in decisionmaking, including the ability to change. Although government agencies are by their nature constrained from acting as quickly as private plans, decisionmaking can be accelerated, as for example in the time it takes the HCFA to issue new regulations or make decisions on demonstrations.

Some of the more promising elements of managed care that might be considered are the following.

—Identify high-cost areas and procedures. In those areas, institute programs of provider profiling, physician incentives, and precertification of services.

—Implement areawide targets in high-cost areas.

—Initiate demonstrations of grants to local agencies (AAAs, public health departments) to institute prevention, particularly tertiary prevention, programs and case management, with limited funds available for off-policy benefits.

—Bring more of a geriatric focus to the Medicare program, perhaps by changing the coverage rules for nursing home visits for long-stay patients and experimenting with "advice nurse" programs.

—Include skilled nursing facility and rehabilitation hospital expenses within DRG payments to hospitals and pay for home health services on a per episode basis.

Notes

1. The distinction of whether the primary focus of a particular intervention is price per unit of service or the more efficient utilization of services is at times a hazy one. This paper, for example, includes options for bundling hospital and physician payments but does not address competitive bidding for durable medical equipment, which is viewed as purely price driven.

2. Health Care Financing Administration, *1996 Data Compendium* (Department of Health and Human Services, 1996), p. 46.

3. Office of Managed Care, Health Care Financing Administration, *Medicare Managed Care Contract Report* (issued monthly).

4. But Medicare risk-enrollment growth would be slowed if federal payment levels were reduced, as is also being discussed.

5. The requirement for prior approval from the health plan or purchaser should not be confused with the requirement that the enrollee obtain a PCP referral. Health plans that require the referral may or may not also require that the PCP obtain approval before authorizing the referral.

6. See Peter D. Fox and T. F. Fama, "Managed Care and the Elderly: Performance and Potential," *Generations*, vol. 20 (Summer 1996), pp. 37–41, as well as various chapters in Peter D. Fox and T. F. Fama, *Managed Care and Chronic Illness* (Gaithersburg, Md.: Aspen Publishers, 1996).

7. Examples of population-based measures are reflected in the Health Plan Employer Information and Data Set (HEDIS) measures developed by the National Committee for Quality Assurance.

8. Political feasibility has not been considered because it can change rapidly.

9. E. L. Hannan and others, "Improving the Outcomes of Coronary Artery Bypass Surgery in New York State," *Journal of the American Medical Association,* vol. 271 (March 9, 1994), pp. 761–66. Based on the New York experience, the authors argue for

combining Medicare data with other data to assess quality. See E. L. Hannan and others, "Using Medicare Claims Data to Assess Provider Quality for CABG Surgery: Does It Work Well Enough?" *Health Services Research*, vol. 31 (February 1997), pp. 659–768.

10. M. R. Chassin, E. L. Hannan, and B. A. DeBuono, "Benefits and Hazards of Reporting Medical Outcomes Publicly," *New England Journal of Medicine,* vol. 334 (February 8, 1996), pp. 394–98.

11. See, for example, N. A. Hanchak and others, "The Effectiveness of an Influenza Vaccination Program in an HMO Setting," *American Journal of Managed Care,* vol. 2, pp. 661–66.

12. One shortcoming of this approach is that beneficiaries may receive inoculations through community organizations that do not submit claims to Medicare.

13. An example of this use of claims data is the 1199 National Benefit Fund, which is one of the largest Taft-Hartley trust funds and administers health benefits on behalf of service workers in the New York City area.

14. See, for example, Center for Evaluative Clinical Services, Dartmouth Medical School, *The Dartmouth Atlas of Health Care* (Chicago: American Hospital Association, 1996) pt. 4, pp. 59–79.

15. There is wide variability in the relationship between Medicare payments and what providers will accept from managed care plans. For example, in some market areas many specialists accept payments that are 20 percent or more below Medicare fee levels, whereas in most markets, Medicare payment levels are viewed as low. This approach would be designed, in part, to achieve savings in markets where Medicare pays more than private health plans.

16. R. E. Hurley, D. A. Freund, and J. E. Paul, *Managed Care in Medicaid: Lessons for Policy and Program Design* (Ann Arbor, Mich.: Health Administration Press, 1993). One caveat regarding the interpretation of research results is that most of the Medicaid experience relates to the AFDC, not the SSI (aged and disabled), population.

17. G. S. Chulis and others, "Health Insurance and the Elderly: Data From the Medicare Current Beneficiary Survey," *Health Care Financing Review,* vol. 14 (Spring 1993), pp, 163–81.

18. For bypasses the HCFA was able to achieve significant savings with no deterioration in quality. See J. Cromwell, *Medicare Heart Bypass Demonstration: Final Report* (Waltham, Mass.: Health Economics Research, 1995). No evaluation of the cataract demonstration has been published.

19. Health Care Financing Administration, *Health Care Financing Review: Medicare and Medicaid Statistical Supplement, 1966* (Department of Health and Human Services, 1966), p. 272.

20. Ibid., p. 296.

21. Most use of the home health care benefit is not associated with inpatient care. See H. G. Welch, D. E. Wennberg, and W. P. Welch. "The Use of Medicare Home Health Services," *New England Journal of Medicine*, vol. 335 (August 1, 1996), pp. 324–29.

22. The data system is referred to as the Outcome and Assessment Information Set and is intended to assist in measuring outcomes and making payment adjustments to reflect case mix or patient severity.

23. For examples of a variety of interventions by HMOs geared to the chronically ill see A. M. Kramer, P. D. Fox, and N. Morgenstern,"Geriatric Care Approaches in Health

Maintenance Organizations," *Journal of the American Geriatric Society*, vol. 40 (1992), pp. 1055–67; P. D. Fox and T. Fama, eds., *Managed Care and Chronic Illness: Challenges and Opportunities* (Gaithersburg, Md.: Aspen Publishers, 1996); and Fox and Fama, "Managed Care and the Elderly: Performance and Potential," *Generations*, vol. 20 (Summer 1996), pp. 31–36. HMOs vary widely in the extent to which they have mounted programs that are focused specifically on elderly or disabled populations.

24. J. G. Zimmer and others, "Nursing Homes as Acute Care Providers: A Pilot Study of Incentives to Reduce Hospitalizations," *Journal of the American Geriatric Society*, vol. 36 (1988), pp. 124–29.

25. See, for example, R. L. Kane and others, "Improving Primary Care in Nursing Homes," *Journal of the American Geriatric Society*, vol. 39 (1991), pp. 359–67.

26. See, for example, J. B. Burl, A. Bonner, and M. Rao, "Demonstration of the Cost-Effectiveness of a Nurse Practitioner/Physician Team in Long-Term Care Facilities," *HMO Practice*, vol. 8 (December 1994), pp. 157–61. David Reuben at UCLA is completing a study of three HMOs with enhanced primary care for long-stay nursing home residents; preliminary findings are encouraging.

27. E. H. Wagner, B. T. Austin, and M. Von Korff, in P. D. Fox and T. Fama, eds., "Improving Outcomes in Chronic Illness," *Managed Care and Chronic Illness: Challenges and Opportunities* (Gaithersburg, Md.: Aspen Publishers, 1996).

28. State of Maryland Diabetes Program, *An Independent Evaluation of the Waiver Granted to the Maryland Department of Health and Mental Hygeine under Sections 1915(b)(1) and (3) of the Social Security Act* (Center for Health Program Development and Management, University of Maryland, Baltimore, 1995).

29. Recognizing this lack of knowledge along with the central role that case management plays in coordinating care, has made evaluating the impact of case management the Robert Wood Johnson Foundation's Chronic Care Initiatives in HMOs program a priority. However, the research is still in progress.

30. *Maryland Medicaid High Cost User Initiative: Case Management and Cost Savings Annual Report, CY 1995* (Baltimore: Center for Health Program Development and Management, University of Maryland, 1996). The savings reported are based on estimates of the costs that would have occurred without the intervention rather than on the experience of a control group. Notwithstanding limitations in the methodology, the order of magnitude of the savings is impressive.

31. See, for example, M. W. Rich and others, "A Multidisciplinary Intervention to Prevent the Readmission of Elderly Patients with Congestive Heart Failure," *New England Journal of Medicine,* vol. 333 (November 2, 1995), pp. 1190–95.

32. To be sure, there has always been lack of uniformity because of variations in the availability of medical resources and differences among fiscal intermediaties in the interpretation of coverage and other rules. However, these differences are of a smaller magnitude than those caused by geographic variations in HMO premiums and benefits, which currently exceed $1,000 per beneficiary per year.

33. J. T. Pacala and others, "Case Management of Older Adults in Health Maintenance Organizations," *Journal of the American Geriatric Society,* vol. 43 (1995), pp. 538–42.

Organizational Models for Restructuring Fee-for-Service Medicare
David G. Smith

THE BALANCED BUDGET ACT OF 1995, although vetoed by President Clinton on December 6, 1995, had some lasting effects. One was to raise to prominence not just Medicare costs and their effect on the budget, but the nature of the program itself: Was Medicare to continue primarily in its traditional fee-for-service form or become increasingly a managed care program, including options for enrolling in private health plans? So far, this description of the issue has stuck, and today Americans find themselves contemplating the most important changes since the program started paying bills in 1966.

An indirect but not unwelcome consequence of this prominence has been to clarify issues and produce some convergence of views. At present, there is a broad consensus that the fee-for-service (FFS) program will continue, even as managed care and HMOs gain a larger share of Medicare beneficiaries. There is also wide agreement among informed groups that the traditional program needs changes, including some managed care practices and private sector adaptations that will save money and improve quality. Disagreements exist about whether the FFS progam should continue to be dominant, whether the emphasis should be on private sector adaptations or public management, and how to resolve such matters. But the basic options would seem to be a modified FFS program with improved management and a procompetition model with broader managed care options, including private health plans.

This idea of improved management for fee-for-service Medicare has a deceptive and dangerous simplicity about it. Improved management may not be the answer, but rather additional legislation. And, recalling recent history, there is more than one devil in the details, especially when dealing with a policy domain as protean as health care. Therefore, a prudent next step might be to consider ways in which improved management could be translated into practice, which is the purpose of the various models I will discuss.

If improved management is the answer to solving Medicare's problems, new powers and more discretion for the Medicare administration may be required. As a traditional and public FFS program, Medicare lacks the authority to manage in ways that private sector health plans can, even private FFS indemnity plans. Among enabling changes that should be considered are exempting the program from some procedural requirements in rule making, permitting it to adopt some private sector managed indemnity techniques, and authorizing it to contract selectively, purchase medical equipment and supplies at "market" prices, and negotiate directly with some providers. Other changes might include reorganization of the Health Care Financing Administration (HCFA) as a separate and more independent agency or even as a government corporation. The possibilities range from incremental changes to fundamental restructuring. And some of the problems or difficulties attending these possibilities also range from minor snarls or pitfalls to matters of constitutional principle. They involve theoretical and practical challenges that could make use of some of the best talents in government as well as the private sector.

Deciding what new powers should be conferred and where more discretion should be allowed is likely to be a perplexing and disputed process. The kind of new powers being mentioned have not been much tested, so their effectiveness as remedies for present discontents is largely unknown. Under America's present circumstances of divided government and strong partisan differences, moreover, persuading Congress to delegate to or to empower an executive branch agency—the HCFA, for instance—may be difficult, especially when Congress has formidable power to act independently and with great effect through the budget reconciliation process. And a prudent administrator will need to be careful about the authority requested, because new powers will have to prove their value in a tough political environment.

The Medicare program will need to be adapted to accommodate an unknown but rapidly growing Medicare HMO and managed care sector. As these entities grow they are likely, at least in the short run, to attract a younger and healthier population, increasing the proportion of high-risk and high-cost beneficiaries in the FFS program. The challenge for the Medicare administration will be to find the program savings or additional funds to keep the traditional program competitive and, at the same time, administer a growing managed care option evenhandedly and effectively. For an FFS program nurtured on social insurance principles, the second part of this assignment may ask too much. In 1995 Congress expressed its view by providing, in the Medicare Preservation Act, for a "second HCFA"to be established within the Department of Health and Human Services (HHS) to administer managed care plans and other private sector options.[1] And the prestigious Institute of Medicine expressed its doubts that the HCFA possessed the requisite capabilities to administer an alternative modeled on the Federal Employees Health Benefits Program (FEHBP) as an adjunct to the Medicare program.[2] Politically, these developments signal a need for persuading doubters. So, as a transition toward managed care moves forward, the Medicare administration will need not only to be fair and effective in dealing with managed care alternatives but be perceived to be so.

Improving management for FFS Medicare will be a technical process but also one that is highly charged politically and will need strong public and private support. Getting that support will demand bipartisan political leadership and public and private advocacy. It will also require forbearance from seeking partisan or tactical advantage and a will to seek out ways of building consensus. The political challenge is perhaps the greatest, for policymakers confront not just radically different visions for the future of Medicare but strongly partisan divisions, distrust between Congress and the administration, and an acute consciousness of the strategic implications of almost any move.

An aspect of Medicare administration that makes strategic implications particularly sensitive is the public-private dimension. Recent discussion has been about whether the FFS program should continue to be dominant or whether managed care would become the norm. But it is also about how the Medicare program should be administered, involving a perennial of American government: the extent to which programs should be privatized or, less drastically, employ market or private sector adaptations. And it is in this respect that the argument for new administrative powers becomes so important: for process often becomes policy, and the way we proceed will largely determine where we arrive. This was at issue in the proposal for a second HCFA. And a proposal based on the FEHBP was opposed by supporters of the FFS program for a similar reason: that it might structure competition unfairly. In a time of transition, process and how it is structured are important.

Considering these complexities leads to the prime emphasis of my discussion: the need for a period of sustained development. Restructuring Medicare will not be like following a blueprint; it will be a matter of learning and devising. Today, the future shares of the FFS program and of managed care are unclear. We do not know how much money managed care might be able to save for the program and still remain acceptable to beneficiaries and the Medicare political constituency.[3] Nor do we know how competitive the FFS program might become with some innovative cost savers and stronger authority. For both options, moreover, specific means for cost saving or quality enhancement are largely unproved, and their practical and political feasibility is yet to be determined. What is needed is an administrative strategy that takes account of these unknowns and is structured for a period of sustained development, one that could last for years, even a decade or more. A requisite for success will be to develop a bipartisan consensus to create a continuing collaboration between Congress and the executive branch similar to that achieved at times for aiding the Social Security program and developing the Medicare fee schedule and the prospective payment system. A close and continuous monitoring of the transition is also essential for midcourse corrections, beneficiary protection, and continuing political support.

This paper discusses these issues, especially as they relate to several possible models for administering the FFS program. It is primarily based on interviews with thirty people (see appendix B) who have or had roles in Medicare administration or participated in activities related to the program. The group includes former and current executives of the HCFA, the Prospective Payment Assessment Commission (ProPAC), and the Medicare Payment Advisory Commission (MPAC), congressional staff and insurance and health plan executives, health policy consultants, and practicing attorneys. The paper has also benefited from discussions with and a review by members of the National Academy of Social Insurance Advisory Panel.

Background for Change

A useful preliminary to considering the various organizational models for fee-for-service Medicare would be to review some of the factors that set practical and legal limits to what can be achieved with present program authority. A highly selective list includes the original legislation, current organizational status, the politics of divided government, and specific constraints or limited authority. A brief characterization of these can help readers understand the limited degrees of freedom and the obstacles to change that characterize the program.

Original Legislation

One of the major achievements of the original Medicare statute was to institutionalize firmly a bill-paying system modeled on FFS indemnity plans of thirty years ago.[4] Changes since 1966 have allowed price setting under the prospective payment system and the Medicare fee schedule but have allowed only limited and mostly experimental initiatives that would change the underlying indemnity approach. Specially qualified Medicare HMOs and competitive medical plans (CMPs) were allowed.[5] And the government experimented with a variety of medical care review organizations.[6] In time, however, the FFS program lagged behind the private sector in innovative adaptations aimed at controlling utilization or improving the quality of care, largely because of provisions in the original statute and a reluctance, mostly on the part of Congress, to change it. Often the reason was that such activities would interfere directly or indirectly with the practice of medicine or beneficiaries' freedom of choice, which were specifically protected by sections 1801 and 1802 of the original statute.[7] HMOs were promoted as an alternative, but only very recently has the idea of modifying the FFS system as such begun to receive serious consideration.

Organizational Status

In considering private sector adaptations that might contain costs or make FFS Medicare more adaptable, it is important to remember that the HCFA is not a government corporation or an independent agency but an administration within HHS and subject to the usual constraints that go with that status, such as civil service rules for hiring and firing, the budget procedures, limits on acquisition and contracting, and the Administrative Procedure Act with its departmental and executive branch clearances and "notice and comment" requirements for rule making. Moreover, health care finance is an arcane, specialized, and politically charged activity, characteristics that make for conflict, delay, legislative and executive branch intrusions, and micromanagement. In a word, change is likely to be difficult, given the form of organization; and for that reason some believe that a nondepartmental, quasi-public status would be preferable.

Divided Government and the Budget Reconciliation Process

Crucially important for health care legislation, especially Medicare, has been the persistence of divided government together with the practice of using the budget reconciliation process for health care legislation. All major Medicare reforms, from the Social Security Amendments of 1972 to the Medicare fee schedule in 1989, were passed under conditions of divided government and, since 1983, as part of budget reconciliation. The Medicare Preservation Act was also part of budget reconciliation: the vetoed Balanced Budget Act of 1995. In considering Medicare administration, this feature of the political environment represents both a danger and an opportunity. On the one hand, divided government and the budget reconciliation process have led to increased politicizing and micromanagement of the administration. They have also widened participation in the policy process, so that initiatives come from many different sources and so too do complaints and peremptory checks on policy development. On the other hand, this same combination of divided government and budget reconciliation can be used for reform: it creates incentives for bipartisan collaboration and allows both experiment with incremental change and passage of large, complex, and controversial legislation.

This argument is not intended to celebrate a development generally regarded as a constitutional pathology but rather to say that it can be turned to good account. The American policy process tends to move slowly and incrementally with occasional spurts of major change. This description is especially applicable to Medicare. Movement is usually incremental because of the hallowed status of the program, the beneficiary and provider interests at stake, the technical difficulties, and the monetary and political consequences of change. Reforms on a grander scale require some major impetus such as inflation or mounting deficits, a program crisis, or political imperatives of the electoral cycle. Reforms that work well, especially for Medicare, may require extras such as bipartisanship and perceptions by beneficiaries and providers alike that the changes are workable and fair. They also seem to be accompanied by repeated attempts, adaptations, learning, and coming to accept the hard choices. In sum, making health policy has often been a learning and devising process sustained over time; and American political institutions are well adapted to this approach. What is needed is to use these institutions creatively.

Limits on Program Authority

One task for policymakers bent on saving FFS Medicare will be to decide how and how much to modify the administrative structure, presumably retaining traditional features such as beneficiaries' freedom of choice and considerable autonomy for providers while strengthening cost containment and quality. For modifying administrative structure the various organizational models can be helpful. But before considering them, it is useful to be aware of some of the ways critics have thought the Medicare program unduly hampered in making constructive adaptations, especially as compared with other government agencies or private sector health plans (see appendix A).

—The program cannot use most managed indemnity techniques.[8] According to present law, preadmission certification, primary care gatekeepers, individual case management, and contracting with preferred provider organizations (PPOs) are not permitted.

—The program cannot select providers or exclude them; the sanctioning process is complex, time consuming, and indirect.

—The program lacks authority to purchase medical equipment or supplies at market prices. It can respond to excessive prices only through a cumbersome and lengthy process.

—The program has limited powers to contract. In general, it must use requests for proposals (RFPs). Medicare cannot use competitive bidding or negotiate with providers. It cannot contract selectively, until recently not even with the carriers and fiscal intermediaries that pay the Medicare bills, audit claims, construct profiles, and perform other acts related to payment. Now the HCFA has more authority, but only in this limited area.

—Many of Medicare's regulatory activities come under the Administrative Procedure Act and are subject to "notice and comment" procedures as well as executive branch clearance and congressional supervision. Regulatory impact or paperwork reduction clearances or both may apply to regulations and required forms or data submissions. One consequence is delay, with three years for a major rule not uncommon. The rule-making procedures also give rise to judicial appeals, occasioning yet more delay.

—The research and demonstration process is lengthy and subject to delays. RFPs must be developed and cleared, responses solicited and approved or rejected, terms and arrangements for the demonstration concluded, and the demonstration completed and evaluated. This protracted process is subjected to varying amounts of executive branch clearance and congressional intervention, with more delays.

—The program is subject to political interference. Inaction or delay is often the result of executive branch or congressional intervention at the behest of clientele or provider interests, holding up a clearance or signaling that a particular demonstration or regulatory provision would be likely to provoke a punitive response. Such actions can hold up particular initiatives for years or lead to their abandonment.

Other items could be added to this list, but these are the most pertinent for consideration here. There is always a danger that such lists are read as an agenda, implying that a remedy must be found for each alleged mischief. That is not the use intended for this list. It points toward some possible modifications in the traditional administration of the FFS program that would allow more discretion or provide additional authority. The organizational models described and evaluated in the next section illustrate various ways to institutionalize such modifications and, it is hoped, provide some guidance in assessing their political prospects, the trade-offs that would be entailed, and the ultimate benefits for the Medicare program.

Alternative Organizational Models

This section sets forth four organizational models with three variants for the last one. The order of presentation of the models is mainly intended to facilitate exposition rather than to show preference or the amount of change involved. They are, arguably at least, workable proposals. Descriptions are based, with modifications, on interviews with past and present Medicare administrators and others in government and the private sector knowledgeable about Medicare. The models embody many of their views about what is possible and desirable in restructuring Medicare administration.

The models illustrate ways additional discretion or new authority might be institutionalized, and they should help in assessing the practicality and desirability of such changes (for a schematic description and evaluation see table 5-2). Presumably, the desirable result is to sustain and improve a Medicare FFS option that can effectively contain costs and achieve high levels of quality consistent with beneficiaries' freedom of choice and the preservation of provider autonomy and viability. Vitally important is sustaining a process of development—of learning and devising—and with that of meeting the main challenges previously described: changes that can earn their way, adaptation to a growing managed care sector, and retention of political support. The long-term goal is an FFS program adapted for improved management but retaining and building on features that have made it attractive in the past. Because a development process is essential to achieving the objective, the contribution these different organizational models can make to that process is important. But long-term schemes can fail, and we also have to live in the present. Therefore, each of these options needs to be considered as a fallback position: Where would it leave the FFS program if the option failed or the development process faltered?

Incrementalism: Full Use of Current Authority with Incremental Changes

Underlying this strategy is a belief that the HCFA has powers that, used creatively, would go far toward putting FFS Medicare in a viable position. It is not a status quo proposal, since it would entail vigorous and adaptive use of existing powers and incremental but strategically important administrative or legislative changes.[9] The restructuring of the HCFA would be minimal, and accountability would present no more of a problem than at present.

PRIORITIES FOR ACTION.   The recent passage of the Kassebaum-Kennedy bill, the Health Insurance Portability and Accountability Act of 1996, increases the attractiveness of this first organizational model. Included in this legislation is a strong antifraud and abuse program establishing severe sanctions; engaging the cooperative efforts of HSS, the Department of Justice (including the FBI), and federal, state, and local officials; and authorizing generous and assured funding. The act also permits the HCFA to contract with "eligible private entities," other than insurance companies, to provide a wide range of activities, including auditing, cost reports, and medical and utilization review. This latter provision—incidentally a good example of strategic incrementalism—removes

Table 5-2.   *Organizational Models for Restructuring Fee-for-Service Medicare*

Models	Major elements	Advantages	Disadvantages
Incrementalism: full use of current authority with incremental changes	Fraud and abuse Incremental additions to purchasing authority Cost savings from HHA and SNFs A Medicare commission; additional savings from PPS and MFS "Fix" the AAPCC; some use of copays and deductibles Use of demonstration authority to experiment with private sector adaptations	Encourages bipartisan collaboration Begins "sustained development," learning and adaptation Important as a fallback Saves money; eases time pressure	Makes little use of private sector adaptations Does not exploit managed care or consumer choice potential Does not address problem of high-cost beneficiaries Lacks strong political appeal, except as a compromise or fallback
Consumer Choice: an FEHBP model	A defined contribution A government agency would administer, provide plan information, and supervise marketing Beneficiary could choose among FFS; managed care, including private plans; and Medicare savings accounts	Institutionalizes a marketlike competition Creates beneficiary incentives for prudent choice Encourages private sector adaptations Reduces opportunity and incentive for administrative or political intrusions Could be phased in	High administrative costs; fraud and abuse Methods needed to protect and inform Medicare beneficiaries Risk segmentation Administration: two HCFAs or not?

Table 5-2. *Continued*

Models	Major elements	Advantages	Disadvantages
Prudent purchasing: reinventing the HCFA	Increased powers for contracting and purchasing Medicare choices expanded; increased information program Managed indemnity, centers of excellence, and other private sector adaptations; special attention to high-cost cases Separate bureaus (or divisions) for FFS Medicare, managed care, and chronically and severely ill	Exploits private sector adaptations and purchasing clout of HCFA Specifically addresses problem of high-cost cases Strong managed care program with beneficiary protection Visibility and accountability for major program development Could approach incrementally; also devolve after development phase	Specific powers or aggregate of powers may be politically unacceptable HCFA control of expanded Choices program may be challenged Separate bureaus not functionally effective Cost savings both unknown and controversial Transition may be perilous
Independent agency Independent status, such as that of Social Security Administraiton		New charter and task assignments Potential for bipartisan support Improved access within executive branch Independence from DHHS policies, constraints, and clearances	Political exposure Lack of allies Little stimulus to change administrative methods

Table 5-2. *Continued*

Models	Major elements	Advantages	Disadvantages
Government corporation, such as U.S. Postal Service		Special personnel authority Relax some constraints of APA More freedom in purchasing, contracting, private sector adaptations	Corporate form an unknown in health care finance Delegations may be limited or have strings Close monitoring essential for "sustained development" Large amount of freedom in rule making or contracting questionable
Partial privatization: Institute of Medicine proposal	Use an FEHBP approach to offer plans, including FFS Supervised by semiprivate market board Quality standards and consumer information system based on best private sector methods	Combines competition, consumer choice, and quality enhancement Facilitates use of best private sector methods More widely acceptable devolution alternative	Would be administratively complex and expensive Risk segmentation Need for development of plan offerings; methods for ensuring universal access and program-wide standards of quality

the long-standing requirement that the Medicare administration must contract only with insurance companies for claims administration and related activities. This change makes possible a much more aggressive use of claims review and auditing. And because an estimated 5–10 percent of program revenues are consumed by fraud and abuse, the dollar savings could be considerable. In addition, data and capabilities developed through this program would support other activities such as physician profiling and quality improvement.

Another possibility would be to use present powers, with incremental legislative changes, to buy some supplies or services at or close to the market price. At present the HCFA cannot, for instance, buy "durable medical equipment" or medical supplies such as surgical bandages on the open market or even by contracting for them because they fall under prescribed payment or reimbursment formulas and are virtually impossible to change except through legislation or a cumbersome administrative process.[10] Consequently, the HCFA often pays three or four or ten times the amount that, say, the Veterans Admnistration does for such supplies. But with a line or two in a budget reconciliation act, the agency might be able to demand the same price for medical equipment and supplies (as opposed to services) that the manufacturer asks from other bulk purchasers, a practice used in state Medicaid programs for drugs.[11] Depending on political feasibility, a next step might be to use bidding and small-purchase procedures, as the Veterans Administration does.

One proposed change that would involve minimum disruption to ongoing programs would be to combine ProPAC and the Medicare Payment Advisory Commission into one commission.[12] With both the prospective payment system and the Medicare fee schedule fully implemented, much of the reason for separate commissions is gone. Nevertheless, their roles in providing a quasi-independent and nonpartisan review of health policy issues and in advising Congress continue to be valuable. And merger seems indicated because a growing number of issues involve both part A and part B or, like managed care, fall under neither part A nor part B. A new charter would also be an opportunity for some corrective legislation or assignments that might generate cost savings or point the way to them.[13]

Much can also be done within the existing administrative framework to save on medical services, and some important initiatives are already under way. For example, home health services and the skilled nursing facilities have been responsible for a large proportion of increased Medicare costs. Getting these costs under control will probably take a variety of strategies, including limited action by Congress, better provider participation standards, bundling or prospective payment or both, some use of copayments, and increased monitoring by intermediaries. These involve incremental changes and in-house capabilities. Promising initiatives, including bundling and captitation, are now being developed.[14]

Some well-designed legislative tinkering could help with the problem of adverse selection that the FFS program is likely to experience as the managed care sector expands. For example, an improved risk adjuster for Medicare managed care entities, combined with some premium contributions or copayments or both, could be actuarily fair and make the FFS program more competitive.[15] Such a project would call for collaboration between Congress, the HCFA, and, possibly, a new Medicare Commission, but it involves mainly traditional tools and methods.

At the same time, there is no reason the incremental organizational model could not be used to experiment with various private sector adaptations. Under the Social Security Amendments, the Public Health Service Act, and various mandates from Congress, the HCFA has a demonstration capability that can be used to develop new modes of health care delivery, alternative methods of payment, and techniques for reviewing and evaluating the quality of care. One promising use of this demonstration authority has been the development of "centers of excellence" that contract with Medicare for heart and liver transplants and bypass surgery.[16] The attraction for the beneficiary, who has free choice in this matter, is to have the procedure done in a center of excellence such as the Cleveland Clinic. For Medicare, there is the assurance of quality and a lower price. A creative adapation of a strategy widely used in the private sector, this initiative is particularly significant as a method of dealing with some of the severe and chronic cases that are a major source of increasing patient care expense for Medicare. Taken a step farther, it might also open up interesting possibilities for competitive bidding or direct negotiation.[17]

Using the demonstration authority and some strategic incrementalism to promote relatively modest legislative changes, the HCFA could experiment with and gradually build up a managed indemnity capability like that widely used by Blue Cross/Blue Shield and large indemnity plans. Managed indemnity could employ such techniques as case management for high-cost cases; fee schedules, bundling, and prospective payment; and provider profiling and educative programs. Done with beneficiary consent and a softer persuasive approach to managed care, such a scheme could retain the best features of FFS Medicare and also save some money.

APPRAISAL. Incrementalism as an organizational model can have a vital role as part of a program of sustained development. The initiatives I have described build on the familiar and accepted, could earn their way, and would engender support and trust for a change in program direction, if needed. This model also provides a good way of testing limits and of deciding, for instance, how to combine traditional regulatory methods with private sector methods to restrain the costs of home health agencies and skilled nursing facilities.

Saving money is important because it is a principal reason for wishing to change Medicare administration: the current program does not and cannot contain costs adequately. But the cost-containment record of Medicare has been on the whole good and, in the past ten years, better than that of the private sector. In addition, the payment formulas for Medicare HMOs need to be amended, and an appropriate accounting must be made for the disproportionate number of high-cost cases in the FFS program. If a combination of legislative and administrative efforts could also bring outpatient surgery, the home health agencies, and the skilled nursing facilities under control, FFS Medicare would become fairly competitive. Or, so this argument goes, it is at least worth exploring this possibility.

Furthermore, if stronger measures are required, this incremental model could provide a feasible method of testing a managed indemnity approach or various component elements of it. Being incremental, the separate steps are more likely to have bipartisan appeal in Congress and would be easier to monitor and to amend or reverse as desirable.

At the same time, there are problems. One is that this first model does not, in its own terms, significantly change the mission of the HCFA and would have little effect on its organizational culture. It might have little bipartisan appeal other than being noncontroversial. Indeed, on the theory that major policy efforts engage much of the energy and talents of an agency, vigorous development of managed indemnity could marginalize the existing HMO and managed care program or at least appear to do so. And, as peacemakers know, appearances are important.

Furthermore, doing fairly well on cost containment is no reason for not doing the best job possible. A major problem with the first paradigm is that it does not take full advantage of private sector methods, possibilities for informing and empowering beneficiaries, market forces and competition, and of the countervailing power that a large purchaser can exert. Each of the next two options illustrates ways in which a different mission and administrative structures can engage these constructive influences.

Consumer Choice: An FEHBP Model

The Federal Employees Health Benefits Program (FEHBP) was created in 1959 and currently covers more than 9 million federal employees, retirees (or annuitants), and their dependents. It is one example of managed competiton and served as the model for Alain Enthoven's original managed competition proposal in 1976.[18] It has been considered as an option for NHI and figured prominently in both the House and Senate versions of the Medicare Preservation Act of 1995.

The two basic elements of this scheme are defined contribution and informed choice. The federal government makes a maximum contribution: 60 percent of a high-option plan, but not more than 75 percent of any plan. The employee pays the rest of the premium and any deductibles and copayments, and so has an incentive to shop among an abundance of plans—400 nationally and about 20 to 40 locally, including an array of HMO and indemnity plans. The Office of Personnel Management, which administers the program with the aid of intermediaries, sets some financial, administrative, and benefits standards but, as a government agency, eschews the provision of extensive consumer information on plans. For that information enrollees must rely on other sources such as privately published reports and associations of federal employees.[19]

MEDICARE ADAPTATIONS.   Proponents of this model generally acknowledge that the FEHBP would need to be adapted to a Medicare population that is on average older and in poorer health than the current plan members. Broadly, such adjustments include an allowance for different health statuses, a more active role in supplementing the information available to beneficiaries, and possibly a larger role in screening plans and in monitoring their behavior.

Plans for organizing such a scheme are broadly similar though they differ in detail. A common feature is the assignment of an OPM-type responsibility to the secretary of HHS, who would oversee the system, collect and disseminate the basic plan information, and organize the annual open enrollment. Traditional FFS Medicare would be one plan offering among a large group that would include Medicare risk plans, private managed care plans, and new Medicare Savings Account high-deductible options. The HCFA would continue to exist, though in the House version of the Medicare Preservation Act, a separate agency would have been created within HHS to administer the managed care options.[20] The conference agreement required the secretary to provide beneficiaries with general election information, a list of plans and a comparison of them, federal contribution amounts, and additional information that the secretary determined would assist people in making their choice.

APPRAISAL.   One merit of this proposal is that it would provide a test on a national scale of a procompetition, managed care alternative to FFS Medicare. Considering the cost pressures on Medicare and the alleged savings of managed care, testing such an alternative may be politically necessary to preserve Medicare. And while we do not know that competititon will save that kind of money, we do not know that it will not. And that is an important unknown that needs investigation.

PHASED INTRODUCTION.   The FEHBP option is one that can be approached incrementally, which would facilitate testing of some of its constituent elements. Estimates for implementing this proposal range from five to ten years, suggesting that phased introduction and testing along the way are feasible. For instance, the consumer education proposals could stand independently and would offer a good opportunity to assess the value of such activities. In its HCFA On-Line initiative, the agency is already exploring the elements of an expanded information program. Similarly, with a growing array of managed care initiatives the HCFA is also planning a small-scale version of the

FEHBP.[21] These initiatives could proceed independently of the HCFA if desirable and would offer additional opportunities to test provisions of the FEHBP option.

MAJOR UNKNOWNS. Possibilities for testing along the way would be a desirable feature of this model, since there are some big unknowns. One is whether such a program would, in fact, generate large Medicare savings without compromising quality or imposing unfair burdens. Experience with Medicare HMOs does not count as strong evidence; but so far as it counts at all, HMOs have cost the program money, not saved it. In any event, a more satisfactory risk adjuster would have to be developed. And although competition in the FEHBP may have worked to contain costs, it is a weakly driven competition, relying largely on individual choice and shifting members to HMOs. Meanwhile, the competitive process has been accompanied by chronic risk segmentation and very high premium differentials and copayments for those selecting indemnity plans, so that the savings represent in part a shifting of costs to the enrollees.[22] There may or may not be satisfactory solutions to these problems, but there is a need for an administrative strategy that includes testing, evaluation, and remediation in the course of development.

A question with the FEHBP model or similar consumer choice plans is the amount and kind of information needed by the consumer and how to monitor and disseminate it. As noted before, the FEHBP supplies general information about the plan but leaves to the private sector the provision of richer descriptive and evaluative materials. Generally, advocates of the FEHBP approach to Medicare recognize that the beneficiaries need more information and different kinds of information from that provided by the OPM, both for their own benefit and to promote competition.

But there are differences over this issue of consumer information that raise questions about implementation. The House version of the Medicare Preservation Act strongly supported beneficiary information to promote informed choice and required quality and consumer satisfaction information along with the usual plan details. The Senate version was less detailed, omitting any mention of quality and consumer satisfaction. The conference agreement said that the secretary might add information that would assist making a choice. An underlying issue is how much the government should or would disclose. Extensive disclosure might almost amount to awarding a government seal of approval. At the same time, unwelcome disclosure could lead to protests and even political intervention. A leading private sector proposal recommended a consumer advisory board to advise the secretary.[23] The whole issue came up later in an Institute of Medicine conference that urged the HCFA and HHS to consider whether this function might not be largely privatized.[24]

ADMINISTRATIVE PROBLEMS.   The administration of an FEHBP alternative is important to consider because the option, offering an array of managed care HMO-type plans, suggests delegation of management and administrative detail. But such a plan, if administered as the FEHBP is, would rely on intermediaries much as the Medicare FFS program does. Since it would involve a large array of plans, administrative costs would be relatively high, several times as much per $100 of claims as either the Civilian Health and Medical Program Uniformed Services (CHAMPUS) or Medicare.[25] And the FEHBP has experienced similar problems with fraud and abuse and in getting the carriers to pursue the issue.[26] If the Medicare Preservation Act mandates were followed, the program would require the development of a large new database with new criteria, standards, and methods of measurement and evaluation. And finally, it would not replace the FFS Medicare program but develop in addition to it. In a word, both the savings and the simplification of administration might be less than anticipated.

Another and larger administrative problem will be protecting Medicare beneficiaries and FFS program interests during a transition to a more competitive system. As a public program, Medicare has a responsibility to ensure access to quality care for all beneficiaries. Practically speaking that will require ensuring that acceptable options are available everywhere in the country and that standards of quality applicable to private health plans and a variety of hybrids are developed.[27] Another transitional problem will be how to cope with shifting program costs if the managed care plans are able to attract a younger and healthier population, leaving the traditional FFS program with a disproportionate share of older, high-risk beneficiaries.

TWO HCFAs?   Extensive cost shifting could bring into bold relief the underlying difference between the social insurance philosophy on which the original Medicare program was based and the market-oriented philosophy underlying the FEHBP proposal. This kind of consideration led the Institute of Medicine to express concern over whether the HCFA as currently structured could effectively manage its own Choices program.[28] One proposal in the House version of the Medicare Preservation Act was that a separate agency be created to administer the Medicare Plus program. Part of the rationale was an alleged bias in the HCFA against HMOs. It was also in part an attempt to institutionalize a competition between the two options and encourage more

Medicare beneficiaries to choose HMOs. Such a plan could be a vehicle for developing a more focused and comprehensive effort to improve both FFS Medicare and managed care and HMOs. The FFS program, for instance, could develop a managed indemnity approach toward cost saving, and the HMO-managed care program could offer attractive PPO and point-of-service options and improve methods for monitoring quality and increasing consumer satisfaction.

But creating a separate agency is a drastic step with significant monetary and organizational costs. Although it avoids direct conflict, it does not resolve the issue of unequal competition, and by institutionalizing separateness it may work against adaptations that could do so. A better solution might be to find ways to institutionalize the separate approaches within the same agency and work toward a fair competition, taking advantage of the existing infrastructure, accumulated expertise, and capacity for exploring adaptations that combined both approaches. This alternative is discussed in considering the prudent purchasing model.

Prudent Purchasing: Reinventing the HCFA

The prudent purchasing option is described as reinventing the HCFA because it contains various private sector adaptations and reforms designed to improve performance and accountability. It goes beyond the first organizational model in seeking significant additional powers to act as a prudent purchaser. And this model would put special emphasis on two groups: the chronically and severely ill and the HMO and managed care enrollees. It is a program designed to preserve a viable Medicare FFS option by addressing both the problem of the high-cost beneficiaries and the growing importance of managed care as a potential cost saver.

EMPOWERMENT FOR PRUDENT PURCHASING. To implement the prudent purchaser concept would require new authority, especially the power to purchase some items (such as equipment or supplies) at or close to market prices and authority, probably selectively bestowed, to use competitive bidding. "Negotiation" may be too alarming a concept, but some of the same results could be achieved through use of the demonstration authority and requests for proposals.[29] A major element of the model would be to seek powers to deal more aggressively with the high-risk, high-cost cases responsible for so much of the Medicare FFS costs. This would be done in part by building on centers of excellence and employing managed indemnity techniques and other private sector adaptations.[30] To make beneficiaries more prudent purchasers, as well as to learn about their interests and preferences, the HCFA has been expanding its information services. Still in a planning phase is an ambitious HCFA On-Line initiative. This program, involving an extensive database and software and communications capabilities, would allow beneficiaries to tap into the HCFA's vast resources of information about health plan and provider characteristics and quality of care, as well as specialized information about managed care and HMOs.

MEDICARE CHOICES. Closely related to this initiative are current HCFA plans to develop a structured enrollment process similar to that administered by the OPM for the FEHBP. This program would build on the HCFA's own Medicare Choices demonstration, under development since 1995. The growing number of Medicare options and the prospect of including private health plans makes such a mechanism increasingly appropriate and even essential. Also, the HCFA On-Line program could add the kind of beneficiary-specific information to make such a system of choice effective and responsive to beneficiaries' preferences. Carefully administered and evaluated, these initiatives could prove invaluable for deciding how best to combine FFS with managed care and competition.

REORGANIZATION. Both politically and for policy reasons, an internal reorganization of the HCFA that would institutionalize some of the underlying principles of this organizational model might be desirable. Politically, it might signal that the HCFA of tomorrow will be different from the HCFA that, rightly or wrongly, some remember without affection. And the developing orientation of the agency, recently described as beneficiary-centered purchasing, would seem to call for a significantly different distribution of functions.

THE HCFA REORGANIZATION PLAN OF 1996. On November 7, 1996, the HCFA announced completion of the design phase of a major reorganization and the beginning of its implementation (see appendix A).[31] In the main this reorganization would institutionalize developments begun in the Strategic Plan of 1994. Especially pertinent in the present context are two organizational changes. One is the creation of a new division of Beneficiary Services and Operations that would be expressly dedicated to beneficiary concerns and well positioned for the development of the HCFA On-Line and Choices programs. A second change is the creation of a new division of Health Plan and Provider Operations that merges the FFS and managed care programs. The purpose of this move is to eliminate outmoded distinctions and integrate FFS and managed care operations throughout the agency.[32]

From a functional perspective, the HCFA reorganization is well suited to implement a prudent purchaser concept. The new Division of Health Plan and Provider Operations would, in the first instance, facilitate the development of multiple choices, including adaptations of both FFS and managed care options. It would position the agency to engage the cooperation of providers, for example, in developing insurance bands or partial capitation models. Combining its efforts with the On-Line and Choices initiatives, the Division of Beneficiary Services and Operations would empower the beneficiary to become a more prudent consumer.

DIFFERENCES FROM THE PROPOSED MODEL.   Despite the merits of this design, it differs in some ways from the underlying philosophy of this paper. From a political perspective, it does not clearly indicate that a managed care approach *as such* will be adequately explored or fully implemented. As to policy, for instance, a continuum of choices might be less effective in containing costs than a strategy that explored the potential of managed care more fully while addressing separately and specifically the deficiencies of FFS Medicare. Lacking agreement on a goal, moreover, the way administrative activities move forward becomes critical. Thus a second vital criterion, in addition to functional efficacy, is how accountable and how corrigible the organizational activity will be, which is especially important when a lengthy period of development under divided government may be needed.

The prudent purchaser model puts less emphasis on functional efficacy and more on political accountability and the representation of specific clientele interests.[33] Underlying this difference are priorities and calculations about the requisites for a sustained course of development. One such calculation is that keeping a Medicare FFS option alive entails finding an appropriate way of dealing with the challenge of high-risk, high-cost beneficiaries. It also requires developing an optimum role for the managed care, procompetition approach. For a period of sustained development, moreover, it is essential to provide assurances that critical priorities and clientele interests are being addressed and that adequate methods for correction exist if they are not being addressed.

A reorganization that would more closely follow these stated requisites might include the following changes. The present Bureau of Policy Development would remain responsible for FFS Medicare and become the Medicare Bureau. The Office of Managed Care would become a bureau with broad responsibility for developing new managed care and HMO options and would be staffed for its increased responsibility. A third bureau for the disabled and chronically and severely ill would be especially concerned with these groups and the delivery of health care for them. All would be committed to prudent purchasing, but this bureau would especially apply "buy right" techniques, managed indemnity, centers of excellence, and other cost savers consistent with FFS Medicare. The specific charge of the associate administrator for policy would be to ensure continuity of care and secure the best trade-offs among cost containment, quality of care, and beneficiary satisfaction.

In comparison with the HCFA reorganization design, this plan is not as good for developing a continuum of health plan options ranging from traditional FFS to managed care plans to HMOs. Nor would it position the HCFA as well for prudent purchasing and contracting with the private sector. And creating a separate bureau for the high-cost cases would risk leaving the frail elderly and disabled as an isolated and politically unpopular clientele, much like the Medicaid population.

Politically, this organizational structure might gain wide acceptance, especially if representative groups were persuaded that new agency powers were being used to develop both FFS Medicare and the managed care options even-handedly and to achieve the best trade-offs between price and quality. The "if" is a big "if," but the organization and bureau missions would make program efforts and accountability for results more visible and more adaptable to a change of administration or of congressional majority. At the same time, by institutionalizing distinctive programs for three clientele groups, this scheme might prove durable and resistant to hasty or inadequately considered change.

A programmatic argument for this particular approach is that it hedges bets by seeking to exploit more fully the potential savings through managed care and HMOs. Some of the criticism of the prudent purchaser model is that there may not be big savings to be had from prudent purchasing, management of high-cost cases, or various other managed indemnity approaches. A part of this skepticism is that inflated prices, unnecessary procedures, and increasing volume are pervasive in the Medicare program but that centers of excellence or managing high-cost cases will do relatively little to address the problem.[34] A further pragmatic question is whether the savings, if there, can be reached: for instance, whether demonstrations of centers of excellence for bypass grafts, cataract surgery, or joint replacements can be widely extended across the nation or whether acceptable methods of bulk purchasing or competitive contracting can be developed and successfully implemented. At present, it is mostly speculation that there are big savings to be realized from either strategy. And should developments prove that the realizable savings have been exaggerated, savings achieved through a vigorous managed care program could provide a welcome offset.

POSSIBLE PROVIDER AND POLITICAL RESPONSE.   Both the prudent purchasing and managed indemnity aspects of this model are likely to encounter resistance from providers and others. Unless carefully implemented, managed indemnity could interfere with the practice of medicine or beneficiaries' freedom of choice, or be viewed as doing so. Prudent purchasing is at present mostly demonstrations. But if, for example, centers of excellence were increased from one in a region to eight or ten, provider interests would be tangibly affected.[35] The experience with competitive bidding provides a striking illustration. Year after year, enthusiasts in Congress and the private sector have advocated use of competitive bidding. Yet repeated attempts to use it for clinical laboratories, durable medical equipment, or HMO premiums have been blocked or impeded when Congress has said, "It may be a good idea; but not in my constituency." Related examples are guidelines for lower back pain, stopped by the House Appropriations Committee; attempts to capitate skilled nursing facilities, delayed by threat of lawsuit; and attempts to buy prescription drugs on more favorable terms, blocked in the courts and more recently delayed by the OMB. Examples of this sort underline the importance of congressional forbearance but also of incrementalism and of new authorizations that can earn their way. Indeed, one reason that the FEHBP option is attractive to many is that they doubt that an alternative, more interventionist policy can be made to work largely because of the many vetoes built into policymaking.

For a number of reasons, this paradigm may be overly ambitious and seek more than providers and Congress would accept or than the HCFA is prepared to undertake. The increased powers and discretion required go against current decentralizing and privatizing trends and would generate anxiety among providers. An expressed concern is that sapping the quantum of available policy energy might prevent Congress and the executive branch from doing well with more achievable options.[36] And, currently, the HCFA is heavily engaged, short of experienced personnel, and facing a number of important retirements in the near future.[37] Regional offices are also unevenly developed and lack experience for some of the kinds of programs being considered.

INSTITUTE OF MEDICINE CONFERENCE.   Concerns that were closely related to the aggregation of powers surfaced in a 1996 conference sponsored by the Institute of Medicine that focused on providing consumer information for Medicare beneficiaries in the coming decade. The conference questioned whether a public agency such as the HCFA could match the sophisticated information and education capabilities in use by Xerox, Southern California Edison, and some health insurance purchasing cooperatives. It recommended that the agency consider putting this activity and its Medicare Choices program under a Medicare Market Board, Commision, or Council.[38] The IOM proposal will be discussed more fully in the next section, but it raises a serious question about the aggregate of powers contemplated by the prudent purchaser option and indicates that privatization or a partial devolution ought to at least be considered.

TRANSITION STRATEGY NEEDED. In considering this organizational model, it should also be apparent that achieving reorganization will be a major problem because a number of controversial steps are involved. For political reasons the prudent purchasing model may require a strategy of privatizing along with strategic incrementalism and sustained policy advocacy. It would also need commitment and strong bipartisan support from both the president and Congress and a resolve to provide the authority needed. Finally, it requires persuading policymakers that FFS Medicare is worth saving, that the way to do that has yet to be developed, and that the HCFA is an essential vehicle for accomplishing the task.

Make the HCFA an Independent Agency

Another way of reorganizing the administration of Medicare would be to establish an independent status for the HCFA for one or more of the usual reasons—freeing it from departmental constraints; gaining independence from nonpolitical or bipartisan control; or getting a fresh start with a new mandate and new powers, such as ability to hire specially qualified personnel or buy and contract more like a business enterprise. The discussion that follows explores this option by considering three examples: the Social Security Administration, an agency that recently acquired independent status; the U.S. Postal Service, a government corporation highly successful in many respects; and the Institute of Medicine's proposal for a Medicare Market Board that would represent a spin-off of one of the HCFA's functions.

INDEPENDENT STATUS: SOCIAL SECURITY ADMINISTRATION. The Social Security Administration is an agency that was, until recently, a part of HSS. In March 1995 it was given independent status with increased powers and authority over personnel, a bipartisan advisory board, and a mandate to address its backlogs in claims processing, slowness to adopt modern technology, handling of disability cases, and other long-standing problems. Other reasons for seeking this reorganization were greater prestige, better access to the executive branch, and more independence from HSS policies and constraints.[39]

In mission and activity the Social Security Administration is similar enough to the HCFA to provide a useful comparison. Its most important activities are rule making, determining eligibility and entitlement, disbursing checks, and informing or counseling recipients. Both agencies must plan for a growing and changing population with differing needs and entitlements depending on whether they are elderly, disabled, or poor. Both have major data operations and problems with staying abreast of the information load and updating the hardware and software. As the HCFA has its problem with Medicaid, so the SSA struggles to maintain equity between Social Security recipients and disability claimants. Both agencies maintain extensive systems for informing their claimants or beneficiaries. With more than 60,000 employees the Social Security Administration is much larger than the HCFA, which has 4,000; but the HCFA deals with a much more diverse and complex set of problems and constitutencies. So the comparison seems at least relevant.

Relevant, but not encouraging. Few if any of the putative benefits from reorganization have been realized by the SSA. Removing the agency from HHS has meant, of course, independence from the agency's policy tendencies, but it has left the SSA more exposed to its various clientele or constituency groups and to congressional and executive branch politics of divided government. In recent testimony before the Ways and Means Committee, the comptroller general observed that the SSA's performance since independence had been disappointing: it was not dealing effectively with its data and software problems, its treatment of disability cases, nor its planning for future demographic and fiscal problems.[40] Others have observed that without independence the SSA would at least have had the protection and aid of HHS. And some have expressed the view that independence was a mistake and should be undone.[41]

Even though removing the SSA from HHS has proved no cure-all, one benefit of independence for the HCFA might be to free it from the necessity to obtain departmental clearances for rule making, paperwork reduction, small business impact, and so forth that slow down and distort policymaking. But however that might have seemed at one time, it is much less pertinent now because of steps taken by the department and the executive branch to streamline clearances. Measures have included delegating more rule-making authority from the secretary to the HCFA administrator, forming joint HCFA-departmental teams to expedite clearances, and reducing the number of regulations that must have OMB clearance. Further simplifications of the clearance process might be counterproductive. Clearances are a part of policymaking, and delays are occasioned by lack of data, unresolved complexities, or legal issues as well as by politics. Shortcuts here could mean resolving a given matter through the intervention of a congressional subcommittee or the federal courts. And independence is not likely to help in this respect.[42]

THE GOVERNMENT CORPORATION: U.S. POSTAL SERVICE. The government corporation is perhaps a more attractive option for two major reasons. First, it provides a way to bestow powers or exemptions on a public or semiprivate organization to operate in a businesslike and market-oriented fashion: powers to contract and acquire property expeditiously; hire more freely and pay market prices; and use special administrative procedures, particularly in budgeting, rule making, and adjudication. Second, the government corporation is a well-understood, reasonably predictable, and legitimate form of organization, so that chartering it implies giving permission for it to do its work and refraining from micromanagement.

The Postal Service was created in 1971 to get rid of a departmental structure and bring more anticipatory, flexible, and market-oriented management to the largest mail delivery service in the world. Like a corporation, it has a board of governors that can remove the CEO (postmaster general) and his or her deputy. It has its own career service and much freedom in hiring executives and specialized personnel. It also enjoys special powers with respect to rule making, contracting, and the acquisition of property.

Despite some grumbling by customers and an occasional scandal, the Postal Service has been a great success. It has adapted to the changing and conflicting needs of a varied constituency, modernized its equipment and data processing, improved its public relations, delivered mail with reasonable accuracy and promptness to every community in the United States, survived the competition of private parcel services and electronic mail, and kept Congress reasonably happy.

Despite its success, there remains the question of which, if any, of the special powers it enjoys would be appropriate or helpful for the HCFA or the administration of Medicare. The most important of these would be the authority to hire, exemptions or modifications of the rule-making process, and increased powers to contract and acquire property. The least important would seem to be special hiring authority.

Special hiring authority for the Medicare administration is of doubtful value and could be harmful. For much of its needed expertise or services, HHS or the HCFA can use consultants or contract out. Moreover, higher salaries are a dubious inducement. Assuming reasonably adequate pay, most good civil servants seem motivated by the opportunity to do important and challenging work. Given the very lucrative outside opportunities available in the health care industry, the modest increments that would be offered under such an authority would be unlikely to attract top-level executives or professionals. There is also the risk that relaxing the entry requirements could open up the civil service to increased numbers of political appointees at the level of deputy assistant secretary or associate administrator and to careerists interested in a line or two on their resumes. In any event the benefits from this power or exemption hardly seem an adequate reason for adopting a special form of organization.

The subject of adopting a special rule-making procedure or some relaxation of the Administrative Procedure Act (APA) is more complex. But it is worth noting that the special provision for the Postal Service applies to rates and is a mixed procedure similar to that by which payments are set under the prospective payment system and the Medicare fee schedule. And the Postal Service rates are still subject to "notice and comment" under the APA. Rule making is unquestionably burdensome for the HCFA, but it seems a burden the agency willingly accepts. Besides, the APA contained an exemption for contracting and benefits that was relinquished in the 1970s on the recommendation of the Administrative Conference of the United States.[43] In other words, passage of the APA was followed by choice. Indeed, the commitment to due process is strong in the HCFA, both as a matter of fairness and because it protects the agency and the beneficiaries as well as providers.

In addition, modifications of the APA, even the procedures for informal rule making, are likely to prove difficult and politically costly. For example, one reason for delay in rule making is the practice of using responses to comments as the basis for appeals on grounds of inadequate consideration. This led, understandably, to more comments and more detailed comments and responses; more high-priced lawyers, actuaries, accountants, and other experts; and enormous expenditures of resources and time. A proposal to change this procedure, however, led to nationwide protests, *New York Times* articles, accusations that the HCFA was abandoning due process, and a quick retreat. A modest proposal that seems feasible and would help with purchasing would be to exempt most purchases from the notice and comment requirements.[44] But in general, amending the APA, at least to make it less constraining, is not a promising option.

Another putative benefit of the corporate form of organization would be the kind of greater freedom in purchasing and contracting enjoyed by the Postal Service, the Veterans Administration, and the Department of Defense in its administration of CHAMPUS. For the Postal Service, such powers are indispensable and have been used to good effect. For health care, especially for FFS Medicare, their importance is less obvious.

First, such powers are not that usable by FFS Medicare in its present form. True, the Veterans Administration can purchase supplies and drugs in bulk, with savings that are both clear and substantial. But for Medicare, which has a limited outpatient prescription drug benefit for drugs administered in physicians' offices, the savings would be small and probably complex to administer. Freedom to purchase durable medical equipment could be more useful, but the prospect of government issue wheelchairs, canes, and crutches does not seem attractive. That leaves surgical bandages. The savings under an FFS program may be so expensive and complex to administer and would likely create so much ill will that they seem scarcely worth the trouble.

Nor is the VA or DoD experience with large-scale contracting for medical services particularly relevant or encouraging for the FFS Medicare program. In the first place, such ventures have primarily involved managed care. But beyond that, they illustrate in classic fashion the difficulties of trying to contract for a complex product where the competition is likely to dwindle to one or two, the other party knows more than you do, the transaction and monitoring costs are high, and replacing the supplier is very expensive financially and politically.[45]

The HCFA has just recently experienced difficulties of this sort with its own elaborate contract administration for the Medicare Transaction System, its new database and software system, that show how taxing such endeavors can be and tend to confirm the wisdom of proceeding incrementally with respect to increased contracting authority.[46] Additional authority may be needed, but the case has yet to be made for a general authority of the sort possessed by the Postal Service, the Veterans Administration, or CHAMPUS.

Neither independent status nor a corporate form of organization would seem especially attractive as a way either to improve policymaking or acquire usable new powers. The complexity and gravity of the interests at stake militate against broad grants of power or large organizational changes with unknown consequences. Nor does either alternative seem to offer an easy shortcut or acceptable alternative to coping with familiar and perennial problems.

PARTIAL PRIVATIZATION: THE INSTITUTE OF MEDICINE PROPOSAL. Another possibility would be to spin off a major activity of the HCFA. The FEHBP proposal is one example of this, but that option would still be under HHS if not the HCFA. An even more dramatic step was proposed in a conference on consumer choice sponsored by the Institute of Medicine.[47] Recommendation 7 of the conference report states:

Serious consideration should be given and a study should be commissioned for establishing a new function along the lines of a Medicare

Market Board, Commission or Council to administer the Medicare choices process and hold all *Medicare choices* accountable. The proposed entity would include an advisory committee composed of key stakeholders, including purchasers, providers, and consumers.[48]

The Conference also questioned whether a public agency such as the HCFA could match the sophisticated information and education capabilities being developed in the private sector and used by corporations and some health insurance purchasing cooperatives. It recommended that the HCFA consider privatizing this activity along with its Choices program.

Three steps are contemplated in this proposal. The first would be to adopt the FEHBP approach, using it to offer both the Medicare FFS option as well as alternative managed care plans and a medigap policy.[49] The second would be to privatize this option, putting it under an independent Market Board. The dynamic element is supplied by a system of "structured accountability," combining state-of-the-art standards and monitoring for quality and a comprehensive and sophisticated system of consumer information using the technology and methods of some of the best private sector organizations.

APPRAISAL. This proposal is likely to be attractive. First, it should quiet the concerns of those who believe that the HCFA lacks the capacity or the requisite neutrality (or both) to administer such a program. It would also provide a better and fairer test of managed competition than would the FEHBP model. Such a proposal might be widely acceptable on that ground, although it could also be perceived as the entering wedge for a largely privatized managed competition model that could be controversial.

The proposal seems well designed to test some of the important elements of managed care. It emphasizes the development of uniform national standards for plans, the further development of such data systems as HEDIS to incorporate measures germane to a Medicare population, and the use of performance standards to bolster informed choice.[50] At the same time, it says little about the problem of risk selection, except that "attention needs to be given to better risk adjusters."[51]

One criticism of the IOM proposal is that it seems more interested in the marketing of plans than with the plans to be marketed, in a sense putting the marketing system before product design. A comparison of this "choices" system with the HCFA group of demonstrations that bears the same name is instructive. The demonstrations would include testing a variety of private sector delivery systems, including point-of-service options, open-ended

HMOs, integrated delivery systems, and primary care management systems. Some demonstrations would also examine mixed managed care and FFS options, the use of insurance risk corridors, and rural adaptations where HMOs either are not available or are not sufficiently well developed. In addition to a central objective of expanding managed care options for Medicare beneficiaries, other concerns seem implicit. One is the recognition that, whatever the dominant model, *all* of the beneficiaries must be served, including the severely ill and those in areas that do not conform well to the modal service delivery conditions. And a second is that Medicare must aim to give each beneficiary a *good* option, not simply the most cost effective for the greatest number.[52]

The recommendation to devolve or privatize the information and education function recognizes some of the potential of private sector approaches. But it loses sight of the public uses of information and the government's proprietary interest in this area. It might make sense to contract out or privatize the development and dissemination of information about health plans, providers, and quality indicators, not only to take advantage of recent advances in communications technology but, perhaps equally important, to get this activity out of politics and guard against bias or the appearance of it. At the same time, the HCFA might wish to keep some consumer information activities in-house, for instance, with regional and field representatives such as the Social Security Administration has done, so that elderly beneficiaries could speak to something that has a pulse instead of getting an 800 number with its baffling and infuriating triage routines. In addition, there is both a proprietary interest in and a public use for much of the information generated by this activity in monitoring managed care entities and HMOs, informing and collaborating with state and local authorities, and jawboning or implicit negotiation with providers.

The IOM proposal would seem to hold forth little to improve the FFS program except to have it compete on unequal terms with HMOs and managed care. One of the important benefits of having Choices under the HCFA is that it can be a vehicle to explore adaptations from the managed care sector, possibly to improve Medicare as well as to test the popularity of these options. Other prospects for cost saving would be carve-outs, partial capitation, and creating subsidized risk corridors. For managed care, systems that make HMOs more user friendly, such as point-of-service, large PPOs or open-ended HMOs, and senior care adaptations, could be explored. In other words, our best prospect is to have two or more alternatives—Medicare FFS, managed care, and various hybrids—that are reasonably attractive and affordable. The IOM proposal could work against this by diverting attention from the most important priority.

Conclusion

However desirable FFS Medicare may be, preserving it is likely to depend on finding pretty quickly some politically acceptable ways of saving money. Tinkering can probably assure trust fund "solvency" for a few years.[53] For the longer term, especially with the impact of costly medical technology and a growing and aging Medicare population, large and sustained savings will be needed. Medicare reform has political appeal and is likely to figure prominently in the new Congress and the second Clinton administration. A widely shared purpose is to devise ways to achieve the necessary savings and yet retain such features of fee-for-service Medicare as individual choice, beneficiary protection, and providers' freedom of practice that make the program worth keeping.

One question important in coming to some conclusions is whether (or why) FFS Medicare should continue as more than a residual program. There may be no conclusive answer, but there are reasons for believing that it should, at least for the near term. One is that most Medicare beneficiaries still prefer or believe that they need the FFS program and are willing to pay to stay with it. FFS Medicare also provides an alternative for providers, especially physicians, who are not only a political force but whose commitment or at least grudging acquiescence is vital for the success of the program. And a strong FFS presence can help sustain quality by providing a competitive yardstick and, in a less obvious way, keeping physicians and other providers active in both FFS and managed care.

Need for a Period of Sustained Development

Reforming Medicare requires sustained development in which the devising of solutions over time is supported by Congress and the president. *Development* is necessary because of the importance of such unknowns as the cost-saving potential of either FFS Medicare or managed care, the adaptability of administrative programs and legal constraints, and beneficiary and political responses to extensive and prolonged change. *Sustained* is emphasized because getting the job done reasonably well will take continuing bipartisan effort, the cooperation and forbearance of elected and appointed officials, and collaboration with and support of providers and other private sector groups.

Importance of HCFA's Role

The need for sustained development makes public institutions such as the HCFA or a new Medicare Commission necessary. The HCFA has extensive experience and credibility with the health care research community and is accustomed to designing inquiries, contracting for the requisite expertise, and evaluating the results. Unlike a private organization, it has the combination of accumulated data, institutional memory, and administrative perspective needed to translate research and policy proposals into institutionally workable and politically acceptable programs. And because it is accountable to both executive branch superiors and Congress, the HCFA can be directed and redirected in the course of sustained development.

Integrally related to development is bestowing additional authority on the agency or agencies taking the lead in development. Neither Congress nor the White House has historically been eager to grant major new powers to any agency dealing with Medicare. Part of the merit of sustained development is that the necessary powers can be conferred incrementally as need is demonstrated. Demonstrated need and repeated advocacy have often gone unheeded in the past. But an early and strong bipartisan commitment to a shared effort should help in some measure. The new Medicare Commission, operating in an advisory capacity similar to that of the earlier ProPAC and PPRC, should also be useful, especially in winning the acquiescence of members of Congress unfamiliar with the technicalities of Medicare or distrustful of the process.

The consideration just mentioned touches on accountability and how best to structure it. A distinction between answerability and responsiveness is useful because it points up some advantages of a public agency such as the HCFA. Being a public agency, the HCFA is *answerable* broadly and with considerable particularity to administrative superiors, elected officials, and the courts. Answerability should, in principle, make the agency more acceptable to lead a process that affects important interests and could become politically charged and divisive. It is also desirable that FFS Medicare be *responsive* to norms such as beneficiary satisfaction and professional standards of quality along with efficiency and cost effectiveness. The agency has a lot of experience trying to do just that. But there is a theoretical point that health care is better when providers internalize these norms rather than being sanctioned after the fact. And like the educative process in general, internalization requires example, peer pressure, reputation, economic incentives, and sanctions or the threat of them. Encouraging this kind of responsiveness entails experience, adaptation, and various approaches. A public agency such as the HCFA with years of experience and an array of administrative tools at its disposal has some advantages.

One reason for concentrating so intensively on the HCFA, particularly in discussing various administrative paradigms, is the belief that restructuring FFS Medicare will require sustained development and that the agency is in a unique position to provide administrative leadership. That said, there remains a question of what role the HCFA should play, along with other agencies, and what new powers should be assigned to it. It would be foolhardy try to answer such questions in detail. But some general conclusions may be useful.

Organizational Models and a Comprehensive Strategy

The first model, described as "full use of existing authority with incremental changes," would require the least change. Included would be vigorous enforcement of the fraud and abuse legislation, cost containment for skilled nursing facilities and home health agencies, urging that the HCFA be given selective powers to buy at or close to market prices, and unification of ProPAC and PPRC.

The problem with this option is what is left undone. It does not address the problem of high-cost cases as such; it does not aggressively promote managed care or consumer choice; and it does little to change the organizational culture of the HCFA. Still, an incremental model might be all that Congress or the administration will accept, at least until costs and the deficit mount considerably. Cost containment with marginally strengthened controls could prove effective enough in the short run to soften demand for more vigorous measures. And Congress might largely ignore the recommendations of the HCFA and push for its own priorities, relying for advice on a newly constituted Medicare Commission and exploiting the budget reconciliation process.

The prudent purchasing model differs from the incremental option in its aggressive approach toward managing high-cost cases and procedures and its expanded managed care and HMO program. Prudent purchasing would be promoted with new powers assigned to the HCFA to engage in competitive contracting and purchasing at or near market prices and through a major program of consumer information. Beneficiary choice would be expanded by additional options and through a program similar to the FEHBP. A separate bureau for managed care and another for the disabled and chronically and severely ill would give prominence to these groups and their needs.

The model would seem best designed to keep FFS Medicare both viable and popular by taking aggressive measures to contain costs, making the FFS and managed care options more competitive, creating options that combine features of both, and increasing beneficiary choice and protections. The organizational changes would tend to mollify both liberal and conservative critics of the HCFA. But providers might not fare so well. And the program could overreach by requiring too many new powers and taking on large and complex new tasks, such as administering a nationwide HCFA On-Line program or an expanded Choices initiative.

Considering the array of new powers and their controversial nature, it is difficult to imagine that Congress would readily cede them to the HCFA. At the same time, there may be strategies for moving by increments that could augment support for the prudent purchaser model while avoiding or reducing opposition. For instance, a concerted attack on rising costs for skilled nursing facilities and home health services would gain wide support and provide an opportunity for the HCFA to work cooperatively with Congress on a number of incremental changes. Complementing this effort, the use of centers of excellence could be expanded, not wholesale but with an authorization from Congress to add to the procedures included (such as joint replacements or diabetes management) and to create a limited number of centers in regions around the country with price benchmarks included in the requests for proposal. Buying at market rates might be approached by starting with some standardized items and authorizing the government to buy at the bulk prices vendors give to their most favored customers.[54] Similarly, a limited version of competitive contracting could be developed through adaptation of the RFP process.[55] In moving beyond experiment and incremental change, the future Medicare Commission can be an important source of independent appraisal and expertise for Congress and to help build bipartisan support. Of course, in pursuing development, much will depend on political leadership, the strength of bipartisan commitment, and the quality of proposals that the HCFA and other sources generate.

Questions have been raised about whether the HCFA should be marketing managed care offerings, especially as the program grows in size and diversity. The Institute of Medicine intimated in its report that this task might exceed the agency's capabilities; and congressional critics have doubted the HCFA's ability to administer such a program fairly. These issues need to be resolved, at least partly, in the development process. The HCFA is experimenting with HMO and managed care options and seeking to enlarge HMO enrollment. That activity ought to precede or grow apace with marketing an FEHBP model. Eventually this activity could be devolved and administered through a semiprivate agency—as much of FFS Medicare is—to decentralize decisions, reassure critics, and increase competition.

Amidst the profusion of organizational alternatives and the welter of detail, it is important to keep in mind the guiding purpose: to preserve the best from the past and adapt to an unknown future. With modifications the original Medicare principles of beneficiary choice and provider freedom are worth striving for. But designing a Medicare program for the next generation is much more difficult than it was in 1965 because of the importance of cost containment. Managed care adaptations are essential, although how far to go in this direction and how to adapt health care delivery and the management of Medicare have yet to be discovered.

How lengthy a course of development and discovery will be is hard to predict. Major issues could well be decided early, then years could be spent working out the details; or elements of a final solution could evolve incrementally. Either way, success in this venture will depend on the sustained and intelligent adaptation that can be achieved. Let us hope that when a next generation looks at this work, it will pronounce it good.

Appendix A: The Health Care Financing Administration

The Health Care Financing Administration was created in 1977 by the merger of the Medicare and Medicaid programs, together with their related medical care quality control staffs. It is a small agency with about 4,000 employees, most of whom work at one end of Security Boulevard outside Baltimore or in regional offices, although a number of its top officials have second offices in Washington, in the downtown complex of the Department of Health and Human Services. The HCFA oversaw the expenditure of about $300 billion in 1996, and is responsible for a varied and highly technical array of programs. Activities that relate especially to Medicare can be summarized under three major headings.

Implementation of the Program

The HCFA is responsible for keeping Medicare running. Its duties are to:

—Develop the policies and write the rules and manuals governing beneficiary entitlements and relations with providers and parties contracting with the HCFA.

—Maintain quality of care; develop standards of quality and performance; set agendas for PROs; work with state and private accreditation agencies; monitor quality in a variety of subordinate programs, such as skilled nursing facilities, home health care organizations, and clinical laboratories.

—Oversee claims processing and the monitoring of fiscal integrity by the carriers and fiscal intermediaries; make recommendations for sanctions to the inspector general.

—Supervise the settling and adjudication of disputes; support activities of the Provider Reimbursement Review Board.

—Implement mandates of Congress, especially those contained in new legislation or the budget reconciliations.

Providing data, information, or policy recommendations to others

The agency is also charged with various communication and information activities:

—Inform beneficiaries and providers about benefits, program activities, and responsibilities.

—Provide data, information, and policy recommendations for other HHS component agencies.

—Develop annual update recommendations for the PPS, the MFS, and other payment schedules.

—Respond to requests for testimony, reports, or policy advice from Congress or congressional agencies.

Planning and Development

The agency must also maintain its research functions. It is expected to:

—Track actuarial, demographic, and macroeconomic trends, and assess their impact on beneficiaries, providers, the health care industry, and the national economy.

—Perform research and development, especially into new service delivery modalities and methods of payment, including HMOs and other managed care entities.

—Develop and implement strategies for updating and expanding data and information systems.

As the list suggests, the HCFA engages in little direct administration. Mostly, it plans, develops, and monitors. In keeping with its responsibility for estimating and responding to future needs, it has its own actuarial staff and research and demonsration capability. It also maintains a huge database and automated information system, an invaluable resource in itself. But much of the program is carried out by contract or liaison with consultants and research enterprises, provider groups and health care plans, state agencies, medical schools, and universities. This mode of adminstration has some disadvantages: delay, dependence on what is available, and various transaction costs. At the same time, it gives the HCFA flexibility in development and access to a great deal of outside expertise and capability.

In addition to the Baltimore and Washington offices, the HCFA has one regional office in each of the ten HHS regional cities. About 1,400 of the 4,000 HCFA employees are in the regions, with activities divided among supervising the carriers and fiscal intermediaries, helping implement and monitor the HCFA's managed care activities, especially Medicare and Medicaid HMOs,

Figure 5A-1. *Proposed HCFA Organization*[a]

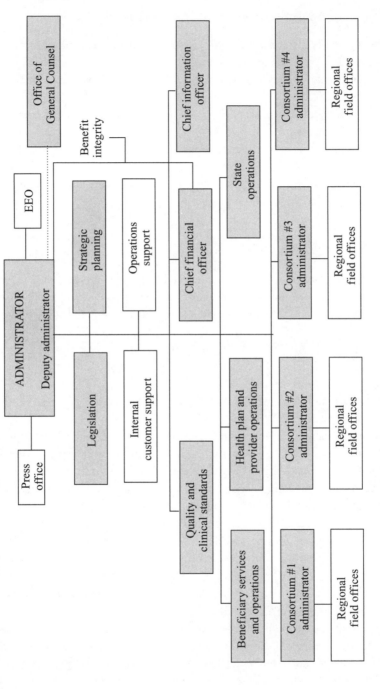

a. Shaded boxes would be members of the Executive Council.

Figure 5A-2. *Health Care Financing Administration Organization as of 1996*

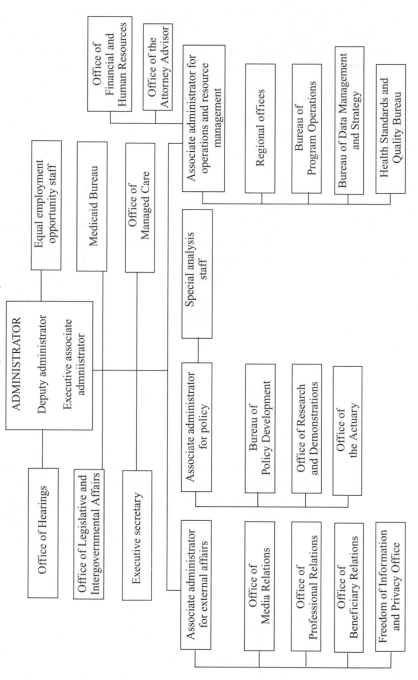

working with state and private agencies on accreditation and on Medicaid state plans, and providing information to beneficiaries and providers. Unlike the Social Security Administration, the HCFA has a very few field representatives working outside the regional offices, although the SSA helped until recently with enrollment and information for Medicare beneficiaries. The Baltimore office sets policy and keeps in touch with frequent communication, including telephone conference calls. Opinion differs about the quality of the regional offices, but there is a consensus that, generally, quality is lower than that in Baltimore and that performance varies from region to region.

On November 7, 1996, the HCFA announced a plan for reorganization. Figure 5A-1 shows the details of this reorganization, and figure 5A-2 shows the existing organization. The major changes include combining managed care and fee-for-service administration under one division of Health Plan and Provider Operations; strengthening relations with beneficiaries and combining this function with the existing Bureau of Program Operations; putting Medicaid and regional activities under a new division of State Operations; and upgrading clinical and quality standards and putting responsibility for them in a new division. The Office of Research and Demonstrations was abolished as a separate entity, although the activities continue.

Appendix B: Persons Interviewed

I wish to express my debt and gratitude to the individuals who gave generously of their time and resources in interviews during 1996 and 1997.

David P. Baine, Director, Federal Health Care Delivery Issues, General Accounting Office.

Alec Peter Bouxsein, Associate Director, Office of Managed Care, HCFA.

Kathleen A. Buto, Associate Administrator for Policy, HCFA.

Harry Cain, Vice President for Strategic Planning, Blue Cross/Blue Shield Association, Washington, D.C.

Terry Coleman, former Deputy General Counsel, DHHS; attorney, Fox, Bennett, and Turner, Washington, D.C.

Elizabeth Cuzack, Director, Office of Physician and Ambulatory Care Policy; Director of the "HOT" Team (HCFA of Tommorow), HCFA.

Lynn Etheredge, private consultant, Washington, D.C.

Paul Ginsburg, Center for Studying Health Systems Change; former Executive Director, PPRC.

Alice Gosfield, attorney, Gosfield and Associates, Philadelphia, Pa.

George D. Greenburg, Senior Medicare Program Analyst. Office of the Secretary, DHHS.

Leslie Greenwald, Special Assistant, Office of Research and Demonstrations, HCFA.

Leslie M. Hash, Principal, Health Policy Alternatives, Washington, D.C.

Thomas Hoyer, Director, Office of Chronic Care and Insurance, HCFA.

Charles N. Kahn, III, Chief of Staff, Subcommittee on Health, Committee on Ways and Means, House of Representatives.

Jerry L. Mashaw, Professor of Law, Yale University School of Law.

Alfred F. Meyer, consultant and HMO executive, Independence Blue Cross, Philadelphia, Pa.

Marilyn Moon, Senior Fellow, Urban Institute, Washington, D.C.

Judith D. Moore, Acting Director, Medicaid Bureau, HCFA.

Steven A. Pelovitz, Associate Administrator for Operations and Resource Management, HCFA.

Elaine Raubach, Director, Office of Information Resources Management, HCFA.

Paul Rettig, Association of Osteopathic Healthcare Organizations, Washington, D.C.

Leonard D. Schaeffer, Chairman and CEO, Blue Cross of California; former Administrator, HCFA.

Janet L. Shikles, Assistant Comptroller General, Division of Health, Education, and Human Services, General Accounting Office.

Edwin P. Strupko, Associate Director, Division of Health, Education, and Human Services, General Accounting Office.

Mary Ann Troyanovich, Executive for Regulations Management, DHHS.

Bruce C. Vladeck, Administrator, HCFA.

Carol Walton, Director, Bureau of Program Operations, HCFA.

Gail Wilensky, Project Hope; former Administrator, HCFA; former Chairman. PPRC.

Craig A. Winslow, Senior Attorney, Office of General Counsel, General Accounting Office.

Donald A. Young, Executive Director, ProPAC.

Notes

1. *Balanced Budget Act of 1995,* H. Rpt. 104-350 (Government Printing Office, 1995), pt. 2, p. 1097.

2. Institute of Medicine, *Improving the Medicare Market: Adding Choice and Protections* (Washington, 1996), esp. vol. 1, p. 105 ff.

3. Assuming, for example, a modified risk adjuster and private health plan participation, with suitable provisions for ensuring access and beneficiary protection.

4. See Robert Ball, "What Medicare Had in Mind," *Health Affairs,* vol. 14, no. 4 (1995), pp. 62–72. Also National Academy of Social Insurance, *Reflections on Implementing Medicare* (Washington, 1993).

5. Social Security Amendments of 1983, P.L. 98-21; and Tax Equity and Fiscal Responsibility Act of 1982, P.L. 97-248, known as TEFRA.

6. Especially the experimental medical care review organizations (EMCROs), the professional standards review organizations (PSROs), and the peer review organizations (PROs). The Social Security Amendments of 1972 authorized the PSROs, and TEFRA established the present-day PROs.

7. Social Security Amendments of 1965, P.L. 69-97.

8. *Managed indemnity* refers to managed care techniques employed by many large indemnity carriers such as Blue Cross/Blue Shield. Techniques include case management, preadmission certification, and physician profiling. Some or even most of these techniques might be used along with free choice of physician and informed consent by the patient to the use of such procedures. Zachary Dyckman and Aaron Knowlton, "Cost-Effectiveness Initiatives by Private Payers in Fee-for-Service Environments," paper prepared for the Physician Payment Review Commission, Center for Health Policy Studies, Columbia, Md., 1996.

9. The idea of strategic incrementalism was one that several HCFA administrators found useful to describe some of their approaches to policy change. One person likened it to finding the log that would break up the logjam and start processes moving.

10. General Accounting Office, "Testimony of Janet L. Shikles," in *Medicare–Private Payer Strategies Suggest Options to Reduce Rapid Spending Growth,* GAO/T-HEHS-96 (April 1996).

11. Interview with Bruce Vladeck, HCFA administrator, August 12, 1996.

12. Proposed in the Medicare Preservation Act and endorsed by present and former directors and Commission members of PPRC and ProPAC.

13. For instance, the volume performance standard for the Medicare fee schedule. See Physician Payment Review Commission, *Annual Report to the Congress, 1995* (Washington, 1995).

14. U.S. Department of Health and Human Services, Health Care Financing Administration, "Ways and Means Draft Testimony on SNF/HHA Payment Reform," Baltimore, August 15, 1996.

15. Interview with Leonard D. Schaeffer, chairman and CEO, Blue Cross of California and former HCFA administrator, December 16, 1996.

16. Health Care Financing Administration, Office of Research and Demonstrations, *Research in Health Care Financing—Active Projects,* 1995, HCFA 03381 (Baltimore: Department of Health and Human Services, 1996).

17. A former HCFA administrator believes, for example, that even within existing authority, demonstrations might be used to establish reasonable prices applicable for purposes of discussion and then set rules of engagement for subsequent requests for proposal. Interview with Gail Wilensky, Project Hope, August 5, 1996.

18. Alain C. Enthoven, *Health Plan: The Only Practical Solution to the Soaring Cost of Medical Care* (Reading, Mass.: Addison-Wesley, 1980).

19. Stuart M. Butler and Robert E. Moffit, "The FEHBP as a Model for a New Medicare Program," *Health Affairs,* vol. 14, no. 4 (1995), pp. 47–61; and A. Evans, *The*

Federal Health Benefits Program, Managed Competition, and Considerations for Medicare (Washington: National Academy on Aging, 1995).

20. In Butler and Moffit, "FEHBP as a Model," traditional FFS Medicare would be be offered through a separate not-for-profit corporation. The FEHBP part would be administered by HHS, but with supervisory powers only.

21. As mandated by the Health Insurance Portability and Accountability Act of 1996, P.L. 104-199.

22. Evans, *Federal Health Benefits Program,* note 20; and *The Federal Employee Health Benefits Plan—Possible Strategies for Reform,* Committee Print, House Committee on Post Office and Civil Service (GPO,1989).

23. Butler and Moffit, "FEHBP as a Model," note 20.

24. Institute of Medicine, *Improving the Medicare Market.*

25. General Accounting Office, *Federal Health Benefits Program—Stronger Controls Needed to Reduce Administrative Costs,* GAO/GGD-92-37 (1992)

26. General Accounting Office, *Fraud and Abuse—Stronger Controls Needed in Federal Employee Health Benefits Program,* GAO/GGD-91-95 (1991).

27. Interview with Kathleen A. Buto, associate administrator, Health Plan and Provider Operations, HCFA, January 3, 1997.

28. Institute of Medicine, *Improving the Medicare Market,* note 29.

29. Many within the HCFA spoke of the problem of the "seven hundred pound gorilla": the HCFA has so much market power that aggressive use of it would seem oppressive.

30. A frequently cited number is that 10 percent of the Medicare beneficiaries account for 70 percent of the health care costs. Less commonly known is that about 5 million dual eligibles (poor and disabled beneficiaries eligible for both Medicare and Medicaid) account for roughly 50 percent of Medicaid costs and 20–30 percent of Medicare costs. Because of the multiple funding streams and their special circumstances, they are difficult to provide for except through a special program.

31. For the present organization of the HCFA see appendix A.

32. Statement to the press by Bruce Vladeck, HCFA administrator, November 7, 1996.

33. Borrowing from Leonard Schaeffer's concept of organizing by market segment. See J. K. Iglehart, "Inside California's HMO Market: A Conversation with Leonard D. Schaeffer," *Health Affairs,* vol. 14, no. 4 (1995), pp. 131–42. Also, interview with Leonard Schaeffer, December 16, 1996.

34. Interview with George D. Greenberg, senior Medicare program analyst, Office of the Secretary, Department of Health and Human Services, July 23, 1996.

35. Interview with Mike Hash, Health Policy Alternatives, July 24, 1996; and interview with Gail Wilensky, Project Hope, former HCFA administrator, August 5, 1996.

36. Interview with Charles N. Kahn III, staff director, Subcommittee on Health, House Ways and Means Committee, August 15, 1996.

37. To this statement should be added that the HCFA is aware of the problem and is actively assisting staff development with training and mentoring programs.

38. Institute of Medicine, *Improving the Medicare Market,* pp. 105–06, note 25. Leonard Schaeffer, former administrator of the HCFA, also expressed some reserva-

tions, saying that consumer information provided by the government tended to be "late, wrong, and terribly confusing." Telephone interview, December 16, 1996.

39. *Establishing the Social Security Administration as an Independent Agency,* Hearings before the Senate Committee on Finance (GPO, 1993); and General Accounting Office, statement of Charles A. Bowsher, comptroller general of the United States, in *Social Security Administration—Effective Leadership Needed to Meet Daunting Challenges,* GAO/TOCG-96-7 (1996).

40. *Establishing the Social Security Administration,* Hearings.

41. Interview with Gail Wilensky, Project HOPE, August 5, 1996.

42. Consider in this respect Title II of the Unfunded Mandates Reform Act of 1995 (P.L. 104-4), the Paperwork Reduction Act of 1995 (P.L. 104-13), and the Contract with America Advancement Act of 1996 (P.L. 104-121), all of which would make rule making more complex and burdensome for administrative agencies. But many believe Congress will act when it believes administrative clearances are inadequate so that "independence" could mean less protection and even less freedom. See J. L. Mashaw, "Reinventing Government and Regulatory Reform: Studies in the Neglect and Abuse of Administrative Law," *University of Pittsburgh Law Review,* vol. 57, no. 2 (1996), pp. 405–22.

43. Sec. 553(a)(2); interview with Terry Coleman, former deputy general counsel, Department of Health and Human Services, August 15, 1996; and interview with Jerry L. Mashaw, Yale University Law School, Sepember 20, 1996.

44. L. Etheredge, "Reengineering Medicare: From Bill-Paying Insurer to Accountable Purchaser," paper prepared for the Health Insurance Reform Project, George Washington University, June 1995.

45. Interview with David P. Baine, director, Federal Health Care Delivery Issues, General Accounting Office, July 30, 1996. See also General Accounting Office, *Defense Health Care: Issues and Challenges Confronting Military Medicine,* GAO/HEHS-95-104 (March 1995); GAO, *Health Security Act: Analysis of Veterans' Health Care Provisions,* GAO/HeHS-94-205FS (July 1994); and John P. Donahue, *The Privatization Decision: Public Ends, Private Means* (Basic Books, 1989), esp. ch. 5.

46. General Accounting Office, *Medicare: New Claims Processing System Benefits and Acquisition Risks,* GAO/HEHS/AIMD-94-79 (January 1994).

47. Institute of Medicine, *Improving the Medicare Market,* note 25.

48. Ibid., vol. 1, p. 105.

49. Ibid., vol. 1, p. 72.

50. Ibid., vol. 1, p. 46. But note in volume 2 the article by Joyce Dubow, "Medicare Managed Care: Issues for Vulnerable Populations," pp. 190–231. She, a senior analyst for the AARP, is much concerned about this issue. See pp. 220 ff.

51. The medigap element derives from the HCFA "select" initiative, which would offer a medigap policy with incentives for beneficiaries to choose cost-saving plans.

52. Interview with Kathleen A. Buto, associate administrator for health plan and provider operations, HCFA, January 3, 1997.

53. Marilyn Moon and Karen Davis, "Preserving and Strengthening Medicare," *Health Affairs,* vol. 14, no. 4 (1995), pp. 31–46.

54. Following a suggestion of Bruce Vladeck, HCFA administrator. Interview, August 12, 1996.

55. As suggested by Gail Wilensky and others.

Comment by Alan Nelson

We have heard two elegant papers, but one might infer from them that managed care and fee-for-service are mutually exclusive. This is not necessarily the case. In the private sector there are a host of combinations, including some in which the capitation payment is made to a medical group that distributes the payment among its members on a fee-for-service basis.

One might also infer from the papers that utilization control through some sort of external bureaucracy is necessary to keep down costs. This is also not necessarily true. In the private sector, perhaps the most effective utilization control is internalized and comes at the local level through the group.

I am going to refer to these points a bit more, but first I want to step back and look at some of the public's attitudes that are deeply ingrained and not transient and that will govern the nature and the pace of change we are about to encounter. I will also give reasons why I believe that transition to a consumer-choice model—something like that suggested by the Institute of Medicine—is likely to occur and will occur more rapidly than most people expect.

The dominant attitudes that will be reflected in any seriously considered legislation are going to be, first, the desire for choice and, second, the desire on the part of the beneficiaries for a system that is simpler and entails less paperwork.

Choice has driven the health care debate for the past five years. It shows no signs of getting weaker. This should not be forgotten when we talk about ways to cut costs, such as by using centers of excellence or restricted formularies or limited physician panels or bureaucratic obstacles to care. Choice is deeply ingrained. The public will continue to insist on it. And it is also reflected in an explosion of proposed state legislation (and some federal legislation as well) that is directed at the managed care industry and that attempts to make certain that choice is not unduly restricted by gatekeepers, that enrollees can easily go outside a plan to see a specialist of their choice (although they may have to pay additional out-of-pocket costs to do so), and that patients have access to all approved drugs and devices. These assurances are currently being proposed by a consortium of state legislators. We should take that seriously.

The attention to drive-through deliveries, outpatient mastectomies, and gag clauses all reflect concerns that financial considerations are going to undermine the integrity of the health care system, whether they are financed through the public or private sector. We are, of course, committed to strategies to cut or eliminate wasteful and unnecessary care. However, for physicians taking care of patients one at a time, the cost-containment strategies can sometimes create real dilemmas. Let me give you one example.

There is substantial evidence that oxygen is being used by some patients who do not need it. Some of this use may be a result of marketing by unscrupulous vendors of oxygen. However, virtually all primary care physicians have patients who are given oxygen because of heart disease or chronic lung disease and who have low blood oxygen levels and clearly require oxygen therapy. Often these patients improve. They may, however, still have certain periods of the day or night when they feel they are smothering and that oxygen will make them feel better. The doctor has a hard time refusing their request for authorization of oxygen equipment just because their blood gases on the day that they ask for the equipment happen to be normal.

The call for better administration of state program costs is always reasonable, but I am not sure that piling on additional layers of utilization review is the answer to the cost problem, if the review is the kind that we have tried for the past thirty years and does not appear to be working very well. It does, however, make sense to invest in demand management in which beneficiaries are provided information on self-help and prevention strategies, and trained personnel are available by phone, day or night, to assist them with decisions on what services might be necessary to deal with their particular problem. Some employers are seeing a substantial return on investment with these strategies, and even more impressive is the fact that they have about a 95 percent level of high satisfaction from the consumers.

As to my second point, many Medicare patients hate the paperwork in the current program, and so do doctors, of course. Doctors hire additional staff to deal with the coding requirements and the increasingly complex documentation requirements that have to be met before they are paid. Often they have to put in a code for a patient who "has something wrong" without knowing exactly what the problem is. They may do some laboratory work to try to clarify the problem and are required to provide a code so the carrier can determine whether the test was necessary. How does the carrier know whether the test is necessary when the doctor does not? Sometimes the bureaucracy forgets that patients do not come in with the diagnosis written on their heads.

Various observers contend that the vast majority of Medicare beneficiaries will be enrolled in traditional fee-for-service Medicare in the foreseeable future. I question that assumption. If it is true, it means that government did something wrong when it had an opportunity to change provider incentives, to move accountability to the level of the provider and plan and, simultaneously, deal with the problems in the current Medicare system that beneficiaries object to most: deductibles and copayments, paperwork, and a wrong-headed refusal to provide preventive services and screening that are now expected to be part of any decent insurance plan.

I support those who believe that beneficiaries should have a voucher that is risk adjusted for an amount set by Congress and should be allowed to enroll in any one of a number of qualified plans that provide a uniform package of benefits. The beneficiaries should be given information so that they can include measures of quality in making their decision. The plans can compete by adding additional benefits, such as drugs or dental coverage, if they are able to do that for the voucher amount. Plans that charge in excess of the defined contribution would have to justify their additional cost to the beneficiaries, who would have to pay for it out of pocket. Beneficiaries should also be able to go outside the plan to purchase a point-of-service rider. In this kind of scenario, the control of utilization would be internalized and local and, presumably, more sensitive to individual circumstances, although not less rigorous because all required services must be covered by the voucher amount.

"What about maintaining traditional Medicare?" you might ask. Some will also ask, "What is to keep?" We have had thirty years to try to simplify it, and it has become more complex; to reduce its costs, and it is going bankrupt; to provide necessary preventive services, and each additional benefit has been added only after a major fight.

We should value more properly primary care services and the component of practice expense in the payment to physicians. Currently the expense component for 120 office visits equals one coronary bypass graft that is done in the hospital anyway. Is the answer to excessive utilization to impose prior authorization and concurrent review or require beneficiaries to have a gatekeeper? Isn't the private sector abandoning some of these strategies?

Is cracking down on fraud the answer to the cost problem? I fully support cracking down on fraud wherever it is found and to the full extent of the law, but I doubt that that is the answer to the long-term problem with Medicare financing because most providers, after all, are honest.

Is prevention the answer to the cost problem? Prevention, like virtue, is its own reward. It is justified because the quality of life is better and, presumably, people are more productive if they are healthier. But, ultimately, we get sick and die; and the longer we live the more health care resources we will consume. Business loves wellness programs because they may defer the final expensive illness until the patient is eligible for Medicare. If we find a cure for cancer and heart disease, according to Joshua Lederberg, the largest single cost item will be nursing home care for the population of the very, very old.

What is the answer? Bite the bullet and enact legislation that will speed a transition to a restructured program that provides choice, less hassle, and market-based incentives to provide quality care at lowest cost.

Comment by Kathy Buto

Will fee-for-service Medicare survive in a managed care world? The answer is yes. There are three reasons for this: the nature of Medicare managed care, the changes that fee-for-service care will undergo, and the expansion and aging of the population. Elements of traditional fee-for-service care will remain, but it will not be FFS Medicare as we know it today.

Let me start with managed care. Most people think of managed care as it exists in the private sector. In Medicare it is not that kind of managed care. It is not a program with great flexibility so that the government can go out and purchase the best plan, or array of plans, for beneficiaries. It is, in fact, an administered price capitation program set with a very detailed formula in statute.

It is true that Medicare managed care has experienced 30 to 40 percent growth in the past few years, but that has probably occurred because HMOs can and do offer such benefits as prescription drugs and services that Medicare does not cover and offer them at the same cost that beneficiaries pay for traditional Medicare. That these extras are available "free" is due in large part to the fact that, on average, Medicare HMO payment rates are high. So, managed care plans are a good deal for beneficiaries. The other thing to note is that medigap premiums are increasing, and beneficiaries are finding Medicare managed care to be more cost effective by comparison.

Based on recent analyses, even if all other things were equal, there is still favorable selection into Medicare risk plans. The program is overpaying plans to provide services because the payments are based on an average. Even though Medicare pays HMOs 95 percent of the average per capita amount in fee-for-service care, HMOs can make a very good profit even as they offer attractive additional benefits. If this year payment reductions are part of legislation affecting the Medicare managed care program, there will be at least a slowdown of plans entering the Medicare managed care market. There will also be some reduction or slowdown in extra benefits, and they may be eliminated in some markets.

So, the real future growth in Medicare managed care is yet unknown. Health Care and Financing Administration actuaries predict that in ten years most beneficiaries will receive care through the fee-for-service system. But it is obvious to all of us in the agency that Medicare managed care has made important changes in the way we think about the care we pay for. We believe the managed care plans in Medicare are leading our efforts to look at measuring quality and to begin to look at outcomes. They are providing a good laboratory for the kind of flexibility and substitution of cost-effective alternatives to care that we do not provide as an alternative in the fee-for-service system. Even in an environment in which most services are paid through fee-for-service financing, Medicare FFS needs to adopt some of the flexibility of managed care plans: substitutions of more cost-effective alternatives to care and packaging of services to allow extra benefits to be offered.

The second reason that fee-for-service Medicare is likely to survive is that it is being reengineered. There are payment reforms. That gets to the issue of cost. Often people confuse cost savings with restructuring. They are not the same thing if you look at CBO's scoring and the HCFA actuary's scoring. Medicare does not get a lot of savings related to managed care right now because of the formula-driven way we pay plans and favorable selection in enrollment. Nevertheless, the HCFA is proposing reforms both in traditional Medicare payment areas and in restructuring.

Savings in payments occur mostly in home health and skilled nursing facility care and outpatient hospital services. Medicare intends to move very quickly to prospective payment systems for those services. The HCFA has also begun payment demonstration programs—at least the design phase—to purchase some high-volume items such as durable medical equipment and lab services competitively. In some areas Medicare is, in fact, being cost shifted to from the private sector, and we believe we need to experiment with ways to purchase items and services more prudently. We hope to have demonstrations up and running in 1998.

The HCFA is also examining such important concepts as bundling payments for postacute care. It is a very difficult area. The agency will first have to build the blocks of home health prospective payment and other prospective payment systems and then look at a rational system for paying the same amount for postacute episodes regardless of site of service, case-mix-adjusting the payments.

As for restructuring Medicare to offer more options, we need to look at greater choice of managed care and fee-for-service options. The HCFA has Choices demonstrations at seventeen or eighteen sites. Six became operational as of January 1, 1996. The idea behind the demonstrations was to go to areas where there was high managed care penetration by the private sector and very low Medicare managed care penetration, but where Medicare capitation payment rates were better than average, to find out what alternative managed care delivery options Medicare needs to start offering beneficiaries. The demonstrations will be working with preferred provider organizations, point-of-service plans, provider-sponsored networks, or HMOs that are partnering with other entities. Choices is also experimenting with different payment methods: risk sharing, total risk, and capped fee for service. In the second year HCFA hopes to be testing some risk adjustors in these demonstration sites.

The agency is also interested in providing better consumer information. This is critical to a new and restructured program, both in fee-for-service and managed care. We need to provide plan comparisons, but comparisons that also include information to beneficiaries on their out-of-pocket fee-for-service costs, including medigap choices in an area. So the HCFA is beginning work on an HMO competitive-pricing demonstration to try to have HMO prices competitively bid in several areas and to provide beneficiaries with a comparison chart, as the Federal Employees Health Benefit Program does.

I will say little about Medicare centers of excellence. Everybody has mentioned them. They are very successful. The HCFA has saved more than $40 million on the heart bypass centers of excellence demonstrations and is planning to expand them. When plans were announced to expand the demonstrations to cover more cardiac and orthopedic services in the Chicago and San Francisco areas, the agency received more than 500 applications from hospitals wanting to participate. They obviously want this as an option in Medicare: they can receive bundled payments for cardiac or orthopedic hospital and physician services that are covered by the demonstration.

In January 1996 the HCFA put out a solicitation to do what it calls "partnerships." This will involve interested physician-hospital organizations and will bundle physician-hospital payments for all DRGs. Although the demonstration is being proposed only for New Jersey, New York, and Pennsylvania, the agency received more than 170 requests for the application kits. So, there is a lot of interest there.

I also want to mention anticoagulation monitoring, which the HCFA plans to do under current law, looking at case management as a way to prevent strokes in at-risk patients. There, the agency intends to pilot-test the method in a couple of areas. It is looking very aggressively at case management in areas such as anticoagulation to see how the regular Medicare program can take advantage of some of the protocols that have worked for managed care.

The agency is also looking at disease management, for example with congestive heart failure. But we are at an early stage there. The issue is, with geriatric patients who have more than one disease process or clinical set of problems, whether a disease-by-disease approach makes sense or whether Medicare should be providing information on a range of chronic conditions to physicians who are managing the whole patient.

Let me go to the third reason why Medicare fee-for-service will survive, which is the beneficiary population of the future. I think David Smith mentioned that the dual eligibles are a growing segment, both of Medicare and

Medicaid, and represent some of the most expensive patients in both public programs. While we are making changes in fee-for-service Medicare, the real question is how the system can provide appropriate care to very old, disabled, chronic-care individuals who in many cases will be living longer and consuming a larger share of health care. How can managed care and fee-for-service systems meet the changing needs of this population? At the moment, neither the managed care nor the fee-for-service sector has stepped up to this challenge in a major way. But the agency is beginning to see a lot of interest, particularly if payments can be risk adjusted, in actually caring for and setting up special targeted programs for those populations. In fee-for-service, particularly, we need to look for better ways to provide incentives for better connectivity and care management.

My point is that both fee-for-service Medicare and managed care Medicare have to change, and we think we have a better chance to promote a third way if the two are changing simultaneously and feeding back to each other. This evolution is crucial because most of the options of the future, I believe, will be somewhere in the middle.

Comment by Thomas Scully

I am the president of the Federation of American Health Systems, which represents investor-owned hospitals. I am also on the board of Oxford Health Plans, an HMO. I am going to say a few things that both of them will hate, as I often did in the old times when I was associate director of the Office of Management and Budget in the Bush administration, where I oversaw Medicare and Medicaid programs.

The most important issue I can comment on is quality, quality, and quality—and the frustration I feel when people talk about managed care versus fee-for-service plans. I agree with Alan Nelson that the issue is just not that straightforward. There are not three categories that you can split things into.

What is managed care? Managed care is the ability to not pay every provider the same amount—to tell somebody, "you are not very good." Medicare should get charged less. There can be a fee-for-service program that can say to a caregiver, "Look, you are a rotten provider. You are not a good provider. You are a low-quality provider. We are going to pay you differentially." The flaw of the fee-for-service system is that it has to pay every provider the same amount in every community. As soon as that common payment is the law, the program inevitably will be a disaster. That is the fundamental flaw of fee-for-service programs. Providers, obviously, do not like to hear that.

The Health Care Financing Administration, Medicare, and the existing fee-for-service system unfortunately will be around forever in some shape. So the system has to be made to work. Looking at the model David Smith brought up: Why don't we make it look more like the Postal Service? If the problem is the HCFA is not structured to manage fee-for-service care and trying to pay rotten providers less and trying to have more flexible rules, the Postal Service might work well as a model. Fannie Mae has, arguably, worked pretty well for housing. I am not a big fan of government-sponsored enterprises because nobody seems to watch the money going out of the Treasury. But there is a model there that works and, if you are HCFA Administrator Bruce Vladeck, you could probably use it to screw my hospitals. But there probably is an argument that if what is wanted is flexibility along with a government-run system that is going to be a giant insurance company spending $180 billion a year, an independent government corporation would work. Why does it have to be a program that is run the way the Social Security Administration or the HCFA is? I do not think that Medicare has to operate like that.

My greatest frustration comes when one asks what the options are for rationally changing to more consumer-driven health care. What is Stuart Butler in favor of? What is Gail Wilensky in favor of? Uwe Reinhardt? Robert Reischauer? Senator Ron Wyden? Senator Bob Kerrey? They cover the political spectrum from liberal Democrat to conservative Republican. What are they for? Some type of a Federal Employee Health Benefit Program (FEHBP) hybrid? And how do they want to accomplish that? One can argue about the details, but what Congress did in 1995 was a great start. I screamed as much as anybody else did about big Medicare cuts—$270 billion. But I challenge anybody to spend the rest of the week debating what was wrong with the bill. There are some things I did not like, such as the PSO provisions, but it was a very good bill.

The reason the Republicans got crushed was the $270 billion in cuts, not because their reform policy was wrong. The policy was great. They are feeling burned that they were trounced in the last election because lots of people ran Medicare campaign ads against them. Still, nobody ran a campaign ad saying the reforms were bad. They ran campaign ads saying the numbers were too big. And now we have an administration and a Congress that agrees that $100 billion in cuts is probably the right amount, but everybody is scared to tough out the reforms. Two years ago, Richard Davidson, head of the AHA, and I and our chairmen said, "We will take Congress's entire package, its whole bill, and $165 billion in cuts, and we will be 100 percent behind Congress." The American Medical Association would have supported the same thing. Unfortunately the leadership did not take our offer. I bet they wished they had that deal back. They said, "$270 billion or bust; see you later." And it did not work out. I think it is unfortunate, but it is a shame to throw away their entire bill.

In the past ten years there have been two great travesties in health care reform. First, America blew the chance for universal coverage. Whether one looks at the George Bush plan or the Bob Dole plan or the Bob Kerrey plan or the Bill Clinton plan, the fundamental idea was to take 11 percent inflation in Medicare and Medicaid, reduce it to 5 or 6 percent, and turn around and spend the savings on universal coverage. I happen to champion deficit reduction, but most rational people would have said four or five years ago, "Let us take half the money and spend it on deficit reduction and half of it on health care." Now the chance at universal coverage is gone. The money all went to deficit reduction, and nobody paid any attention. Universal coverage is gone for twenty years.

The second travesty is the failure to hold to the reform effort. Congress came up with a great reform bill two years ago that got caught up in the politics of $270 billion of budget cuts. It was a very good package. It can be tinkered with and argued about. There is lots of room for compromise. You can talk about reducing the AAPCC and different HMOs and you can beat each other's brains in. Still, two years ago, at the end of the day, most people could have lived with a compromise. Lots of people in the provider community beat each other up on PSOs and other things. Most of us could live with some compromise. We had a very good bill with vastly excessive, by political standards certainly, Medicare cuts.

Why throw that away? But when I talked to members of Congress in the past few weeks, no one was talking about reforms. Most people could probably agree on the 1995 bill as a platform to build on, and we ought to go ahead and get a bill passed this year. Yet, that seems to be off the political agenda. And it is a shame. I will leave you with that point. Can we change fee-for-service care? Yes. Is there a basis for such reform? Yes, it was created two years ago, it got caught in over-excessive budget cuts, and it is a shame we cannot all agree to go back. Look at that bill of two years ago. The president and Congress are going to agree on the numbers. Let us take $100 billion in cuts and not miss the chance to finally reform the system.

6

Leadership and Politics: Four Views

ALTHOUGH THE AUTHORS in earlier chapters focus on the basis and substance of reforming the Medicare program, those in this chapter look at the political environment, including the role of political leadership, that makes change possible or impossible to achieve.

View by Anthony Beilenson

THE POINT OF VIEW of many observers concerning what should be done about Medicare has been how best and most equitably to solve a fixable problem, a program in need of some adjustments, using some combination of the several available means of fixing it. The perspective of Congress and the president will be this: Is there some way we can resolve this problem, either wholly or in part, without hurting ourselves politically in the process? More directly, members of Congress will be asking themselves, "Can we act usefully and responsibly on Medicare without losing an appreciable number of votes at the next election"—one must remember that it is just a year away for all the members of the House of Representatives and for a full third of the Senate—"and without jeopardizing our access to money we will need to finance the campaign?"

It is not entirely their fault that this is the perspective they bring to national issues such as this, although of course there are things they could have done about financing elections and still can do to improve the situation in which they find themselves. But to be fair about it, if you were a public official who had to stand for election frequently, you would probably consider these matters in much the same way that they do because our election process has become daunting, an obstacle course through which we now put our politicians.

Having recently read David Donald's book, *Lincoln,* I was reminded what it was like in President Lincoln's time. The things said about perhaps the greatest of our American presidents by his critics were outrageous. And, of course, I can remember the vituperation Franklin Roosevelt endured. But today, running the gantlet of America's political process is even more difficult.

First, the cost of campaigns has risen enormously, which means that candidates have to raise far more money than they would have just twenty years ago. When I first ran for the state legislature thirty-five years ago, we raised and spent $20,000 in a district about half the size congressional districts are today. But in my final two congressional campaigns we had to raise $720,000 and $500,000, and many members of the House of Representatives raise and spend much more.

A candidate cannot raise that kind of money from regular folks who think he is a nice representative or who support him because he is a Democrat or Republican. Most of the candidates from both parties rely on political action committees, on special-interest, on single-interest groups. And that leads, of course, to problems.

Members of Congress are naturally very careful to please or at least not to offend these important sources of campaign funding. When members vote on an important bill or issue these days, they do not raise the questions in their own minds that one would expect and hope they would: "Is this good for the country?" "Is this good for my district and the people I represent?" Instead, they ask themselves, "Will this offend or please group A, group B, group C?" This question can be extended to cover perhaps twenty or thirty special-interest groups from which they may have sought and received financial help in the past and to which they will have to go again.

Second, there has also been a spectacular increase in the number of special-interest pressure groups, which hardly existed three decades ago. There are now about 4,500 registered organizations of this sort in Washington. Most have their own fund-raising capabilities. All have communicating techniques that bring down on every office on Capitol Hill a cascade of faxes and phone calls and letters and postcards whenever anything important is afoot.

If, for example, a member of Congress is soon to vote on a matter of interest to the American Association of Retired Persons, he will hear within twenty-four hours from thousands of citizens who live and vote in his district. The sad fact is that a member cannot even consider a proposal without thousands of messages flooding his office, precluding the chance to think through what might be best for his country, constitiuency, or the system he is trying to fix. If he does what may be a right but not a popular thing, thousands of voters in the district will be very aware and not terribly happy about it.

Third, politics has changed because campaigning consists mainly of nasty personal attacks on candidates and, in the case of incumbents, distorting or taking out of context their positions and votes on many issues. And it works. Pollsters tell us that candidates are foolish to waste money on ads singing their own praises. Why? Because the people who watch the ads do not believe them. You say that "Tony Beilenson is a wonderful and honest politician, and he has been around for twenty years and you ought to vote him back in office." Nobody will believe that. They will not believe that he should be reelected or that he has been honest all of this time.

Anyway, the votes of members of Congress are, to an extraordinary extent, now used as political weapons against them, not only by political opponents but by special-interest groups that often represent thousands of one's constituents. And there is no better subject for effective negative campaigning than a vote to slow the growth of the Medicare program with whatever cost cutting or benefit denying or premium increasing it may involve.

Any member knows that however good or decent a Medicare reform bill may be, his opponent in his next campaign will use a vote for that bill against him. It does not take a clairvoyant to see what the television commercial will be: "When he had the chance to protect Medicare, the program that provides health care to all of us in our vulnerable old age, our congressman, Tony Beilenson, voted instead to protect the special interests by increasing the premiums." Forget about all the cuts in payments to doctors and hospitals, which pay for 90 percent of the funding changes. "He voted to protect the special interests by increasing the premiums we all must pay for doctor and hospital care." An opponent has to be an idiot not to make campaign hay with that vote.

The principal reason, of course, that a vote to reform Medicare is so potentially damaging is that it affects 38 million people, many of them middle-class citizens. These people are likely to vote, and almost all are older citizens, who are especially likely to vote. Reforming Medicare is vastly more difficult than and different from, in the political sense, reforming welfare, which Congress did last year or reforming Medicaid, which I hope will be done soon, because those programs, although they affect huge numbers of people, generally affect poor people and often younger people who vote in much smaller numbers than those who are richer and older.

Finally, the voters themselves, most of whom do not belong to any special-interest group, are nonetheless very difficult. Members of Congress do not know if the electorate knows less or is less well educated than it used to be, but it certainly is more incitable. The frustrations and fears of the public are more easily directed and taken advantage of than in the past when people were, to be frank about it, more passive and left the government alone to do its work. Whether one likes it or not, the truth is that the government usually did a better job when not everybody was watching so closely and letting their representatives know every moment whether they wanted them to do this or that and thinking only of their own interests instead of whether the representative should do something good for the country.

Here is what politicians in Washington and across the nation have to deal with, and one must understand this when one is dealing with Medicare. Pollsters say that only 1 or 2 percent of the people we represent know very much about any of the issues with which we are dealing. Another 10 or 15 percent know something about one or two issues. Health care professionals know about medical issues; others involved with health care know about insurance and Medicare. But most people—75 to 80 percent—do not know anything about any of the issues on which Congress spends all its time every day.

For example, even though probably only 1 percent of the U.S. budget is spent on welfare, the average voter believes that 20 percent goes to welfare and is upset about it. If 20 percent went to welfare, I would be upset. The average voter thinks that 15 or 20 percent of all federal monies goes to foreign aid. It is actually about two-thirds of 1 percent. Most important of all, the average voter thinks that at least 20 percent of the federal budget is spent on waste, fraud, and abuse, as if waste, fraud, and abuse were a line item in the budget. So obviously, the average voter does not believe that we have to cut Medicare or any other program to balance the budget because all we have to do is just cut out the waste. Unfortunately that is what politicians have to deal with.

Finally, what is the political outlook for at least some Medicare reform this year? The answer is surprisingly good. We always have politics with an issue like this. We seldom have the leadership. We seem to be getting some leadership at the moment, both from the president, whose support is absolutely necessary to give political coverage to members of Congress and especially to Democratic members of Congress, who have been demagogueing this and the Social Security issue to death for the past two years, most of them. We will see if this leadership remains decent and constant. We also seem to be getting some decent bipartisan legislative leadership, especially from the Republican leaders. One of the reasons for the leadership is that both the president and many people in Congress really do want to reach an agreement on a four- or five- or six-year budget-balancing plan and, of course, slowing the rate of growth of the Medicare program is the single biggest and most important piece of that particular puzzle. For those who wish to protect as much as possible the so-called domestic discretionary programs that already have been cut too deeply, it is absolutely necessary to involve some of the big entitlement programs such as Medicare.

It also may be that members of Congress have enough sense to want to solve the Medicare problem before it becomes a crisis. They hope to be in the House or the Senate four or five years from now when the trust fund is projected to run out of money. They do not want to be required at that point to do something to the system that is far more drastic than what some gradual and less radical steps would accomplish if they were taken now.

The final and, perhaps, the biggest reason we are getting political leadership at this time may be that it does not require very much courage. In the president's proposal, the savings would come mostly by reducing the amount of money the government pays hospitals, health maintenance organizations, home health agencies, skilled nursing facilities, and to a lesser extent physicians who treat Medicare patients. It would also, of course, cancel the planned reduction in premiums under part B that would have the effect by 2002 of raising by about ten dollars a month the amounts that some beneficiaries would have to pay.

But with the exception of the physicians and those who may have to pay a modest amount more in premiums, what all the other groups that have received less funding have in common is that, however upset the hospitals and the HMOs and the home health agencies are about this proposal, they are not very frightening entities to the average congressman. Not many voters are members of these groups, nor are they particularly large. And with the exception perhaps of the doctors in some areas, they are not significant contributors to political campaigns.

So, whether or not you believe that the president's proposed changes in Medicare or something very like them is what we should be seeking, they are likely to look a lot like what the folks in Washington eventually come up with later this year because they are about as politically palatable as any proposals can be.

View by Sheila Burke

I PREPARED for this program by reviewing the past nineteen years and the opportunities that Congress had and the issues it confronted that appeared at the time to be unresolvable. Among the things that I thought at the time were insurmountable but, in fact, were resolved was the Tax Equity and Fiscal Responsibility Act (TEFRA). I looked at the 1983 bailout of Social Security, the 1988 welfare reform legislation, the Kassebaum-Kennedy insurance reform bill, immigration reform, the early tax reform legislation, the Americans with Disabilities Act, the Civil Rights Act, the Clean Air Act, and the telecommunications bill (TELCOM). And, in the case of those efforts in which Congress failed miserably, one, of course, starts the list with the failure to pass a bill guaranteeing catastrophic health insurance, followed very quickly by a bill for health care reform, followed by some of the hospital cost containment initiatives and some of the health insurance efforts for the unemployed.

Common threads in the successes include public support, bipartisan commitment, a fair amount of risk taking on all sides, honesty in people's dealings with one another, some early establishment of trust in terms of how we would approach these issues, a common language that we could agree on and use throughout the discussions, and clearly articulated common goals. When we failed miserably, those elements were almost always missing.

Historically, Republicans and Democrats approach these issues very differently. They approach health care very differently. Republicans have been less than enthusiastic about massive overhaul of America's health care system and have tended to be in favor of more incremental changes. The American people also seem to view these debates from very different angles but with some very strong values.

In 1994 Robert Blendon tried to articulate what some of the public's core values were. One was a strong concern for the uninsured, but it was not strong enough for people to become engaged in urging a new national health insurance system if it was not their specific problem. The second was that they were somewhat fearful about their own health care coverage and its security, worrying that at some time it would be inadequate.Third, people did not believe that the existing problems of the health care system were their own doing, or that they, in fact, were responsible for any of the difficulties they were facing. Fourth, they were very unwilling to expose themselves to higher costs or higher risk. Fifth, they generally distrusted government and believed that the private sector was better at doing things with the exception, and tempered by their distrust, of the insurance industry. Finally, they were very cynical about the system itself and believed that most serious problems were, in fact, caused by the greed of most institutions.

Although there is a case that many of those observations are still accurate, with Medicare reform one looks at a somewhat different picture and can learn from experience.

Republicans across the board seem to be more interested and aggressive about major reforms and reconsidering the structure of these programs. Democrats seemed to be, generally, more reflective and more insistent on incremental changes and no major overhaul.

The public seems to hold a strong commitment to the elderly and the disabled. Some of the commitment is, in fact, personal because people worry about their parents, and for those in my age group, fear that they will be us before too long. Unlike the uninsured, there is a real voting block among these people so that, in the case of the commitment to the elderly, they can make a huge difference this time around. People are concerned about their peace of mind. In addition there continues to be a lack of self-blame. "It is never my doctor. It is never my congressman who is the problem. It is always somebody else's. I am not to blame for the kinds of problems we see now in terms of use and so forth." There continues to be a remarkable lack of willingness to sacrifice much of anything in terms of personal benefits or protection.

As I noted earlier, there is an extraordinary distrust of all aspects of government, although there seems to be less distrust of Medicare because there is this sense that, in fact, that is something that the government may have done well and people want the government to stay involved. Then, finally, there continues to be the cynicism about the system and the firmly held attitude that most major institutional providers are providing services that are subject to waste, fraud, and abuse.

Given the public's lack of detailed knowledge, conflicting values, and ambivalence about what America should be doing with its health care system, it is a little early to tell what the outcome of this debate will be. But I think the critical battleground for proponents and opponents will be one critical question for the public, and that is whether they will be better off or worse off at the end of Medicare reform. A complicating factor is that although most people want to preserve Medicare, as they do Social Security, very few understand the program or the issues. Someone once suggested it was rather like a Swiss bank: "We knew that it worked, but we were not quite sure about how it worked or why." Anyone who has been a staff member or has sat in committee hearings in the House or Senate has known the experience of sitting in front of a committee and watch its members' eyes glaze when Medicare is discussed.

We want the program to be above politics. We know that goal is impossible. If Social Security is an 800-pound gorilla, Medicare weighs in at about 750, but again, admitting that Medicare is inherently political is also something that scares people.

There are people who say that those who talk about a Medicare crisis simply want to do away with the program and want to highlight the very tough things that have to be done. Those who suggest simple changes and incremental changes are accused of, essentially, wanting to hide the tough choices and decisions that have to be made. It is, in fact, the political process that has to bring some balance to the two sides.

If Medicare is complex, it is also expensive. But whether one is concerned about the financial future of Medicare, the growing cost of care, the availability of long-term care, the health-related economic risks to the elderly, or the ethical choices surrounding the allocation of health care resources, the large policy issues facing the elderly can rarely be understood by simply saying that there is a Medicare problem.

So, as we begin this discussion and look at what the politics will be, we have to remember that there is a diverse population, an elderly population that is growing rapidly, and a very turbulent environment in America's health care industry.

Backing up for just a moment to my examples of past battles and what worked and what did not, everyone has a piece of this action in terms of the kinds of things that have to be done. The politics of division that we have seen over this issue, particularly in the past few years, have to come to an end if we are going to take on Medicare reform. The effort has to begin with an agreement on the common language. It has to begin with establishing some common goals.

Two groups will be instrumental in achieving the common language: the press and the American Association of Retired Persons (AARP). Words such as *gutting* and *slashing* and *devastating* and the kinds of language that we saw in the last campaign cannot be allowed to continue. The kind of language used then is what frightened people away from discussions and decisions that should have taken place. The press will be important, as will the groups of elderly in talking to their members, who will look to them for some guidance as they have in the past.

Our common goal has to be something beyond the next election. We have to begin to look at policies that are not driven by two-year cycles, that are driven by a longer-term goal. It will get no easier. The days of being able simply to slip the periodic interim payment a day, which some of us did more than once, are gone, and the decisions that are left are not simple decisions.

We have to begin with what we can agree on. There has to be time spent in rebuilding trust because there currently is no trust between the two parties on this issue. To be able to go forward, there must be a bridge between the two parties. The way to do that is to see what there already is in common, what it is that we can understand and can appreciate and agree to and build on that.

It is clear to me, as was the case with Social Security in 1983, that this will happen only if the effort is bipartisan. I can remember vividly a conversation between Bob Dole and George Mitchell at one point during the debate on catastrophic health insurance. None of us forgets Dan Rostenkowski being chased down the street by a group of elderly voters, I am sure. None of us ever wants to see it repeated. But I can remember Dole and Mitchell talking about their need to stick together, essentially holding hands and going over the cliff together. In fact, they did. We can only move this reform forward if the effort is bipartisan. There is no way in this political environment that members of either party will take a risk that puts them out in front of the other. They cannot afford to.

Unfortunately, the headlines in the *Washington Post* do not suggest that we are moving very quickly. There is now bipartisan criticism—maybe that is progress—of administration proposals.

To go back to my earlier point, it is critical to educate members of Congress as well as the public. No one gains from ignorance in this environment, but that is what we have bred in the conversations about Medicare in recent years. There is, clearly, an absence of understanding; people do not understand what they get and how it is paid for. It goes from that to the complexity of the financing to the problem of long-term solvency. Each of those issues has to be discussed and understood. There is no reason why people cannot understand these issues anymore than they can anything else.

So, we must begin to put some emphasis on the press and on the associations and people who have stakes in Medicare reform, whether they are the teaching hospitals, physician groups, or specialty groups, in helping people understand. The secret language of acronyms that we all talk must be forgotten. What we have to do is help people understand the issues they are confronting and the choices they have to make.

In the end it can be done. In the end it absolutely should be done. In the end will it be done? I am not at all clear. We have to be able to keep the goal, saving the program, in mind and not get tied down and lost in some of the internecine battles that are likely to occur. But simple solutions that never begin to challenge us to look at the structure of the program cannot be the answer. The promises we are making, given the demographics we face, constitute a failure to treat people the way they should be treated—certainly a failure in honesty in terms of dealing with one of the most difficult issues we will have to confront.

If we develop common goals and a common language and begin to build on the things that we can agree on and do it in a bipartisan way and rebuild trust, we will be on our way to solving a very tough problem

View by Haynes Johnson

I WAS DOING a biography of William Fulbright in 1967–68 when he was leading the dissent against the Vietnam War, and he opened up his office to me and I spent two years going through all his files. I remember vividly the day that his chief aide, Lee Williams, introduced us and said: "Haynes, we have somebody we want you to meet, who has just joined the staff." He was a fat-faced kid from Arkansas, and it was Bill Clinton. I worked out of that office for the next year. Everyday it was Haynes and Bill. He was exactly the way he is now, a little slimmer, eager, earnest, full of information, always at your shoulder asking questions and smiling and wanting to be pleasing and ingratiating and that is how I did begin to watch that fellow and later on, when Fulbright became, sort of, a father to me, I regarded him second only to my own father as someone I felt close to.

When Arkansas University named a college in honor of Fulbright, I gave a speech, some black-tie thing, and young first-term governor Bill Clinton introduced me. But I did not keep up with him until he came to Washington, and it really was not until his health care reform efforts began that I started following his activities almost daily.

I am not a health policy expert. When David Broder and I set out some years ago to do the book that became *The System,* our idea originally was to do three books on how well the system was working or not working. The first was going to be on the cities, going inside four city halls around the country and seeing what really happens there. What are the pressures and how well does the local government really serve the people it is supposed to serve? Second, we wanted to have it translated into the states, four different capitals, and finally here in Washington.

After hiring people and taking money from a publisher for this grandiose idea, we happily scrapped it, because it was clear that we probably would not live to finish it and that David and I, who go back to the 1950s together—we worked on the *Washington Star* in those days—probably would never speak to each other again. So we chose health care reform as a way to tell that larger story of how much one issue touches everybody in the country and every entity of government from the White House to Congress to the press and down to the states and county commissioners and city halls. That was the story we set out to tell.

We got quite an education in the process. Health care reform is not just a policy question. It is a political question. The problem was not arriving at the perfect policy formulation. It was how one gets the policy that will be enacted politically in a very difficult time

The first big book that I did was on the Bay of Pigs. Later on, the historians described that as the perfect policy failure. It was. This health reform effort was the perfect political failure. Perfect in every respect: as President Clinton said to us in the Oval Office, acknowledging his own mistakes to an astonishing measure,

> I tried to do too much, too fast. I did not realize and appreciate that Hillary would be such a lightening rod, not only among the public but among my own staff. I should have reached out to Republicans earlier. I should have embraced Dole from the very beginning. I should have been more modest. When I realized it was not going to go forward, I should have made a speech to the country and said that it was not going to happen this year, and not in one hundred days, but it is going to happen in a year or two. We are going to keep on going. It failed and set the stage for the Republican takeover of Congress. I should have made another speech to the country. I should have honestly said that "here is what we need to do."

"Yes, it failed. Here is what we are going to try to do," and he did none of those things. It was an astonishing concession of mistakes that in our history a sitting president, then facing reelection on an issue that led to the takeover of the Congress, has ever acknowledged so publicly. And, he was right in every particular. It was also a failure of Congress, both parties, the interest groups, and not least the press. I agree with what Sheila Burke has said about the failure of the press to take on and explain, as carefully as possible, a very complicated issue; but in the end it was, by far and overall, a classic political failure.

What is interesting now is that the story that we began to chronicle then is an even greater story with a more unfinished ending now. It is at the center of our public political debate and will be for years to come. When David and I went on our book tour, we were stunned that everywhere we went, there was the anger, the fear, and the insecurity of citizens, everywhere, about health care. Whatever the pollsters may have said, this fear, this apprehension, this anxiety, not only has failed to abate, it has intensified at every measure, and for good reason. There is the growing sense that the system is not going to be there to work for the people it is supposed to.

This is the great challenge of our political times. It is akin to the civil rights struggle in that it is an old issue that can tear us apart because it touches every life in the country. It goes to the heart not only of our values as a society, but who we are, whether we are up to taking on major changes.

I agree that we must have bipartisan support and incremental change. I remember saying to Hillary Clinton at one of our sessions in the White House in the first few months of the administration. "You are erecting the Taj Mahal, but you are doing it overnight. You do not even have the foundation laid, and it is going to be this grand wonderful thing, but that can't work."

I remember Robert Reischauer making the point in one of our many conversations when he headed the CBO that there have been three great efforts in our country's history in recent years where the government accomplished enormously difficult things, and it took the widest consensus in the public to do it. The first was the Manhattan Project, which even though secret had to enlist all the thinkers of the country—the military, the economists, the scientists—in putting together this extraordinary effort, and, of course, it was helped because there was a war.

Second was the Marshall Plan, maybe even more stunning because one forgets that this was not a country that wanted to spend its money to rebuild its enemies. In fact, we were disbanding the armed forces left and right, which led four years later to Korea when we had no force, and that was a stunning singular act of bipartisanship that, carefully put together, worked and transformed all of the history of the past fifty years.

The last, of course, was the space program, when John Kennedy set a goal of putting a man on the moon within a decade. It was one of those things that, again, required enormous efforts across the board, but it excited the country.

Those were all easier than reforming Medicare, and they came at a time when one could use the cold war or various enemies abroad to justify the efforts.

So, I think the lesson for the policymakers is to be much more modest and set the goals clearly. Yes, they will be torn by dissent and misinformation, but if they set out a long-term approach to a problem that everyone knows (and this is the key—that they know in their hearts) will affect their lives and their children's lives, the policymakers can begin to make the steps that will lead to a more secure future.

I am fascinated watching the Republicans and the Democrats almost changing clothes in the past few years. The rhetoric is stunning. The same language that was used by the Republicans in the first years of Clinton's first term has been used word for word in the past two years by the Democrats. I mean, word for word. And what about the public? Do they know less? No, they know more, but they believe less. This is part of the problem.

So, I think I would be even much harsher today about the policymaking that went into the health care debacle. But the hope is that the lessons are there, and we are now at one of these extraordinary moments when we are poised to go in a very positive direction, but it is a moment that is extraordinary because both political parties have been chastened. Neither one has any assurance of inheriting the future.

The 1996 election was the most interesting and important in at least sixty years and, not by happenstance, the outcome mirrored exactly the way the public feels. It gave back-to-back presidencies to the Democrats for the first time since 1936, a rather fateful year in our history. And, it gave the Republicans control of successive Congresses for the first time since the days of Calvin Coolidge and Herbert Hoover. This did not just happen. It was a clear check on the powers of each with a clear message: "Let us get on with our business and with what has to be done." No one expects perfection or the perfect policy, but our citizens do expect an end to the rancor and getting on with the business. This is where we are at the moment. Whether the détente lasts or whether it breaks apart, it is going to define our politics and our public life for years to come.

I thought I would share with readers the way David and I concluded the paperback edition of *The Afterward* because it may have some pertinency as to where we are at the moment in our political system.

We have been lucky enough, throughout our history, to avoid open political conflict between the generations.

There is no guaranty that truce will last forever. The last time Americans were deeply divided by an issue that affected everyone in the land—the institution of slavery—a new party emerged. Republicans replaced Whigs and wrested control of the national government from the Democrats. If the Republicans and Democrats who now share power narrowly and uneasily in Washington fail to deal with this growing entitlement issue centering around health care, another political crisis could confront our political system.

Very possibly it could lead to the emergence of a new governing party. It is not difficult to imagine moderate Republicans and Democrats joined by political independents forming a coalition around the issues of fiscal discipline and generational equity, a Concord Coalition writ large.

Such a party, shunning the ideological extremes and operating from the political center, could find a powerful secondary appeal by contrasting its own aloofness from interest groups.

It would have an opportunity really to reform the way money flows in our politics by casting off the obvious tethers that the interest groups place on both Republicans and Democrats to preserve the advantages they already enjoy.

Such a new centrist party could draw strength from the energy and anger of millions who feel the system does not work for them. It would instantly pose a serious and sobering threat for all those now in power if it convinces them that they have no choice but to deal with the questions of entitlements, fiscal responsibility, and money in politics now. It will be a boon to the country.

Otherwise, the new century may bring greater changes in the system than we have seen in our lifetime or, perhaps, even in that of the nation.

I really do believe that that is where we are. This is not a normal time. Politics as usual or policy is regular. This is a different period with great stakes that are yet to be resolved.

View by John Rother

I AM GOING to propose seven rules that should inform the long-term debate over reform of Medicare.

First, for the short-term Medicare debate, my advice to Congress is just to enact the budget agreement quickly. But for the long term, my advice is quite different. I would start with a point that Sheila Burke made, which is the fundamental need for a real effort to educate the public. The last campaign to reform health care in this country generated a lot more heat than light. If anything, the public may be more confused than it was earlier. For example, after talking to members of the American Association of Retired Persons (AARP), I understand that most people do not know that 75 percent of part B payments are subsidized by general revenues. They do not understand how much the program does not cover. If a person does not know these facts to start with, all the discussions about changing financing or benefits for part B might as well be in Greek.

Most people do not know how the program interrelates with Medicaid or with supplemental insurance, except in their own experience. They do not have the view of the overall health insurance financing system and, when people talk to them in terms of making changes in the system, they do not easily translate it to their own experience. We need to get out consistent public education efforts before this debate heats up again. I would even propose that Harvard could sponsor some education efforts, and we at AARP will be doing a lot. Perhaps C-Span would carry a few programs designed to help the public understand what the basics of the program are and what challenges the program faces and let people interact with that and lay the foundation for reform.

Second, start with a commitment to a gradual approach. It would be foolish to do otherwise, given how important this program is in people's lives. Talk of revolution or radical change scares people, and once they are scared they will resist efforts to move them. We have to admit that there is no magic bullet, that even managed care is not going to be the solution to Medicare's financing problems, that we are going to have to probably confront the problems many times in a series of adjustments. Once people hear that solutions will be applied gradually, the anxiety level will fall and policymakers can then start to engage people on the merits of the reforms.

Third, we need to get people personally engaged in the effort to do something about waste, fraud, and abuse. There has been a lot of talk about waste, fraud, and abuse in the program. People know from their own experience that there is unnecessary care and overcharging, and they are angry about it. The Clinton administration has launched Operation Restore Trust. It is terrific that the Kassebaum-Kennedy bill allocated new funds for stepped-up enforcement, and it is terrific that we are going to have a presidential commission examining quality in health care and consumer protection in managed care. But we are just beginning to pursue this matter seriously. So, we need to get people involved.

Why? Not just because this kind of action is going to save a lot of money. Unless we first deal with the perception of waste, fraud, and abuse, it is difficult to deal with other things. If people believe that waste is the problem and that nothing is being done about it, they are not going to listen to anything else policymakers have to say.

Fourth, we need to distinguish between program cuts and program savings. Policymakers should stop this debate now. We ought to say that the measure of an appropriate growth rate for Medicare expenditures is some kind of per capita risk-adjusted rate of growth equivalent to the growth in the private sector and stop the confusion about what is a cut and what is a savings. We should simply say that Medicare should be expected to grow at about the same rate as private health care, adjusted for the fact that the risk pool is different and that the program is enrolling more people.

Fifth, we need to develop a common language. Unless there is a common language, people are only going to be confused. In a similar vein, what people respond to more than anything else is not the details of policy proposals but their perception of the intent of the proposals. People listen to the language and they say, "Is this person caring more about reaching a balanced budget or about maintaining a good-quality health care system?"So the language is important. We should not talk about money so much. Yes, we have to make the program work financially, but the public should be informed more about health care and how to keep a quality health care system affordable while it is being made more efficient.

If people hear that quality is what reform is about, they can say, "Okay, I can relate to trying to keep my health care system effective." But if they hear only talk about costs, it looks as if the people in charge do not care about health care and that they will do something in the name of the budget that will damage it.

Sixth, do not always deal with Medicare in the context of budget reconciliation. One of the things that badly injured the Republican effort to change Medicare in 1995 was putting the changes in the same bill with massive tax cuts. Reconciliation has become the easiest way to deal with complex legislative changes in Congress, but we would be better off, in terms of the public debate, if we talked health care and what is good health care in the long run without necessarily linking it to tax cuts and other parts of the budget. It is damaging to have Medicare costs being presented in the context of a balanced budget as if cost cutting were the overriding goal. Again, what the public needs to hear is that the debate about Medicare reform is a debate about health care and how to make health care better and more efficient.

I remain impressed with the success of the legislative effort to preserve Social Security in 1983. That matter was presented on its own terms. The Greenspan Commission did not solve the entire problem with the system's funding, but it did help educate the public. It did define the options. It did identify the common goal. And it made bipartisan action more likely. I am not saying that a Medicare commission is necessary, but I do agree with Sheila Burke that we need to keep the debate bipartisan and we need to have a common goal. We must have a common definition of the problem for the public and the press; and we must identify those matters on which we agree— that would get us part of the way there. Ultimately, of course, some of the questions must be resolved politically; an expert commission can never resolve those issues.

Finally, the public must know that the burden of change will be shared. People know that there is no painless way to resolve the ills of the Medicare program. There will be sacrifices. Again looking back to 1983 and looking at deficit reductions since then, it is very important to say that the sacrifices will be shared broadly, that everyone has a stake in a strong Medicare system, and that no one part of the population will be asked to bear more than its fair share of the sacrifice. That is after we have made Medicare more efficient and after we have squeezed payments to health care providers where appropriate. But there is a point—and we may be reaching it—at which providers have made as many efficiencies as they can consistent with maintaining quality.

So the message of shared sacrifice involving workers, providers, and retirees is very important and needs to be backed up with a specific proposal. Congress was able to do that in 1983 with Social Security. And many of the deficit-reduction packages since then have met that test.

The public may be more prepared than one might think for small steps that move Medicare in the direction of offering more choice and greater individual responsibility. But this movement will occur only if there is a common language, if policymakers can talk to people in terms that allow them to be part of the debate and not push them away from it, and if leaders can somehow reassure the public, particularly older persons, that what they are trying to do is to strengthen the health care system, keep the quality, keep it affordable, and not just reach arbitrary ways of balancing the budget to free up money for other purposes. Ultimately, reform is all about clarity in values and intent.

If this can be done, there will be ongoing opportunities, not to enact some radical omnibus bill to fix Medicare once and for all, but to take a series of steps toward restructuring the program that will keep it vigorous for generations to come.

7

Public Opinion and Medicare Restructuring: Three Views

THIS CHAPTER examines the significance of public support and public opposition to Medicare reforms. In focusing on the public, the authors emphasize generational and gender differences that complicate the consideration of reform options.

View by Karlyn Bowman

A FEW WEEKS AGO, as an exercise in historical curiosity, I decided to go back to the Gallup Polls of the 1960s to see what kinds of questions had been asked about the new health insurance program known as Medicare. The results were surprising. In 1965, the year that Medicare legislation passed, Gallup polls did not ask respondents a single question about it. In 1964 only one question was asked about a social insurance program like Medicare: Gallup found 63 percent of respondents approved a compulsory medical insurance program covering hospital and nursing home care for the elderly. Twenty-eight percent disapproved.[1]

In the last three months of 1996 alone, the Roper Center at the University of Connecticut, the largest archive of survey data in America, added to its polling database sixty-nine questions about Medicare. The database includes nearly all the surveys conducted by Gallup, Harris, Robert Blendon at Harvard, ABC News, CBS News, *Washington Post, New York Times,* and so forth. Only nine of the sixty-nine questions, by my rough count, were substantive. The largest number dealt with the politics of Medicare; what is called the horse race in presidential election-year polling. Over and over the pollsters asked a variant of "Who is winning on the Medicare issue, the president or the Republicans in Congress?" Over and over we learned that the Democrats were maintaining or enlarging their historic advantage as the party better able to deal with the Medicare issue.

Perhaps it is not surprising that during an election year the emphasis of survey work in the public domain would be largely political, but the intensity of the political coverage by the public media–polling group partnerships in 1996 did little to deepen policymakers' understanding of public opinion about Medicare, and it may have done some harm. More about that later. Fortunately, much useful polling has been done about Medicare, and it can guide legislators and others who have an interest in addressing the program's problems. Robert Blendon has summarized a great deal of that work in his presentation.

Although answers to questions on specific aspects of Medicare reform bounce around depending on how the questions are worded, the direction of sentiment is usually very clear. First, and perhaps it is too obvious to mention, the Medicare program has strong public support. In a survey that Bill McInturff of Public Opinion Strategies did for the Cato Institute in 1996, some 72 percent had a favorable view of Medicare. By contrast, only a quarter had a favorable impression of the welfare system and 28 percent a favorable impression of the federal income tax system.[2]

But beyond favorable impressions, people believe that this social insurance program is essential. One hears a great deal about economic anxiety these days, and although it would be foolish to dismiss anxiety, I am not certain the level of anxiety is significantly higher today than it was in the past. Still, it is certainly true that people cannot begin to imagine paying for their retirement health care costs. In a survey done by Matt Greenwald and Associates for the Employee Benefits Research Institute, Americans were more worried about paying for their retirement health care than they were about covering basic expenses of retirement.[3]

The strong support that the program has can be seen in many questions that ask people to rank Medicare reform and other important public policy issues, including one that has traditionally been a top goal: balancing the budget. Poll after poll shows that people think it is more important to protect Medicare than to balance the budget. Medicare's virtual sacrosanct status is demonstrated by a question that Gallup has asked a number of times: Is it only fair to consider cuts in Medicare along with cuts in other programs, or is Medicare a special program that should not be cut even if there are increases in the deficit? Fifty-nine percent describe Medicare as a special program that should not be cut; 37 percent say it is fair to consider cuts in Medicare along with cuts in other programs.[4]

The view expressed in many polls during 1995 and 1996 that the Republicans were pushing Medicare reform too fast is another indication of the deep public commitment to this program. The commitment may explain the answers given to a question in one of the Kaiser-Harvard surveys. When asked which of two descriptions came closer to their view about what Medicare should look like in the year 2000, sixty-four percent described a program that would remain as it is today with a fixed set of benefits and with government providing individuals with a single insurance card. Only a third thought that the program as we know it would no longer exist and that people would instead receive a voucher or a check for a fixed amount and and would buy their own policies.

I do not like that question; the alternatives are not balanced. But the surveyors revised it and asked people which of these more balanced alternatives was closer to their opinion: "Medicare should remain as it is today with a defined set of benefits for people over age 65 and the government providing them with a single insurance card," or "Medicare should be changed so that people over age 65 would receive a check or a voucher from the government each year for a fixed amount they can use to shop for their own private health insurance policy." The numbers were not too different. Sixty-four percent agreed with the first formulation; 32 percent with the second one.[5]

One of the most important issues that needs to be addressed is how serious the public believes Medicare's problems are. Unfortunately, the polls have often provided more confusion than clarity. I confess to being confused by a certain kind of question that I saw first during the health care debate in 1993 and later in the debate about Medicare reform. The questions ask people whether the country has a health care or Medicare crisis, and many people say that, in fact, the country does. From the answers, one might infer that the public would be receptive to significant changes in the program or to some serious restructuring. But that is not so. For the past decade polling data confirm that people have believed the system is in crisis. In a poll conducted more than a decade ago, only 35 percent of respondents had confidence that Medicare would be around for them; 54 percent said that it would not. Those results are very similar to a Concord Coalition poll done by Bill Hamilton and Bob Teeter.[6] About 60 percent of those surveyed said that Medicare would not be around for them.

The view that the system is in crisis, then, seems to be a constant. Saying the system is in crisis is simply a way for people to say to their elected legislators: "Pay attention. This issue is important to me." But there is another explanation for why people would suggest there is a crisis but then choose mild responses. In the polls of the past few years, it is possible to find questions about an education crisis, a crisis in the criminal justice system, a crisis in race relations and, of course, that hearty perennial, the budget crisis. When everything is a crisis in the public's mind, nothing is; that makes political progress on Medi-care reform particularly difficult.

The crisis formulation does not capture the way people are thinking about Medicare, but it will still make headlines and continue to mislead policymak-ers. Approaching Medicare reform and other matters in a less sensational way is likely to yield more useful results. It is also helpful to compare responses about Medicare with responses people give on other matters the government may take action on.

When Bill McInturff's firm asked in its 1996 survey for the Cato Institute about views on a handful of government programs, 41 percent of respondents said that the welfare program needed radical changes, and nearly a quarter believed the income tax system did too. But only 13 percent said that Medicare needed radical changes, and 16 percent that Social Security did.[7] When asked about the next fifteen to twenty years, however, 27 percent thought that Medi-care would need radical change, and 40 percent thought that it would need major changes.

A *Los Angeles Times* question had produced similar results.[8] When asked to look ahead ten or fifteen years, 80 percent of respondents said that Medicare would be in financial trouble. Only 10 percent thought it would be financially sound. These responses clearly show that people are aware the system has problems, but at least at this point people do not have a sense of urgency about them.

Short of a major overhaul, what kind of responses to Medicare's problems are people willing to consider? At the end of 1996 NBC News and the *Wall Street Journal* surveyed Americans about changes that might be made in the Medicare program. The results confirmed what many other polls have shown. I cite these because they are some of the most recent surveys asking about Medicare. In the NBC News/*Wall Street Journal* poll, 60 percent of those surveyed said that they believed Medicare beneficiaries with incomes of more than $40,000 a year should pay for some of their health care coverage. Thirty-six percent rejected means testing.[9]

A much longer question asked by the *Los Angeles Times* a few months earlier reminded respondents that all Medicare recipients pay the same premium, regard-less of income. Then it went on to explain a new proposal that would increase Medicare premiums for people with higher incomes and found 60 percent support-ing means testing when described this way.[10] The Hamilton/Teeter poll for the Concord Coalition found that three-quarters of respondents supported the idea that people with incomes of more than $50,000 a year should receive full benefits, while those with higher incomes should have to pay proportionately more.[11] Means testing appears to be an idea that the public will accept.

In the NBC/*Wall Street Journal* polls the public rejected by a margin of two to one a proposal to gradually raise the eligibility age for Medicare from 65 to 68.[12] This is a familiar finding to those who have examined public attitudes about raising the retirement age for Social Security: the public does not go along. But another idea may be more acceptable. The Concord Coalition's poll found 60 percent of respondents endorsing a sliding scale of benefits based on age, with higher premiums and copayments for those who elect to receive Medicare earlier than for those who elect to receive it later.

Those surveyed by NBC News/*Wall Street Journal* in December 1996 also rejected by 52 to 42 percent the idea of raising the Medicare payroll tax for all employed people. Other questions have produced similar results, and it is probably fair to say that the public is very skeptical of raising the payroll tax. The resistance to a tax increase can be seen in the responses to the 1995 Concord Coalition poll question. People were asked about doubling the 1.5 percent Medicare payroll tax "to allow Medicare to be fully funded and elderly Americans to continue to draw all the same benefits they do now." Even in this formulation, only a bare majority endorsed the idea, and 46 percent rejected it.

In the NBC/*Wall Street Journal* survey, 50 percent of respondents favored keeping premiums at current levels for those who agree to join HMOs and increasing premiums for those who choose to continue seeing private doctors. A Harris poll from 1995 found 72 percent supporting the idea of providing incentives to recipients to join less expensive HMOs or other managed care plans.[13]

I am not sure that most people understand the implications of reducing the fees that Medicare pays to hospitals and doctors for services. Responses vary to questions about this. The NBC News/*Wall Street Journal* poll found 45 percent in favor and 47 percent opposed. In a September 1995 Gallup poll question the public was evenly divided about whether doctors and hospitals would find ways to deliver the same services more efficiently if their fees were reduced. Majorities of respondents believed that prices would be increased to make up for health care providers' lost income, that many Medicare patients would be refused treatment, and that providers would reduce the quality of care available to Medicare patients.

A voucher system described in different ways in various polls seems to attract the support of about 30 percent of the population. It is not clear from the data I have seen exactly how firm that support is. Do these respondents reject the system we have now? Is the response simply a message to do something to save the system? Or is the 30 percent a measure of actual support for a voucher system or some alternative? I am not sure that we know the answers judging from the current questions in the public domain.

Nearly all the survey results decisively reject reducing benefits to seniors, although many of the same surveys show that people believe that Medicare as it is currently designed encourages people to run to a physician for everything.

As a final consideration, how does the Medicare debate compare to the health care reform debate? There is one crucially important difference. Health care reform, in the words of the Gallup Poll's David Moore, is a civic issue, important for the nation but not necessarily important for individuals themselves.[14] What Moore means is that during the health care debate people believed the country would be better off with significant reforms, but they themselves would not necessarily be better off if reforms were enacted. Most people, after all, are pretty well satisfied with the health care that they have. Medicare, Moore says, does not elicit the civic response. With Medicare, Americans are more likely to believe that the country, the elderly, and they, personally, would be worse off rather than better off under reforms. This is an important distinction, and it makes the job of those interested in addressing Medicare's problems much more difficult.

That brings me back to the concerns I have about the horse race coverage of Medicare reform. People are cynical about politics and distrust politicians. The pollsters are helping to feed the cynicism and distrust by their incessant focus on who is winning the Medicare issue. In the report on its 1995 bipartisan poll the Concord Coalition said that when people are educated about the seriousness of the problems of entitlement programs, they respond seriously. It is hard to explain the need for reform when the issue is treated as a political football, when the pollsters and the media emphasize the horse race and report the polling stories that way.

Polls can be a very useful tool to understand a complex public. When carefully designed they can provide guidance for policymakers. When they focus almost exclusively on the competition of politics, as they did in the last three months of 1996, polls are a much less valuable tool.

Notes

1. *The Gallup Poll Public Opinion, 1935–1971,* vol. 3 (Random House), p. 1915.

2. Public Opinion Strategies for the Cato Institute, Social Security Reform National Survey, June 12–16, 1996.

3. 1996 Retirement Confidence Survey, Wave IV, conducted by Matthew Greenwald and Associates, Employee Benefit Research Institute, and American Savings Education Council, 1996, p. 15.

4. Gallup poll for CNN and *USA Today,* May 11–14, 1995.

5. Survey of Americans on Health Policy by the Kaiser-Harvard Program on the Public and Health/Social Policy, July 30, 1996, p. 11.

6. Public Opinion toward Entitlements and the Federal Deficit by Hamilton & Staff and the Coldwater Corporation for the Concord Coalition, June 1995.

7. Social Security Reform National Survey, 1996.

8. *Los Angeles Times* poll, September 16–18, 1995.

9. NBC News/*Wall Street Journal* poll, December 5–9, 1996.

10. *Los Angeles Times* poll, September 16–18, 1995.

11. Public Opinion toward Entitlements and the Federal Deficit, June 1995.

12. NBC News/*Wall Street Journal* poll, December 5–9, 1996.

13. *The Harris Poll,* May 31–June 5, 1995.

14. David Moore, "Polling on Health Care and Medicare: Continuity in Public Opinion," *Public Perspective* (October-November, 1995), p. 13.

View by Robert J. Blendon

IN THE 1996 national exit polls done by the television networks, voters were asked to choose the most important national issues. They picked Medicare–Social Security as the second most important. Rounding out the top five were the economy and jobs, the federal deficit, education, and taxes. About 50 percent of those who cited Medicare–Social Security were older than age 60.[1] Almost no one younger than age 30 voted according to their concern for this issue. To put this in context, those older than 60 represented 24 percent of the voters, and 50 percent of those chose Medicare–Social Security. Those younger than 30 chose not to concern themselves with this problem. They chose public education, economy, and jobs as their most significant concerns. The biggest splits in public opinion on Medicare and how or whether to fix the program are between people 60 and older and and those younger than 30. In our analysis of the polls, it is important to note that the younger people did not choose to exercise their voting franchise on this particular issue. They have very strong views, possibly, but not on this.

The majority of voters who ranked Medicare–Social Security as one of their top three priorities voted for President Clinton. In an earlier survey my colleagues and I gave people who indicated they were going to vote on the basis of a candidate's stance on the Medicare issue a variety of choices. They opposed major reductions in future spending on the program. Thus, those who voted on this issue were people who did not want significant reductions in future spending.[2] Although this does not tell us where the rest of the public stands, it is important to know who the voters are on Medicare and Social Security.

To the public, there are three primary spending issues: balancing the budget, preventing short-term trust fund bankruptcy, and preserving Medicare for future generations. In Washington, the mentality is that a dollar saved for Medicare is a dollar saved regardless of the reason for the savings. The Congressional Budget Office projects it as a reduction in future spending.

To voters, the rationale behind reducing the spending matters a great deal. In our analysis of the polls, we found that voters oppose balancing the budget using Medicare savings (figure 7-1). A large part of the public does not realize Medicare is part of the consolidated budget.[3] They think the budget is either totally or partly separate, like a highway trust fund, and thus do not understand why trade-offs are even being discussed. In addition, although many elite

Figure 7-1. *Share of Voters Who Favor Major Reductions in Future Medicare Spending, by Reason for Favoring, January 1997*

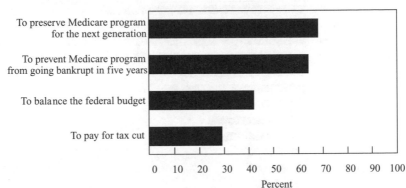

Source: Kaiser/Harvard/PSRA Post-Election Survey of Voters' 1997 Health Care Agenda, January 1997.

groups feel strongly about the need to deal with the entitlement crisis, this is not the case for the public at large.

The real issue is the American public's preferred trade-off for the federal budget. Surveys have shown that when people are told they have to confront choices over the deficit, regardless of what is on the list, Medicare and Social Security always rank as programs that should not be substantially cut. People want to ensure that these programs are the last to be reduced (figure 7-2).

It is important to understand that a large share of the people interviewed do not consider Medicare and Social Security to be a part of the consolidated budget, and they do not want program funding reduced in favor of increasing funding for other programs. This means that every time reducing spending is discussed, there are different responses from those addressing the other two issues—Medicare bankruptcy by 2005 or the task of saving the program for the next generation—that involve the program.

Why are there these differences? A 1995 article in the *Washington Post* suggested it was all "spin."[4] In fact, it is not just spin. This is the way people think about the issue. They recognize that the government does not have enough money to deal with an aging population and the fact that people are retiring earlier. They also realize that American government may not have adequately funded Medicare and may not be able to meet future obligations.

This concern is different from having to trade off Medicare funding for funding other items in the federal budget. When people discuss reducing future spending to save Medicare from near-term bankruptcy or from longer-term

Figure 7-2. *Voter Opinion of Where Government Spending Should Be Cut to Reduce the Deficit, 1995*

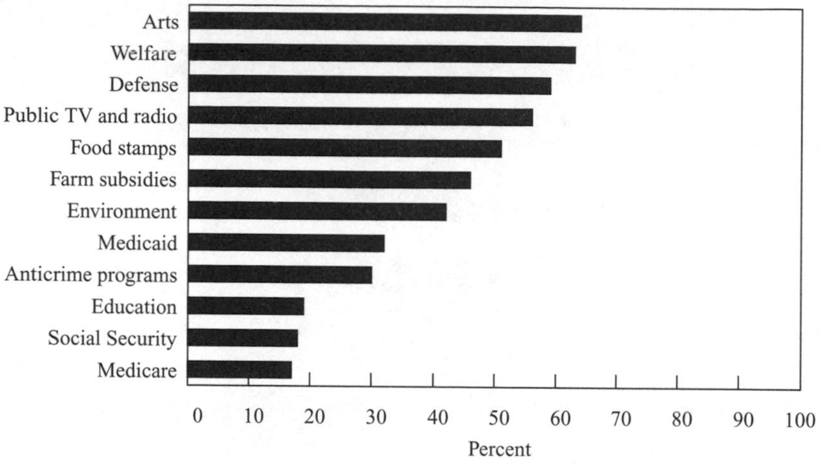

Source: ABC News/*Washington Post* poll, 1995.

problems, there is a wider acceptance of a range of policies than there is in the budget debate alone. My recommendations will be to balance the budget with the least controversial approaches to Medicare and not try to have a broad public debate about tough choices or restructuring the program at this time.

Additionally, there is some misunderstanding about the longer-term issues. There is what I call "simplistic polling" that has been done by a variety of survey groups on questions related to Social Security and Medicare. Respondents are given a chance to answer, "Are you worried that the program won't be there or are you not worried?" And predictably, the majority of the people answering are worried. But careful polls have offered another choice of thinking about Medicare in the future: "What do you think it is going to be? Medicare as it is, benefits cut back, or no program at all?" Most respondents envision fewer benefits as the likely future. They see the same thing happening with Social Security.

The only group in which half the population picks the bankruptcy of Medicare as likely is people younger than age 30. Most Americans believe that there will be fewer benefits for them in the future in both Medicare and Social Security. However, most Americans do not favor making these changes soon. In the short term the average citizen rejects the solution of reduced spending.

Why are people in complete denial on the issue? It is because they are not saving enough for their retirement and do not believe they will have enough income to purchase an adequate private insurance supplement to Medicare. When people are asked how they expect to support their retirement, the first thing they say is "my private savings," the second is "my pension," and the third is "Social Security." If the subject is how they will pay for health care, the third is then "Medicare." If they are asked, "Are you worried that Medicare won't be there in the future and are you worried that you will not have enough savings when you retire?" 77 percent of adults say they are worried that they are not saving enough for retirement. Then, if they are asked how much they are saving, one in three adults reports having saved nothing for retirement. The remainder report that they have saved half of what they need. They know that they are going to have to save. They know their benefits are going to be reduced in the long term. It is, "Next year, I will save; next year we will reduce the benefits."

The public is misinformed about two important topics. First, they believe that welfare and foreign aid are larger items in the budget than Medicare. Second, they believe that the poverty rate, or the number of elderly who live in poverty, has grown in the past twenty years. These two beliefs, although false, are widely held, and therefore they make it extremely difficult to discuss restricting Medicare benefits now or making budgetary cuts.

On managed care the jury is still out about the potential long-term cost savings. People who have been in managed care systems for a long time find them acceptable and get used to the fact that their choice of providers is restricted. So, if those under age 30 had a choice, Medicare would be principally managed care. That is what they know, and they would not have difficulties accepting policies that favor such care.

Managed care is spreading very quickly among the rest of the population. But those who have absolutely no use for it, particularly if it threatens traditional fee-for-service care, are people older than age 60. Thus the largest voting group is the same group that has the strongest ties to the traditional fee-for-service program. This situation has a lot to do with the future and possible change in the Medicare system.

I want to make recommendations for those in public life, and I have great empathy for legislators and staff who work on Medicare issues. The work is difficult because nobody wants to raise taxes or reduce benefits. Polls show that the public opposes significant increases on taxes for Medicare, and a modest increase can barely get majority support. Let us focus on the short term. If I were in Congress, I would try to get out of this budget debate by adopting the Federal Advisory Board's recommendations and offer the most politically acceptable approaches to saving money: paying the providers less, asking wealthier people to pay more for their benefits, and making some administrative changes. The public will not see these changes as very threatening. Thus in the short term, I would save the money by taking what is often called "the usual suspects approach."[5]

But in the longer term, there are more options. First, if a decade from now, the bulk of people who are about to retire are in managed care and have not experienced fee-for-service systems, it would be feasible to move Medicare almost entirely to managed care. There would be a two-tiered program in which people who are due to retire a decade hence are offered a choice of only managed care plans. Those who have already retired may keep the traditional plan. I think such a compromise would be politically acceptable. What would not be acceptable would be to impose managed care tomorrow on those who have already retired.

Whether to adopt managed care exclusively is a crucial issue for the future. We at Harvard no longer have a traditional plan. Younger assistant professors do not know what this Medicare debate is all about. They have no choice between traditional and managed health care plans. But many of the senior faculty are not happy.

I also want to look at the adequacy of people's private savings to support health care in retirement. America needs to develop a national plan to encourage savings beginning at very young ages for moderate- and middle-income people. If no plan is developed, we will never be able to deal with the politics of the benefit issue because the denial is "if I do not start saving now, I know that I am not going to have the benefits in the future." This is true for retirement income as well as retirement health benefits.

There can be no broader discussion unless people see a new type of saving plan that is for everyone, not just for the top 15 percent of American earners. We must have some way to encourage younger people to save for retirement and give them a sense that they will have some private security when Medicare and Social Security benefits are reduced.

In politics and in the press, today's story is the only story. Education, particularly by the president, about the long-term viability of the Medicare program is very important. People know what is going to happen. They say they know that future benefits will be less. They know we may have to face a tax increase, but they do not want to talk about it. It is very important to encourage people to talk about this problem without asking them, necessarily, to solve it immediately. Education is very important for understanding the long-term problems of funding Medicare, but the discussion will never begin if we first have to achieve a balanced budget through major reductions that seem to average citizens to have no political legitimacy.

Notes

1. Robert J. Blendon and others, "Voters and Health Care in the 1996 Election," *Journal of the American Medical Association*, vol. 277 (April 16, 1997), pp. 1253–58.

2. Ibid.

3. Robert J. Blendon and others, "What Do Americans Know about Entitlement?" *Health Affairs* (September-October 1997), pp. 111–16.

4. M. Weisskopf and D. Maraniss, "Gingrich's War of Words: How He and His Legions Marshaled the Forces of Rhetoric to Change Medicare," *Washington Post,* national weekly edition, November 6–12, 1995, pp. 6–8.

5. Robert J. Blendon and others, "The Public View of the Future of Medicare," *Journal of the American Medical Association*, vol. 274 (November 22–29, 1995), pp. 1645–48.

View by Celinda Lake

I AM AS CONFUSED about what we should do about Medicare as other people are. But I believe I am a good pollster. I can share their misunderstandings. This political football will be thrown back and forth a great deal more. That is because reforming the program is an issue of enormous importance to some constituents such as seniors and voters 50 to 60 years old that are going to be a battleground between the parties in the 2000 elections.

I would like to discuss how we got here. What was the campaign that was waged in 1995 and 1996, at least from the perspective of a pollster? What did that do to the agenda? The battle is not just about Medicare from a political standpoint or the way that some of us think about it. It is having a bigger change in terms of the broad agenda out there that has to do with retirement, security, the economy, families, and values.

The early Democratic press victories diminished rapidly by the fall of 1996. The Republicans were very astute in their Medicare strategy, moving the issues from a clear Democratic advantage closer to a draw and establishing that their goal was to reform the system to save it. They will try to replicate part of the Medicare strategy in 1997 in the education area by redefining the debate. From a political standpoint, the very interesting comparisons are not Medicare and health care reform, but the difference between the Medicare debate and the education debate (that is, the debate around the federal role in and priorities for education) in terms of what happened.

The Democratic advantages were substantial early on and then diminished, and that has had some impact on support for different solutions. Democrats drew the line early on affirmative action to protect Medicare for seniors, while the Republicans were willing to cut Medicare along with other programs to provide tax breaks for the wealthy. However, the Democratic strategy was too static, allowing the Republicans to change the definition. They said that Medicare needed to be reformed to save it. Voters became concerned. The Democrats never responded, and their message ended up sounding like just more politics. I also want to talk about where that has left the debate in the public's mind, in terms first of the budget debate and then in terms of Medicare and the kinds of changes that people are willing to entertain. As Robert Blendon commented, most of the public wants the changes to be somebody else's somewhere else.

Why is this issue important? To understand it from a political standpoint only, one must separate the elderly vote from the rest of the vote to see how the

Figure 7-3. *Congressional Vote among Voters Age 60 and Older, by Party, 1992, 1994, 1996*

Percent

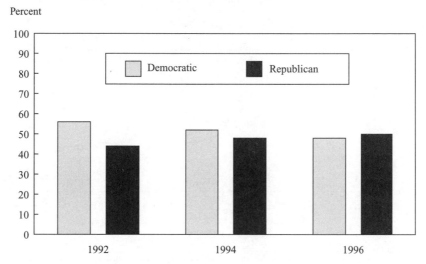

Sources: *New York Times* exit polls, November 1992 and November 1994; and VNS exit polls, November 1996.

two political parties think about it. In 1994 Democrats in the congressional elections lost the vote of the nation's elderly (figure 7-3.) That was devastating because older people turn out, and Democrats had counted on their support. By 1996 support of people older than age 60 for the Democrats had pulled slightly ahead of that for Republicans. In 1995 the Democrats had been even further ahead. The power of the Medicare issue in bringing the elderly back to the Democratic party was very important. By November it was much more a battleground, even among seniors. But the Democrats maintained more of an advantage among them than among others on the issue of Medicare financing.

A new strategy is so important to Democrats that they will continue to run on their support of the system as well as other retirement issues. At least challengers and congressional Democrats will use it in a limited way in part because of the advantage that they maintain among elderly voters. These voters have shown tremendous volatility and, in fact, showed some volatility even over the course of the campaign. In the fall of 1996 they consistently supported President Clinton, but not at the levels they had in 1995. In the congressional races as a whole the elderly were more volatile (figure 7-4). As long as they remain volatile and as long as they constitute a battleground between the

Figure 7-4. *Support of Voters Age 65 and Older for Parties in Congress and Candidates in Presidential Campaign, September–November 1996*

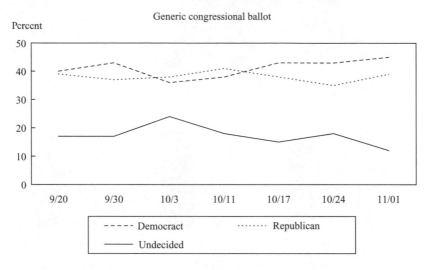

Generic congressional ballot

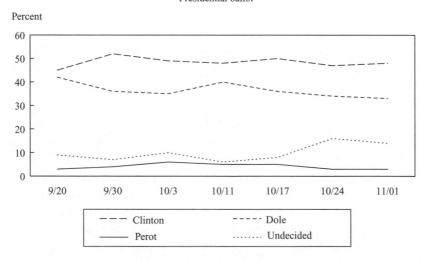

Presidential ballot

parties, Democrats will focus on Medicare reform, at least in the congressional contests.

The second thing the Democrats weigh in their calculation of how to go about Medicare reform is that they did very well with the generation Xers. Of course, most of these young people did not vote, but the ones who did voted overwhelmingly Democratic, giving Democrats a 19-point advantage com-

Figure 7-5. *Matters People Worry about Most, 1996*

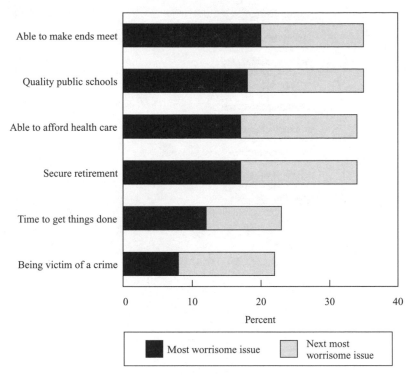

Source: The Tarrance Group, *U.S. News & World Report*, XXV, #7418.

pared to a 6-point lead with the rest of the electorate. If the Democrats had had the advantage among the elderly in November 1996 that they had had in 1995 and if generation Xers had turned out at the same rate in 1996 that they did in 1992, the Democrats would have taken back Congress.

The November exit polls showed a decline in importance of health care and retirement as major concerns. However, when measured as a personal concern, retirement and health care are of more importance (figure 7-5). Obviously, this result was very dependent on the questions that were asked, but this question was, "Which issue do you worry about personally most?" Secure retirement and affordable health care were of greatest concern. In 1995 women in particular, especially women older than age 50, made health care and Social Security priorities, but during the fall of 1996, in part, I think, because of a very successful strategy on the part of the Republicans to confuse the issues and redefine what protecting Medicare meant, those concerns became less important.

Figure 7-6. *Priority Concerns about Public Issues, by Sex, 1997*

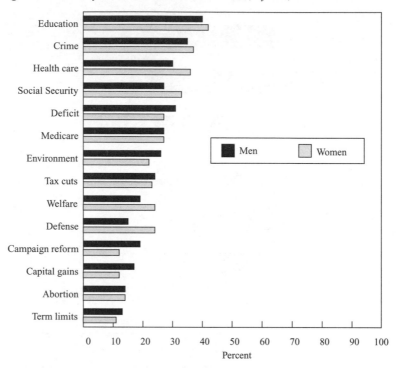

Source: Gallup/CNN/*USA Today* polls, January–February 1997.

Question: Here are some issues now being discussed in Washington. For each one, please tell me whether you think it should be the top priority for Congress and the president to deal with in 1997, a high priority, a low priority, or not a priority at all.

One of the things I noticed is that opinions on health care, Medicare, and Social Security issues tend to move in tandem. When people are talking about Medicare, their health care concerns also become more important. Senior citizens were concerned with Medicare, and younger women expressed their concerns more in terms of general health care. The other thing that the Medicare debate has done is to increase enormously people's general anxiety about retirement. It also probably increased their denial that there is a problem with Medicare that requires fundamental changes in their benefits. This nexus of issues connected to retirement is one of the sleeper issues for the twenty-first century and a reason affordable and accessible health care will reemerge on the agenda.

Women are much less concerned than men about deficits and government spending and more concerned about education and social issues (figure 7-6). In

Figure 7-7. *Issues of Importance to Voters, by Presidential Candidate They Supported, 1996*

Percent

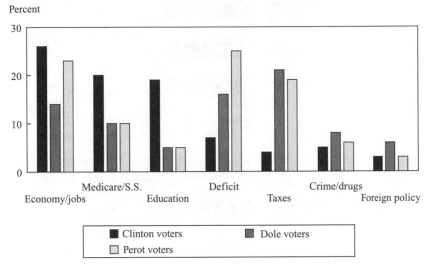

Source: VNS exit polls, 1996.

1996 the difference between men and women's voting choices became particularly prominent. Basically, men and women chose different Congresses and, by 1 percentage point, chose different presidents.

And they belong, in their minds at least, to different parties. The gender gap came down even among some married couples. Traditionally, it had reflected the behavior of single voters, not married voters; but this difference in agenda and in opinions about the role of government affected men and women in their voting choices as well. Women concluded 53 percent to 45 percent that the Republican budget cuts were going too far; men, particularly those who were college educated, believed 47 percent to 35 percent that the cuts had not gone far enough. The issues also made a difference in terms of which candidate a person chose. Clinton voters worried about the economy, education, Medicare, and Social Security. Dole voters worried about taxes and the deficit. Perot voters worried about the deficit and the economy (figure 7-7).

So, Medicare reform came onto the agenda in 1995, but the agendas of men and women and the agendas of the candidates' coalitions were very different. Still, Medicare reform has some potential to sway voters if approached by Democratic candidates to include protection as well as reform.

In the *Campaign for America's Future*, Stan Greenberg ranked various topics in terms of what people thought were important things to do; at the very

Figure 7-8. *Highest Priorities for Federal Action, November 1996*

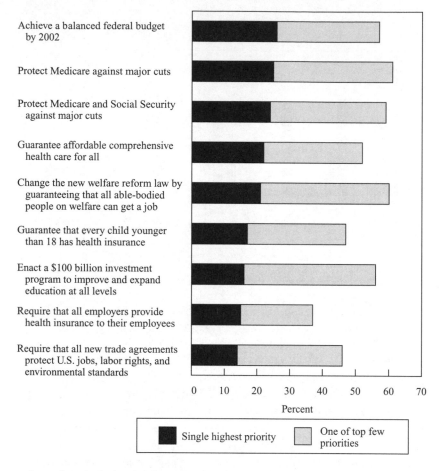

Achieve a balanced federal budget by 2002

Protect Medicare against major cuts

Protect Medicare and Social Security against major cuts

Guarantee affordable comprehensive health care for all

Change the new welfare reform law by guaranteeing that all able-bodied people on welfare can get a job

Guarantee that every child younger than 18 has health insurance

Enact a $100 billion investment program to improve and expand education at all levels

Require that all employers provide health insurance to their employees

Require that all new trade agreements protect U.S. jobs, labor rights, and environmental standards

0   10   20   30   40   50   60   70

Percent

■ Single highest priority   ☐ One of top few priorities

Source: Campaign for America's Future, Greenberg Research, November 1996.

All questions asked of half the sample:
Question: For each issue I mention, tell me if you think it should be the single highest priority, one of the top few priorities, but not the highest, near the top of the list, in the middle of the list, or toward the bottom of the list of priorities for the new Congress and the president.

top, their priorities were balancing the budget, protecting Medicare against major cuts, and protecting Medicare and Social Security against major cuts (figure 7-8). A number of matters such as entitlement reform that appear in political debates are not at all on the public's agenda. In sum, Medicare and Medicaid reform still have a great deal of potential energy among women and seniors and could easily emerge as a top political issue. Homemakers have

Figure 7-9. *Lowest Priorities for Federal Action, November 1996*

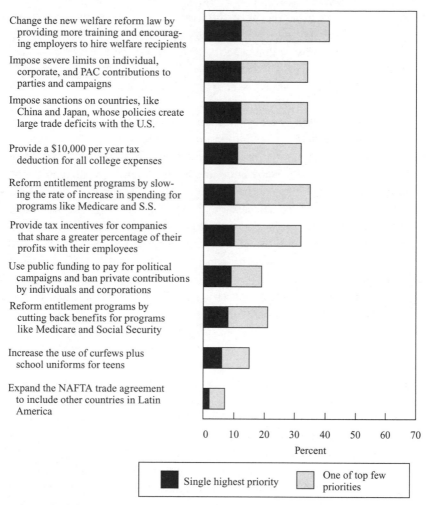

Source: Campaign for America's Future, Greenberg Research, November 1996.

All questions asked of half the sample:
Question: For each issue I mention, tell me if you think it syould be the single highest priority, one of the top few priorities, but not the highest, near the top of the list, in the middle of the list, or toward the bottom of the list of priorities for the new Congress and the President.

traditionally been a swing group that has not been very favorable to Democrats, but it is a group worried about retirement matters, very afraid that their husbands are going, the pension is going, and Medicare is going, and what will people be left with?

The concern about Medicare reform does not lead people to favor a broader reform of entitlements. The way the policymakers are thinking and talking about this issue could not be more different from the way that most other people are thinking about it. For example, as figure 7-9 shows, reforming entitlement programs by cutting benefits for Medicare and Social Security are generally of low priority. Even when one talks about reforms and specifically mentions the programs that people are worried about, entitlement reform still ranks low.

If that is where people were on election evening in 1996, how did they get there? The pattern started in fall 1995 among swing voters. Crime and the economy had become matters that were less important to them and Medicare and Social Security had become more important. When Medicare and Social Security were discussed together, the effect on the voters was much stronger than when they were discussed separately. And when a Democrat wanted to create the pattern or the appearance that a Republican member of Congress was trying to cut back Medicare, listing the representative's votes on Medicare and Social Security matters made his or her opponent much more believable than when only the votes on Medicare were listed. A list of issues about Medicare and Social Security created a sense that this member must really mean what he says.

The people who were most worried about cuts to Medicare and Social Security were those without a college education and the elderly, particularly elderly women (figure 7-10). Those are also the most traditional voters on Medicare issues. In some key congressional districts the AFL-CIO and other unions and groups had started to run ads condemning the efforts to cut Medicare and provide a tax break for the wealthy. Even in the fall of 1995, half the voters said that they had seen these ads, and older voters were again the ones overwhelmingly the most likely to have paid attention. Voters 50 to 64 years old were also likely to pay attention (figure 7-11).

The Republican strategy of saying, "We are trying to reform Medicare to save it; we are not trying to cut it," disaggregated the coalition that had been very energized on this issue, separating out those who were 50 to 64 years old from the voters older than 65. The older voters remained very suspicious of the Republicans, even toward the end. The 50- to 64-year-olds were much more likely to agree with the Republican argument, thinking that "this program is going to disappear, and I am in a situation where I do not have enough time to put together the money or the retirement plan to save myself and this program."

The 1998 elections will have an overwhelmingly higher turnout among voters older than 50 (younger voters do not turn out very much in an off-year election). These voters may respond very differently to proposals for reform. Those age 50 to 64 may be much more sympathetic to the argument that

Figure 7-10. *Swing Voters' Attitudes on Threats to Social Security and Medicare, by Educational Attainment and Age Group, Fall 1995*

Percent who say they have serious doubts

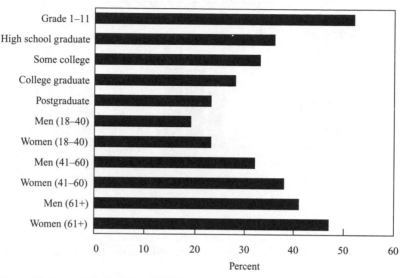

Source: Lake Research, The '95 Project, Fall 1995.

Medicare must be saved through significant reform. Voters older than age 64 should be much more sympathetic to arguments for making only minor changes or for leaving the program alone entirely. Again, after seeing the ads in 1995, voters, particularly older women voters, believed that the Republican cuts were going too far.

One may well wonder at this point why the Democrats did not take back Congress in 1996. One reason is that when voters were asked, "Do you think the cuts that are being made are being proposed mainly to preserve Medicare from bankruptcy or mainly to provide a tax cut for the wealthy?" the districts were very much divided in their responses. Less affluent populous districts such as the tenth district in Ohio, which is Cleveland, responded that "politicians are doing this to provide something for the wealthy." The ninth district in Washington, which includes Tacoma in Seattle's suburbs, was much more split. This debate about whether the Republicans were proposing cuts in Medicare to provide a tax cut that would mainly benefit the wealthy—the Democratic argument—or whether they were proposing cuts to save the program became part of the major battleground in 1996. While the Republicans made more progress in this debate, swing voters were still undecided by various

Figure 7-11. *Share of Voters Who Saw or Heard Medicare Ads, by Age Group, Selected Congressional Districts, 1995*

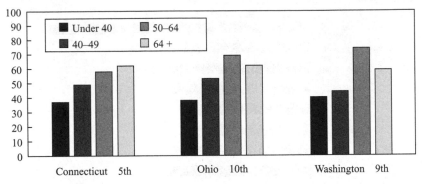

Percent

Legend: ■ Under 40 ■ 50–64 ■ 40–49 □ 64+

Connecticut 5th   Ohio 10th   Washington 9th

Source: AFSCME, Fall 1995.

Question: During the last few weeks have you seen or heard any ads on the TV or radio concerning Medicare?

margins that the Republicans' efforts were more about providing a tax cut for the wealthy than about saving Medicare.

Many voters knew about the assertion that the Republicans were out to cut Medicare, but they did not connect this position to their representative in Congress. In the fall of 1996, where the Democrats had been able to identify an incumbent as someone who had voted to cut Medicare, they were successful, but the connection was very difficult to establish. A lot of Republicans had both individual and group strategies for trying to disentangle the connection. For example, Representative Jack Metcalf (Republican of Washington) ran ads featuring his senior citizen brother and sister saying, "Jack would not cut my Medicare. Jack would not cut *your* Medicare." Jesse Helms's ads announced: "I am a senior citizen; would I cut social security and Medicare?" Voters believed that senior citizens in general would not cut Medicare and Social Security.

In early 1995 voters were convinced that the Newt Gingrich Congress had gone after Medicare and had intended to cut it. They thought it was very suspicious that the Medicare cuts matched the intended amounts of the tax cut for the wealthy. By the end of 1996, Republicans were running ads proclaiming that they had supported record spending on Medicare. That confused voters. By 1996 they were much more divided in their opinion. In twelve swing districts they were asked, "Which position comes closer to your view? We need to make changes in Medicare. The drastic cuts will end up hurting our families, or Medicare is in serious trouble, and we must reform it by capping rising medical

Figure 7-12. *Share of Voters Who Favor Major Reductions in Future Medicare Spending, by Party, Age Group, and Reason for Favoring, January 1997*

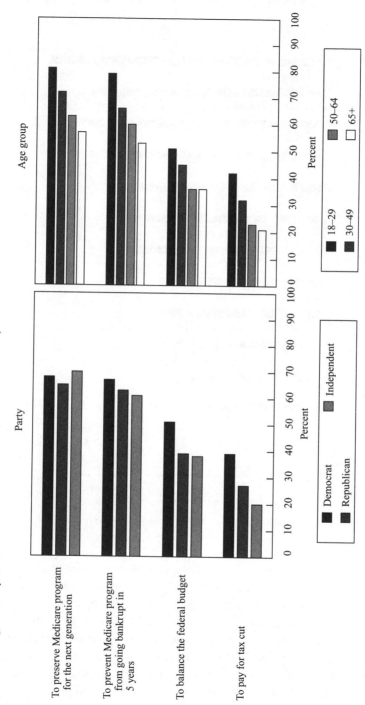

Source: Kaiser/Harvard/PSRA Post-Election Survey of Voters 1997 Health Care Agenda, January 1997.

Figure 7-13. *Party That Voters Trust More, by Issue, 1996*

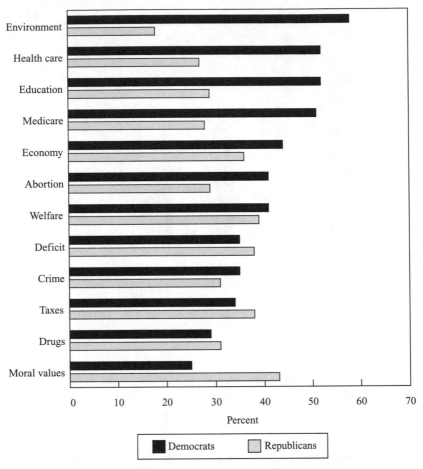

Source: Lake Research & Greenburg Research for Emily's List, March–November 1996.

costs and eliminating waste and fraud." The respondents now split, 47 percent believing proposed cuts went too far and 40 percent that costs must be contained. The twenty-point swing meant that the Republicans pulled ahead among ticket-splitting voters on the matter of Medicare reform.The Republicans, however, never fully won back the support of the elderly. Thus voters younger than age 65 agreed with the Republican argument while those older than 65 still favored more conservative strategies and arguments (figure 7-12).

Democrats found that one piece of their strategy, which will probably continue to be used, is not to just talk about Medicare alone but to talk about it

Figure 7-14. *Voter Allegiance in Partisan Disagreements over Medicare and Medicaid, by Sex, November 1996*

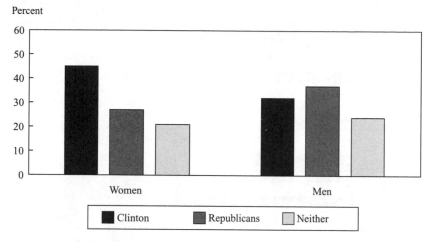

Percent

Source: Empire State Poll, November 1996.

as part of a broader agenda. In many congressional districts they broadcast or printed ads saying that the Republicans had tried to make spouses and adult children responsible for the costs of nursing home care. It was a very strong argument in the abstract. But voters were still skeptical of its truth, skeptical that anyone would be politically stupid enough to take on citizens. They wanted to know what the motivation would be. The Democrats also argued that the Republican incumbent had allowed employers to raid pensions. This argument also worked well, even in the fall of 1996, awakening voter alarm in part because there seemed to be an actor on the other side, that is, corporations. Democrats will continue to use this issue politically and discuss it politically, but more often in a broader constellation of health care and retirement issues.

Where did that leave voters? What were their final conclusions? First, it left them concluding that the Democrats would do a better job in dealing with Medicare. When voters were asked, "Which do you prefer, the Democrats or the Republicans?" on a number of topics, Medicare reform was part of a constellation of economic issues on which voters favored Democrats, but the Democrats did not have the same advantage that they had earlier in the fall (figure 7-13). When a poll asked respondents whether they were more likely to side with President Clinton or the Republicans in partisan disagreements over Medicare and Medicaid, the Democrats' advantage shrank from 20 points to 10 points. Women were much more likely than men to favor the president and the Democrats (figure 7-14). Again, when questions included Medicaid men

Figure 7-15. *Share of People Who Believe Medicare Will Be Able to Provide for Them in Their Retirement, by Age Group, December 1996*

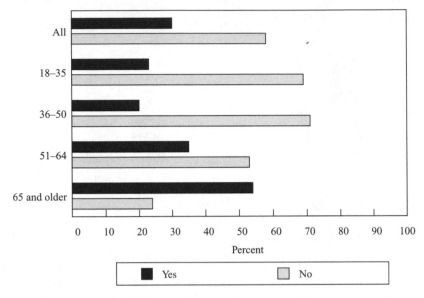

Percent

Source: NBC News/*Wall Street Journal* poll, December 5–9, 1996.

Question: Do you think the Medicare program will have the money available to provide the benefits you expect in your retirement?

slightly favored the Republicans, but women followed Democrats two to one. Response to the Medicare issue when specific reforms are discussed has enormous gender and age variations. Younger voters, for example, favor putting seniors in HMOs and oppose raising the retirement age. Seniors hold the opposite opinions.

Voters have also come to some conclusions that are mutually exclusive in policy terms. Except for those 65 and older, they believe Medicare will not be able to provide for them in their retirement. This belief is solid among baby boomers and generation Xers (figure 7-15). They have also concluded by three to one that there is no reason the budget cannot be balanced. This result occurs because they believe that Medicare is not part of the budget, or at least it ought not to be. As people in one focus group said, "it would not be part of the budget, except that they kept stealing the money." Even when politicians talk about Medicare as being part of the budget, there is a sense that they are saying so to cover up other sins and they are moving money that ought to be sacrosanct and in a trust fund. And because people get Medicare and Social Security mixed up,

Figure 7-16. *Share of People Who Favor or Oppose Medicare, by Age Group, June 1995*

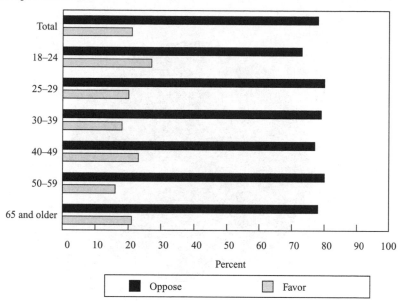

Source: Harris Poll, June 8–11, 1995.

Question: Do you favor or oppose making cuts in the Medicare program—which pays for health care for people age 65 and over, and some people with disabilities—to reduce what the government will spend on Medicare in the future?

it is a potent argument for politicians to say, "Leave that money untouched. Keep the trust fund absolutely untouched."

Across the political spectrum and across age groups voters entered the 1996 election opposing Medicare cuts (figure 7-16). If they were to be forced to accept cuts, they would drag their feet at every stage saying that they want modest cuts. People also believe that most of the Medicare crisis could be dealt with by cutting waste, fraud, and abuse in government, particularly if the congressional pay raise were added to Medicare money. Some 65 percent of voters are convinced that enough money could be cut from other less desirable programs to save Medicare (figure 7-17).

Women and senior citizens, who care most about Medicare reform, are willing to make some incremental changes. Other voters, younger voters in particular, already show a willingness to consider managed care and HMOs (figure 7-18). People are also fairly positive about paying doctors and hospitals

Figure 7-17. *Voter Attitudes toward Ways to Maintain Medicare Benefits, December 1996*

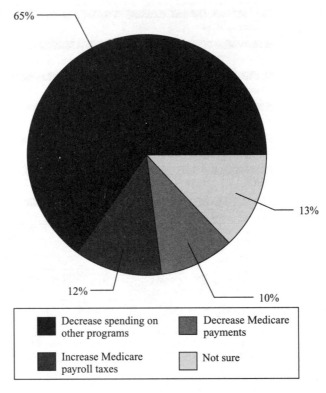

65%

13%

12%

10%

■	Decrease spending on other programs	■	Decrease Medicare payments
■	Increase Medicare payroll taxes	▢	Not sure

Source: NBC News/*Wall Street Journal* poll, December 5–9, 1996.

Question: In future years, it is expected that revenues for the Medicare system will not be enough to cover expenses. Which do you think is the best way to deal with this situation: increase Medicare payroll taxes, decrease Medicare benefits, or decrease spending on other programs to maintain Medicare benefits at current levels?

less as long as medical care is not compromised. They feel comfortable, particularly voters in the 50- to 64-year-old group, with having those people who have higher incomes pay more. Finally, nobody in any cohort favors requiring the elderly to pay a larger share of Medicare cost (figure 7-19).

In short then, I would say that we are in some ways in for the worst of all worlds. First, Medicare reform is a very potent political issue and a battleground between the parties. And when it is made part of a bigger agenda, it is still very important to voters, particularly the elderly and women. Second, the

Figure 7-18. *Voter Attitudes toward Ways to Keep Medicare Financially Sound, by Age Group, January 1997*

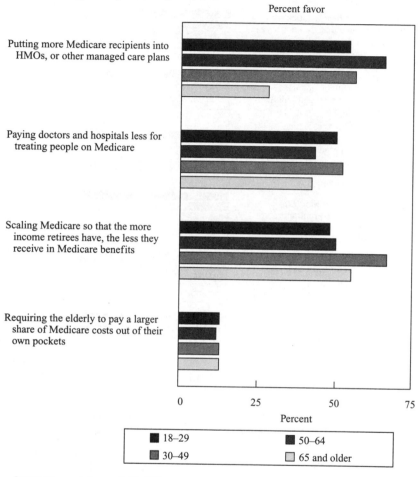

Percent favor

Putting more Medicare recipients into HMOs, or other managed care plans

Paying doctors and hospitals less for treating people on Medicare

Scaling Medicare so that the more income retirees have, the less they receive in Medicare benefits

Requiring the elderly to pay a larger share of Medicare costs out of their own pockets

Percent

■ 18–29   ■ 50–64
▨ 30–49   ▢ 65 and older

Source: *Newsweek*, January 9–10, 1997.

Question: I'm going to read you some proposals to change Medicare to keep the system financially sound in the future. Please tell me whether you would generally favor or oppose each change that I read.

voters who care the most about Medicare reform and are most likely to focus on it are by far the most conservative. Third, voters deny that the program must be reformed and are also very antipolitical about reform. They believe that they are being asked to make tough choices that they do not want to make and in

Figure 7-19. *Voter Attitudes toward Medicare Funding Proposals, December 1996*

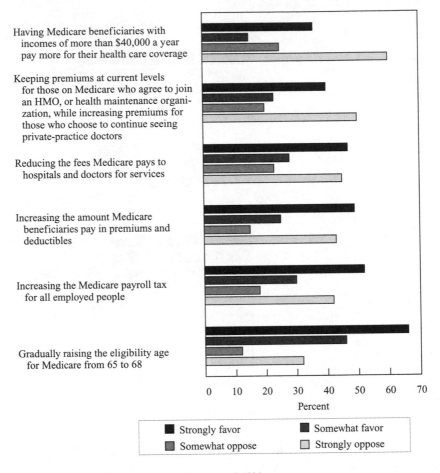

Source: NBC News/*Wall Street Journal*, December 5–9, 1996

Question: The following are some proposals that are being considered in Congress to deal with Medicare's funding problems. For each one, please tell me whether you strongly favor, somewhat favor, somewhat oppose, or strongly oppose this proposal.

some ways do not accept by a rotten political system that has raided a trust. There are dramatic cohort differences in attitudes, but in the short run this is a very incendiary political issue. It will be hard to create the political will for the kinds of changes we need.

Contributors

Joseph R. Antos is Assistant Director for Health and Human Resources at the Congressional Budget Office.

Robert M. Ball is a consultant on Social Security, health, and welfare policy to many organizations and elected officials and was Commissioner of Social Security (1962–73) and Administrator of Medicare during the program's first seven years.

Anthony C. Beilenson is a former Representative for California.

Robert J. Blendon is Chairman of the Department of Health Policy and Management at Harvard University School of Public Health.

David Blumenthal is Chief of the Health Policy Research and Development Unit at the Medical Practices Evaluation Center of Massachusetts General Hospital.

Karlyn H. Bowman is a Resident Fellow at the American Enterprise Institute.

Melinda Beeuwkes Buntin is a doctoral candidate in health policy, Harvard University.

Sheila P. Burke is Executive Dean and Lecturer in Public Policy, Harvard University.

Stuart Butler is Vice President and Director of Domestic and Economic Policy Studies at the Heritage Foundation.

Kathleen Ann Buto is Deputy Director, Center for Health Plans & Providers, Health Care Financing Administration.

E. J. Dionne is a syndicated columnist.

Bryan Dowd is Professor of Health Policy, University of Minnesota School of Public Health.

Judith Feder is Principal Deputy Assistant Secretary for the U.S. Department of Health and Human Services.

Roger D. Feldman is Blue Cross Professor of Health Insurance and Professor of Economics, University of Minnesota.

Peter D. Fox is President of PDF Inc.

Haynes Johnson is an author and syndicated columnist.

Stanley B. Jones is Director of the Health Insurance Reform Project at George Washington University.

Charles N. Kahn III is Staff Director of the Health Subcommittee on Ways and Means, U.S. House of Representatives.

David B. Kendall is Senior Analyst for Health Policy for the Progressive Policy Institute and Director of the Progressive Foundation's Health Priorities Project.

Celinda Lake is President of Lake Sosin Snell Perry & Associates.

Alan R. Nelson is Chief Executive Officer of the American Society of Internal Medicine.

Patricia Powers is Executive Director of Pacific Business Group on Health.

James Robinson is Associate Professor of Health Economics at the School of Public Health, University of California at Berkeley.

John C. Rother is Director of Legislation and Public Policy at the American Association of Retired Persons.

Theda Skocpol is Professor of Government and Sociology, Harvard University.

Thomas A. Scully is President and Chief Executive Officer of the Federation of American Health Systems.

David G. Smith is Professor Emeritus of Political Science, Swarthmore College.

Conference Program

National Academy of Social Insurance
Ninth Annual Conference

Medicare: Preparing for the Challenges of the 21st Century
January 23–24, 1997

Thursday, January 23, 1997

9:00 am–9:45 am   Welcome and Introduction

Opening Address

The Honorable Pete Stark (D-California)

9:45 am–10:45 am   Session I. Medicare's Social Contract: Two Views

A contrast of two perspectives on Medicare's philosophical underpinnings. What is the "social contract" between workers and beneficiaries? Is it relevant as we enter the next century?

Chair: Rosemary Stevens, University of Pennsylvania

Stuart Butler, The Heritage Foundation
Theda Skocpol, Harvard University

10:45 am–12:00 pm   Session II. Financing Medicare: Preparing for the Retirement of the Baby Boomers

How much is needed to sustain Medicare in the coming decades? What are the pros and cons of the basic choices for financing Medicare? How much of

the needed monies will come from workers and
beneficiaries, now and in the future?

Chair: Marilyn Moon, The Urban Institute

Presenter: Joseph Antos, Congressional Budget
Office

Discussants:
Dave Kendall, Progressive Policy Institute
Judy Feder, Georgetown University
Charles Kahn III, Health Subcommittee, House
Ways and Means Committee

12:15 pm–1:15 pm   Luncheon address: How Did Medicare Come About?

A historical assessment of what Medicare's
architects intended, the compromises forged in its
passage, and the choices made during its
implementation.

Introduction: Karen Davis, The Commonwealth Fund

Robert M. Ball, former U.S. Commissioner of Social
Security

1:30 pm–3:00 pm   Session III. Building a Sound Infrastructure for Choice

As managed care becomes a larger component of
Medicare, what structures and safeguards are needed
if beneficiaries' choice of health plans is to be
increased? How might such choice be structured?
How do we minimize "favorable selection" by health
plans?

Chair: Geraldine Dallek, Families USA

David Blumenthal, Massachusetts General Hospital
Roger Feldman, University of Minnesota
Stanley Jones, George Washington University
James Robinson, University of California, Berkeley

3:15 pm–5:00 pm   Session IV. Will Public Opinion Help or Hinder Medicare
Restructuring?

Polling experts review public opinion about
Medicare and health care systems generally. What
are Americans' hopes, fears, and expectations for

Medicare? What information do they rely on? What trade-offs do they see?

Chair: Martha Phillips, The Concord Coalition

Panelists:

Robert Blendon, Harvard University

William McInturff, Public Opinion Strategies

Karlyn Bowman, American Enterprise Institiute

Celinda Lake, Lake Research

6:30 pm–8:30 pm   Dinner and Heinz Dissertation Award ceremony

Dinner speech

E. J. Dionne Jr., Syndicated Columnist

Friday, January 24, 1997

8:45 am–10:00 am   Roundtable Discussions

Teaching and Talking about Social Security Reform

Current Issues in Social Security around the World

Disability, Return-to-Work, and Health Care

10:00 am–10:45 am   Opening Address

The Honorable William M. Thomas (R-California)

10:45 am–12:15 pm   Session V. Can Fee-for-Service Medicare Survive in a Managed Care World?

Despite a greater reliance on managed care, most beneficiaries will remain in Medicare's fee-for-service (FFS) component well into the future. A restructured Medicare program may require bold administrative innovations to maintain FFS as a viable choice for beneficiaries. What are the ways in which the Health Care Financing Administration might manage FFS? What opportunities exist for FFS to adopt some of the cost-control and quality-assurance tools of managed care? What are the political and institutional barriers and risks in such changes?

Chair: Janet Shikles, General Accounting Office

Presenters:

Peter Fox, PDF Inc.

David Smith, Swarthmore College

Discussants:
Alan Nelson, American Society of Internal Medicine
Kathy Buto, Health Care Financing Administration
Thomas Scully, Federation of American Health
    Systems

12:15 pm–1:15 pm   Luncheon Address

Introduction: Gerald M. Shea, AFL-CIO

The Honorable Bruce C. Vladeck, Administrator,
U.S. Health Care Financing Administration

1:15 pm-3:00 pm   Session VI. Leadership and Politics: What Next?

Even when experts agree about reform, quick or
significant change is often difficult. What are the
political constraints to health policy change? How
might Congress move toward Medicare restructuring?

Chair: The Honorable Willis Gradison, Health
Insurance Association of America

Panelists:
Sheila Burke, Harvard University
The Honorable Anthony Beilenson (D-California)
John Rother, American Association of Retired
    Persons
Haynes Johnson, *The Washington Post*

3:00 pm–3:30 pm   Wrap Up by Conference Co-Chairs

Stuart Butler, The Heritage Foundation
Judith Lave, The University of Pittsburgh
Robert D. Reischauer, The Brookings Institution

Index